# Color Atlas

## *of*

# Common Oral Diseases

*Second Edition*

# Color Atlas

## *of*

# Common Oral Diseases

## *Second Edition*

**Robert P. Langlais, DDS, MS, FACD**
Professor
Department of Dental Diagnostic Science
University of Texas Health Science Center at San Antonio
School of Dentistry
San Antonio, Texas

**Craig S. Miller, DMD, MS**
Associate Professor of Oral Medicine
Microbiology and Immunology
Department of Oral Health Science, Medical Microbiology and Immunology
College of Dentistry, College of Medicine
University of Kentucky
Lexington, Kentucky

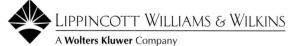

LIPPINCOTT WILLIAMS & WILKINS
A **Wolters Kluwer** Company
Philadelphia • Baltimore • New York • London
Buenos Aires • Hong Kong • Sydney • Tokyo

*Editor:* Sharon R. Zinner
*Managing Editor:* Tanya Lazar
*Marketing Manager:* Rebecca Himmelheber
*Production Coordinator:* Danielle Hagan
*Project Editor:* Jennifer D. Weir
*Design Coordinator:* Mario Fernandez
*Illustration Planner:* Wayne Hubbel
*Cover Designer:* Nick Lang
*Typesetter:* BI-COMP, Inc.
*Printer/Binder:* Everbest

Lippincott Williams & Wilkins
227 East Washington Square
Philadelphia, PA

Accurate indications, adverse reactions, and dosage schedules for drugs are provided in this book, but it is possible that they may change. The reader is urged to review the package information data of the manufacturers of the medications mentioned.

*Printed in the United States of America*

First Edition, 1992

**Library of Congress Cataloging-in-Publication Data**

Langlais, Robert P.
    Color atlas of common oral diseases / Robert P. Langlais,
Craig S. Miller. — 2nd ed.
        p. cm.
    Includes index.
    ISBN 0-683-30173-X
    1. Oral medicine—Atlases.   I. Miller, Craig S.   II. Title.
    [DNLM: 1. Mouth Diseases—pathology—atlases.   2. Tooth
Diseases—pathology—atlases.     WU 17 L282c 1997]
    RC815.L35   1997
    617.5'22'00222—dc21
    DNLM/DLC
    for Library of Congress                                    97-2654
                                                                          CIP

*The publishers have made every effort to trace the copyright holders for borrowed material. If they have inadvertently overlooked any, they will be pleased to make the necessary arrangements at the first opportunity.*

99 00 01
2 3 4 5 6 7 8 9 10

*To our wives,*
*Denyse and Sherry*

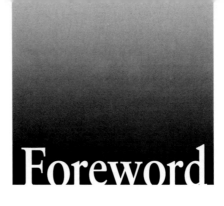
# Foreword

Practicing oral medicine—that is, diagnosing and treating oral manifestations of local or systemic diseases—is often a difficult challenge for the practitioner. This complexity stems from the many conditions that directly or indirectly affect the mouth and adjacent structures and the entailing spectrum of signs and symptoms that often make a differential diagnosis quite difficult.

The organized approach that helps to simplify this aspect of oral health care delivery demands careful history taking, methodical oral examinations, recognition of normal structures and deviations from normal, and the ability to form a differential diagnosis—a priority list of conditions or diseases that the findings suggest. The differential diagnosis forms the basis for performing tests that should lead to a definitive diagnosis and the appropriate treatment plan. These steps are important for standards of care, optimal patient health and function, protecting the clinician from censure, and nurturing meaningful referrals.

An important step of the diagnostic sequence, not to be overlooked, is the dental hygienist, who often sees the patient first. Because many signs and symptoms may represent malignant disease, precancerous lesions, or infectious conditions, it is incumbent upon the dental hygienist to recognize deviations from normal, identify patients who may have these disorders, and inform the dentist of the clinical findings.

The second edition of *Color Atlas of Common Oral Diseases* by Drs. Langlais and Miller greatly assists in the diagnostic process by providing an updated and organized approach to conditions that afflict the mouth. Chapters on normal anatomy, specific tissues, different sites, and clinical features of color and form are presented with many high-quality color illustrations that have been carefully selected to represent features of conditions or diseases. The accompanying text is abbreviated to present concise overviews with emphasis on the clinical description of oral lesions, which allows a useful understanding of the entity in question. The book also includes a brief glossary of useful terms that describe clinical findings, tables summarizing the characteristics of each group of disorders, and a separate listing of prescriptions useful in the management of these problems.

Because it is so difficult to master the complex variations of signs and symptoms associated with the multitude of oral manifestations of disease, a visual approach is one of the most helpful aids. Thus, the second edition of the *Atlas* will be of significant help to clinicians at all levels of experience in creating a differential diagnosis, establishing a diagnosis, and forming a basis for a rational approach to managing and resolving patient problems.

Sol Silverman, Jr, MA, DDS

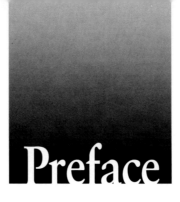

# Preface

The 2nd edition of *Color Atlas of Common Oral Diseases* is a thorough revision of the first edition and promises be a large improvement. We have added more than 100 new illustrations and diagnostic concepts. Sections on normal oral anatomy, tooth-related disorders, gingivitis, periodontitis, caries and caries progression, odontogenic infections, and facial swellings have been added. The sequence of the atlas has been rearranged so that the reader begins with normal anatomy and progresses to disease. Throughout the text, select illustrations have been replaced with better cases that more accurately represent the disease described.

As before, we realize that there are many excellent textbooks available of oral diagnosis, oral medicine, and oral and maxillofacial pathology; we hope that this edition provides students with a high-quality, affordable, practical, and user-friendly color atlas. The goal of this atlas continues to be to provide both high-quality color illustrations and salient clinical features of common oral diseases for those who are studying or attempting to identify oral disorders. We are fully aware that space has limited the scope of the written text, which is not intended to be all-inclusive but rather to serve as a reference for the clinical diagnostic aspects of the more commonly encountered oral diseases. We hope that this edition will be useful to students of dental assisting, dental hygiene, and dentistry, as well as postgraduate dentists and hygienists whose goal is to become more knowledgeable about the clinical appearance of oral disease. This color atlas will also be of great value to practicing dentists, physicians, and specialists. Although many healthcare providers may use this atlas as adjunctive material, we have made efforts to ensure that the text is as current as possible. In this regard, we have extensively researched each disorder and updated all statements so that the text is in concert with the current thinking of the majority of the profession.

This edition continues to arrange the illustrations practically, according to clinical appearance, to facilitate the construction of a differential diagnosis. Each color plate consists of eight illustrations per page so that disorders closely related by appearance or cause can be easily compared. The first two sections provide the reader with the necessary background to understand normal anatomy and properly describe lesions to colleagues. The illustrations selected for specific diseases have been chosen with the intent of showing each disorder in its most typical appearance and location. When several locations are possible, we have included several examples, often from the same patient. On the pages opposite the color plates, the written text discusses the nature of various disease processes, as well as other clinically relevant information such as location and the sex, age, and race affected by the disorder. The emphasis continues to be on the signs and symptoms of common oral diseases. Cause and treatment methods are briefly discussed to provide additional valuable information. It is hoped that by arranging the material in this manner, the reader will be able to integrate concepts of oral diagnosis, medicine, pathology, and radiology.

Of some importance to all students of dentistry are a variety of helpful learning tips or methods. At the back of the text, the reader will find a glossary of terms; several tables of common oral conditions; prescriptions arranged by management of disorders; and a self-assessment test similar to those used in school examinations, state and national boards, and clinical sections of the specialty boards of Oral Medicine and Oral and Maxillofacial Pathology. In this edition, the appendix of prescriptions has been expanded and made easier to read by placing each individual prescription in a box. The most current American Heart Association guidelines for antibiotic prevention of infective endocarditis are found in Appendix II.

We wish to express our thanks to all health care professions who have referred patients to our clinics and provided illustrations found in this text.

Robert P. Langlais
Craig S. Miller

For persons involved in education, the authors have the complete set of illustrations available for purchase as color slides. Details on the purchase of these slides are available by contacting

Craig S. Miller, DMD, MS
MN 118, Oral Medicine
University of Kentucky College of Dentistry
Lexington, KY 40536-0084
cmiller@pop.uky.edu
FAX 606-323-9136

Information regarding an annual summer conference that provides continuing education of material found in this text can also be obtained by contacting Dr. Miller at the above address.

# Acknowledgments

We are extremely grateful to our many colleagues who have graciously provided material for publication in this atlas. Without their contributions, this fine quality text would not have been possible. We are also grateful to all practicing dentists and physicians who have referred patients throughout the years to the Department of Dental Diagnostic Science Referral Clinic.

To Professor Sol Silverman, who completely reviewed this text and wrote the foreword, we extend our thanks for his valuable comments and contributions. In addition, we are grateful for the many illustrations Dr. Silverman has provided, which can be seen throughout this text.

Dieter Karkut and Al Julian of the Photographic Services Section of Education Resources of The University of Texas Health Science Center receive a special thank you for their masterful job of cropping and recreating the proper color balance on our illustrations. We are especially grateful for the incredible efforts made by Dieter Karkut, who personally reviewed each color slide for possible color modifications and/or correction. We are also grateful to Albert Preciado and the entire Photography Unit, whose photography skills are evident throughout this work.

Finally, we would like to thank our wives, Denyse and Sherry, for their continuing support throughout this project. Authorship of a high quality text requires numerous off-duty hours; without the understanding of these two most important people in our lives, this work might never have been completed.

We also wish to express our appreciation to the following persons for contribution of their clinical photographs and radiographs used in this text:

Dr. A.M. Abrams
Dr. Marden Adler
Dr. Tom Aufdemorte
Dr. Bill Baker
Dr. Douglas Barnett
Dr. Pete Benson
Dr. Howard Birkholz
Dr. Steve Bricker
Dr. Dale Buller

Dr. Jerry Cioffi
Dr. Laurie Cohen
Dr. John Coke
Dr. James Cottone
Dr. Robert Craig, Jr
Dr. S. Brent Dove
Dr. David Freed
Dr. Franklin Garcia-Godoy
Dr. Birgit Glass
Dr. Tom Glass
Dr. Ed Heslop
Dr. Michael Huber
Dr. Sheryl Hunter
Dr. J.L. Jensen
Dr. Ron Jorgenson
Dr. Jerald Katz
Dr. George Kaugers
Dr. Olaf Langland
Dr. Al Lugo
Dr. Curt Lundeen
Dr. Carson Mader
Dr. Nancy Mantich
Dr. Tom McDavid
Dr. John McDowell
Dr. Monique Michaud
Dr. Dale Miles
Dr. David Molina
Dr. Charles Morris
Dr. Rick Myers
Dr. Chris Nortjé
Dr. Linda Otis
Dr. Roger Rao
Dr. Tom Razmus
Dr. Spencer Redding
Dr. Michele Saunders
Dr. Tom Schiff
Dr. Jack Sherman
Dr. Sol Silverman
Dr. Larry Skoczylas
Dr. D.B. Smith
Dr. John Tall
Dr. Geza Terezhalmy
Dr. Martin Tyler
Dr. Margo Van Dis
Dr. Michael Vitt
Dr. Elaine Winegard
Dr. Donna Wood

# Contents

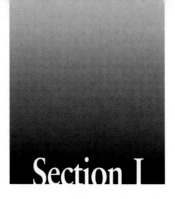

Section I

# Anatomic Landmarks

# Landmarks of the Oral Cavity

The oral cavity has several important functions. It is the portal to the gastrointestinal tract serving to masticate food, initiate digestion, and lubricate the food bolus for swallowing. It serves as an airway for the flow of respiratory gases when the nose is obstructed or otherwise unable to function. The soft tissues of the mouth contribute to speech, facial expression, and esthetics as well as kissing and romance.

**Lips (Fig. 1.1)** The lips are soft tissue structures that form the external border of the oral cavity. They are covered by parakeratotic mucosa, beneath which is fibrovascular tissue that lacks adnexal structures. Deep to the connective tissue are the muscles that control lip movement (orbicularis oris, levator, and depressor oris). The color of lips depends on the pigmentation of the patient. Melanoderms, such as African-Americans, may have pink or brown lips, whereas white persons have pink lips. The junction of the lips with the labial mucosa is the **wet line**. It represents the point of contact of the maxillary lip with its mandibular counterpart. The **vermilion** is the portion of the lip external to the wet line. The **vermilion border** is the junction of the lip with the skin; it should be smooth, well delineated, and slightly raised. The lips should be raised, inverted, and palpated during the oral examination. The surface should be smooth; nonscaly; uniform in color; and free of fissures, ulcerations, nodules, and masses.

**Labial Mucosa (Fig. 1.2)** The labial mucosa is the internal lining of the lip. Thin, pink parakeratotic epithelium covers the region. In melanoderms, the mucosa may be brownish-pink or pink with patches of light brown. Small red capillaries can traverse the labial mucosa; these vessels bring nutrients to the region. **Minor salivary gland ducts** empty multifocally onto the labial mucosa. When the lip is everted, the surface of the 1-mm orifices is covered by mucinous saliva. The labial mucosa is bordered by the alveolar mucosa, which covers the fornix and alveolar bone and the buccal mucosa posteriorly. The muscles that support this region are the levator labii superioris, levator labii inferioris, and depressor labii inferioris.

**Buccal Mucosa (Fig. 1.3)** The buccal mucosa is the inner epithelial lining of the cheeks. It extends bilaterally from the labial mucosa to the retromolar pad and pterygomandibular raphe region. It is composed of smooth, pink parakeratotic epithelium and is similar in appearance to the labial mucosa. The presence of fat within the connective tissue can make the buccal mucosa appear more yellow or tan. Accessory salivary glands are present in this region.

**Parotid Papilla (Fig. 1.4)** The parotid papilla is the terminal end of **Stenson's duct**, the excretory duct of the parotid gland. It is a triangular-configured, raised, pink papule located on the maxillary half of the buccal mucosa, adjacent to the maxillary first molars bilaterally. Parotid function can be assessed by milking the gland.

This is accomplished by drying the parotid papilla with a 2-inch by 2-inch gauze, pressing the fingers below the mandible, and then extending the pressure upward and over the gland. Clear saliva should flow from the duct within the parotid papilla.

**Hard Palate (Fig. 1.5)** The hard palate is the dorsal aspect of the oral cavity. It is composed of squamous epithelium, connective tissue, minor salivary glands and ducts (in the posterior two thirds only), periosteum, and the palatine processes of the maxilla. Anatomically, the palate consists of several structures. The **incisive papilla** is found immediately behind the maxillary incisors. It is a raised, pink ovoid structure that overlies the nasopalatine foramen. The **rugae** are located slightly posterior to the incisive papilla, in the anterior one third of the palate. These fibrous ridges run laterally from the midline to within several millimeters of the attached gingiva of the anterior teeth. Rugae help guide food to the teeth and influence phonetics. The alveolar bone that supports the palatal aspect of the posterior teeth is called the lateral vault. In the center of the hard palate is the **median palatal raphe,** the yellowish-white junction of the right and left palatine processes.

**Soft Palate (Fig. 1.6)** Compared with the hard palate, the soft palate has more minor salivary glands and more lymphoid and fatty tissue. It also lacks bony support. The soft palate functions during mastication and swallowing. It can be elevated by the action of the levator palati and tensor palati muscles; motor innervation is controlled by cranial nerves IX and X. The **median palatal raphe** is more prominent and thicker in the soft palate. Just lateral to the raphe are the **fovea palatinae.** The fovea are 2-mm excretory ducts of minor salivary glands. They serve as a landmark for the junction between the hard and soft palates. At the midline and distal aspect of the soft palate is the **uvula.**

**Oropharynx and Tonsils (Figs. 1.7 and 1.8)** The oropharynx is composed of the anterior and posterior tonsillar pillars and posterior pharyngeal wall. The **uvula** borders the anterior aspect of the oropharynx; the latero-anterior aspect is bordered by the **tonsillar pillars (fauces).** The **anterior pillar** is formed by the palatoglossus muscle, which runs downward, outward, and forward to the base of the tongue. The **posterior pillar** is larger than the anterior pillar, and it runs downward, outward, and posteriorly. It is formed by the palatopharyngeus muscle. The **tonsils** are lymphoid tissue that lie within the pillars. They are dome-shaped structures with cryptic invaginations for capturing ingressing microbes. In healthy persons, they are held within the pillars or extend slightly beyond the borders of the pillars. They enlarge during adolescence (a lymphoid growth period) and during infectious, inflammatory, and neoplastic processes. Islands of tonsillar tissue are seen on the surface of the posterior pharyngeal wall. **Waldeyer's ring** is the ring of adenoid tissue formed by the lingual, pharyngeal, and faucial tonsils.

# Landmarks of the Oral Cavity

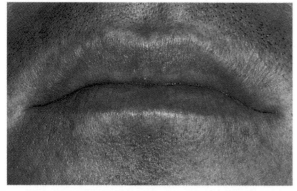

Figure 1.1. **Lips** in a healthy young adult.

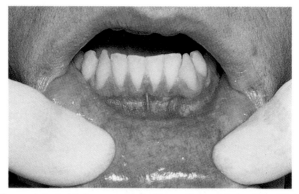

Figure 1.2. **Labial mucosa:** the inner lining of the lips. Pink, moist, and shiny appearance.

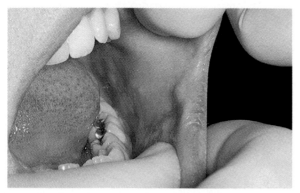

Figure 1.3. **Buccal mucosa:** the oral epithelial lining of the cheek. Caliculus angularis is bump at commissure.

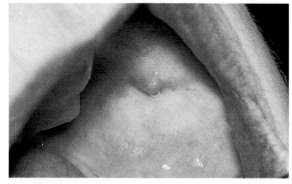

Figure 1.4. **Parotid papilla:** triangular structure that points downward and is adjacent to the maxillary first molar.

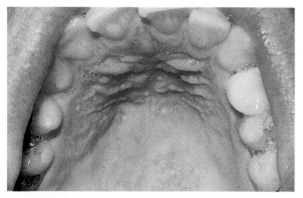

Figure 1.5. **Hard palate:** incisive papilla and rugae in anterior third of the palate, which contains no accessory salivary glands.

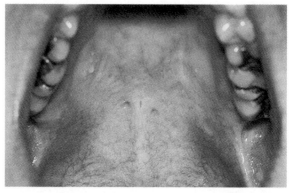

Figure 1.6. **Soft palate:** fovea palatinae seen in soft palate just behind junction with hard palate. Median palatal raphe in midline.

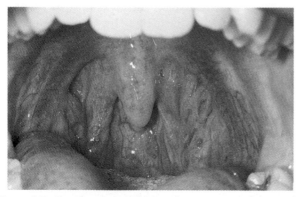

Figure 1.7. **Oropharynx:** pinkish-red appearance of the uvula, tonsillar pillars, and posterior pharyngeal wall with tonsillar tissue.

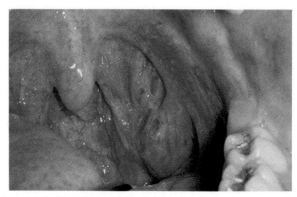

Figure 1.8. **Tonsillar pillars:** cryptic invaginations on surface of tonsils located between the anterior and posterior pillars (fauces).

# Landmarks of the Tongue and Variants of Normal

**Normal Tongue Anatomy (Figs. 2.1–2.5)** The tongue is a compact muscular organ covered by a protective layer of stratified squamous epithelium. It functions primarily in deglutition, taste, and speech. The dorsum of the tongue has numerous mucosal projections that form papillae. There are four types of projections: filiform, fungiform, circumvallate, and foliate papillae. **Filiform papillae** are the smallest but the most numerous. They are slender, hairlike, cornified stalks that may appear red, pink, or white, depending on the degree of daily irritation experienced. In a patient with good oral hygiene, the papillae appear pink. The dorsum contains fewer **fungiform papillae** than filiform papillae; the former are brighter red, and broader than the latter. Fungiform papillae are noncornified, round, or mushroom-shaped; they are slightly elevated and contain taste buds. These papillae are most numerous on the lateral border and anterior tip of the tongue. Fungiform papillae sometimes contain brown pigmentation, especially in melanoderms.

The largest papillae are the **circumvallate papillae.** They appear as 2- to 4-mm pink papules arranged in a V-shaped row along the sulcus terminalis at the posterior aspect of the dorsum of the tongue. They are surrounded by a narrow trench and also contain taste buds. The dorsum contains 8–12 circumvallate papillae, which anatomically divide the tongue into two unequal sections: the anterior two thirds and the posterior third.

If the lateral border of the posterior region of the tongue os examined carefully, the **foliate papilla** can be identified. These papillae are leaflike projections oriented as vertical folds. Foliate papilla are more prominent in children and young adults than in older adults. Corrugated hypertrophic lymphoid tissue (lingual tonsil) extending into this area from the posterior dorsal root of the tongue may sometimes be mistakenly called foliate papillae. The **plica fimbriata** are linear projections on the ventral surface of the tongue. The plica fimbriata occasionally have a brown pigmentation.

**Fissured Tongue (Plicated Tongue, Scrotal Tongue) (Fig. 2.6)** Fissured tongue is a variation of normal tongue anatomy that consists of a single midline fissure, double fissures, or multiple fissures of the dorsal surface of the anterior two thirds of the tongue. Various fissural patterns, lengths, and depths have been observed. The cause is unknown, but fissured tongue is probably developmental, increases with age, and may be associated with xerostomia.

Fissured tongue affects about 1–5% of the population. The frequency of the condition is equal in men and women. Fissured tongue occurs commonly in patients with Down's syndrome and in combination with geographic tongue. It is a component of the Melkerson-Rosenthal syndrome (fissured tongue, cheilitis granulomatosa, and unilateral facial nerve paralysis). The fissures may become secondarily inflamed and cause halitosis as a result of food impaction; thus, brushing the tongue to keep the fissures clean is recommended. The condition is benign.

**Ankyloglossia (Fig. 2.7)** The lingual frenum is normally attached to the ventral tongue and genial tubercles of the mandible. If the frenum fails to attach properly to the tongue and genial tubercles but instead fuses to the floor of the mouth or lingual gingiva and the ventral tip of the tongue, the condition is called ankyloglossia, or "tongue-tie." This congenital condition is characterized by an abnormally short and malpositioned lingual frenum and a tongue that cannot be extended or retracted. The fusion may be partial or complete. Partial fusion is more common. If the condition is severe, speech may be disturbed. Surgical correction and speech therapy are necessary if speech is defective or if a mandibular denture or removable partial denture is planned. The estimated frequency of ankyloglossia is one case per 1000 births.

**Lingual Varicosity (Phlebectasia) (Fig. 2.8)** Lingual varicosities, or venous dilations, are a common finding in elderly adults. The condition has no direct association with peripheral varicosities or with compromised venous return to the heart. The cause of these vascular dilatations is either a blockage of the vein by an internal foreign body, such as a plaque, or the loss of elasticity of the vascular wall as a result of aging. Intraoral varicosities most commonly appear superficially on the ventral surface of the anterior two thirds of the tongue and may extend onto the lateral border and floor of the mouth. Men and women are affected equally.

Varicosities appear as red-blue to purple, fluctuant nodular growths. Individual varices may be prominent and tortuous or small and punctate. Palpation elicits no pain but can disperse the blood from the vessel, thereby flattening the surface appearance. Diascopy causes varices to blanch. When many lingual veins are prominent, the condition is called "phlebectasia linguae" or "caviar tongue." The lip and labial commissure are other frequent sites of phlebectasia. No treatment of this condition is required.

# Landmarks of the Tongue and Variants of Normal

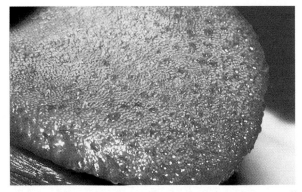

Figure 2.1. **Normal tongue anatomy:** red fungiform papillae are interspersed among the more numerous and whitish filiform papillae of the dorsal tongue.

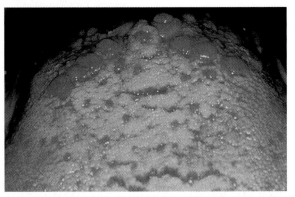

Figure 2.2. **Circumvallate papillae** forming a V-shaped row on the dorsum, at the border of posterior one third of the tongue. (Courtesy Dr James Cottone)

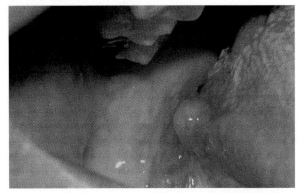

Figure 2.3. **Foliate papilla** on the posterolateral border of the tongue.

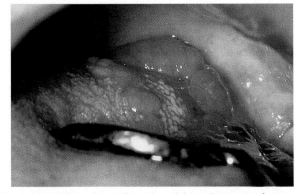

Figure 2.4. **Lingual tonsil** at dorsal lateral aspect of tongue, posterior to the circumvallate papillae.

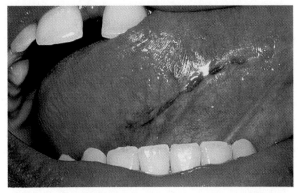

Figure 2.5. **Plica fimbriata,** which in this person is pigmented.

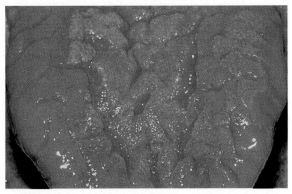

Figure 2.6. **Fissured tongue** and subtle manifestations of geographic tongue.

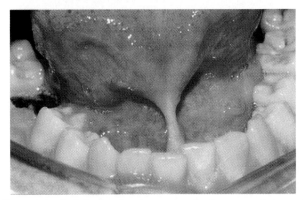

Figure 2.7. **Ankyloglossia;** the patient had no speech impediment.

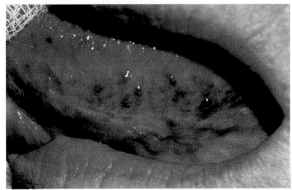

Figure 2.8. **Lingual varicosities;** several purple venous dilatations on the ventral tongue. (Courtesy Dr Linda Otis)

# Landmarks of the Periodontium

**Periodontium (Figs. 3.1 and 3.2)** The periodontium is the tissue that immediately surrounds and supports the teeth in the distal, mesial, buccal, lingual, and apical directions. It consists of alveolar bone, periosteum, periodontal ligament, gingival sulcus, and gingiva; each of these components contributes to stabilizing the tooth within the jaws. The **alveolar bone** is composed of cancellous bone, also known as spongy bone. It is located between the cortical plates and is permeated by blood vessels and marrow spaces. The **periosteum** is dense connective tissue attached to the outer surface of the bone. The tooth is anchored to alveolar bone by the attachment of the **periodontal ligament** to the periosteum and the **cementum** of each tooth root. The periodontal ligament follows the outline of the tooth root and extends superiorly to the base of the gingival sulcus. The **gingival sulcus** is lined internally by a thin layer of epithelial cells called junctional epithelium. This epithelium provides the barrier to the ingress of bacteria. In health, the gingival sulcus is a crevice that is less than 3 mm deep. Colonization of bacteria within the sulcus promotes inflammatory processes that lead to breakdown of the **epithelial attachment**. A **periodontal pocket** is a gingival sulcus that has experienced apical extension of the epithelial attachment beyond 3 mm because of repeated inflammatory insults and poor oral hygiene. Although accumulation of bacterial plaque is the most important factor influencing the health of the periodontium, position of the tooth within the arch, occlusal loading, parafunctional habits, appliances, drugs, and frenal attachments also affect periodontal health and the development of periodontal pockets.

**Alveolar Mucosa and Frenal Attachments (Figs. 3.3 and 3.4)** Mucosa is epithelium covering mucus-secreting glands. The **alveolar mucosa** is moveable mucosa that overlies alveolar bone and borders the apical extent of the periodontium. It is moveable because it is not bound down to the underlying periosteum and bone. The alveolar mucosa is thin and highly vascular. Accordingly, it appears pinkish-red, red, or bright red. Upon close inspection, small arteries and capillaries can be seen within the alveolar mucosa. These vessels provide nutrients, oxygen, and blood cells to the region. The alveolar mucosa blends into the gingiva and the vestibule. As the mucosa rises from the vestibule away from the periodontium, it is generally identified as either buccal mucosa (if it is located posteriorly) or labial mucosa (if it is located anteriorly).

Frenae are muscle attachments at specific locations within the alveolar mucosa. With the lip distended, they appear as arc-like rims of flexible tissue. They sometimes produce several fiber-like attachments. Six oral frenae have been identified. The **maxillary labial frenum** is located at the midline between the maxillary central incisors, about 4–7 mm apical to the interdental region. The

mandibular labial frenum appears similarly below and between mandibular central incisors within the alveolar mucosa. The **maxillary and mandibular buccal frenae** are located within the alveolar mucosa near the first premolar on the right and left sides. Although frenae that attach within 3 mm of the cementoenamel junction of a tooth do not directly contribute to periodontal support, they can pull on periodontal tissues and contribute to the development of gingival recession.

**Mucogingival Junction (Fig. 3.5)** The mucogingival junction is an anatomic landmark representing the border between the unattached alveolar mucosa and the attached gingiva. It is curvilinear and extends around the buccal and lingual aspects of the arches. The prominence of the junction depends on the difference in vascularity and thus the color of the two tissues. It is easily distinguished when the alveolar mucosa is red and the attached gingiva is pink.

**Attached Gingiva and Free Marginal Gingiva (Figs. 3.6– 3.8)** The attached gingiva and free marginal gingiva are close to the tooth. They cover the external aspect of the gingival sulcus. The attached gingiva extends coronally from the alveolar mucosa to the free marginal gingiva. It is covered by keratinized epithelium, is bound down to periosteum, and cannot be moved. In health, the attached gingiva is pink and 2–7 mm wide. Its surface is slightly convex and stippled, appearing like the surface of an orange. **Interdental grooves** can be seen in the attached gingiva as vertical grooves or narrow depressions located between the roots of the teeth.

The **marginal gingiva** provides the gingival collar around the cervix of the tooth. It is pink and keratinized like the attached gingiva. Unlike the attached gingiva, however, the marginal gingiva is not attached to periosteum. Its freely moveable nature allows a periodontal probe to be passed under it during assessment of pocket depth. Accordingly, it is also termed the **free marginal gingiva**. The junction of the marginal gingiva and the attached gingiva is called the **free gingival groove**.

The **interdental papilla** is the triangular projection of marginal gingiva that extends upward between the teeth. The base of the triangle is nearest the attached gingiva, the apex closest to the interproximal contact of the teeth. The papilla has a buccal and lingual surface. In healthy persons, papillae are pink and knife-edge and can barely be moved by the periodontal probe. The presence of inflammation and disease (i.e., gingivitis) alter the color, contour, and consistency of the free marginal gingiva and interdental papillae, causing the marginal gingiva to appear purple, soft, swollen, and tender. Between the buccal and lingual interdental papillae is the **col**, a concave depression of the free marginal gingiva between the teeth.

# Landmarks of the Periodontium

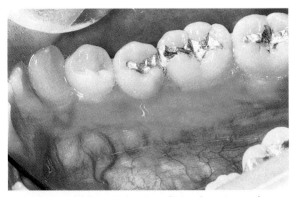

Figure 3.1. Healthy periodontium: anterior view showing prominent gingiva and alveolar mucosa.

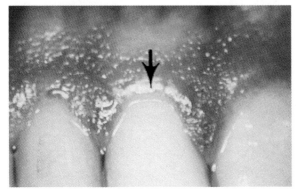

Figure 3.2. Healthy periodontium lingual aspect with prominent small arteries within the alveolar mucosa apical to the first premolar.

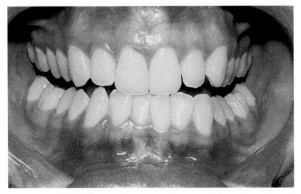

Figure 3.3. Healthy periodontium and buccal frenum: whitish pink regions over canines represent prominent bone and thin gingiva. Maxillary buccal frenum prominent apical to maxillary first premolar.

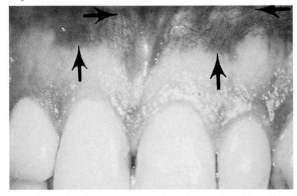

Figure 3.4. Alveolar mucosa: red and vascular, identified by arrows.

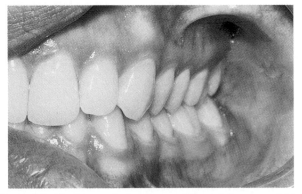

Figure 3.5. Mucogingival junction: identified by arrow.

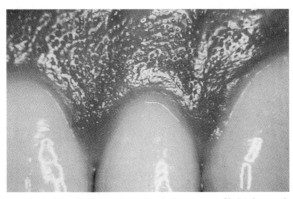

Figure 3.6. Attached gingiva: stippled texture of labial-attached gingiva of maxillary incisors. Interdental grooves between the roots of the incisors.

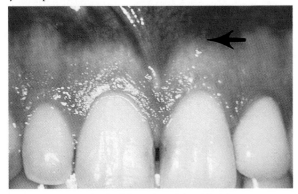

Figure 3.7. Free gingival groove: delineating free marginal gingiva from attached gingiva.

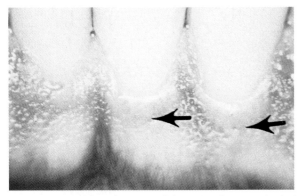

Figure 3.8. Free marginal gingiva: the collar of gingiva adjacent to the cementoenamel junction of the tooth.

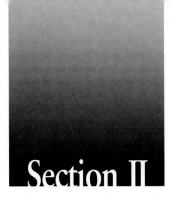

# Section II

# Diagnostic and Descriptive Terminology

# Diagnostic and Descriptive Terminology

**Macule (Figs. 4.1 and 4.2)** A macule is a circumscribed area of epidermis or mucosa distinguished by color from its surroundings. The macule may appear alone or in groups and as a blue, brown, or black stain or spot. The macule is neither elevated nor depressed and may be of any size. The term macule is usually reserved for lesions 1 cm or smaller. A macule may represent a normal condition, a variant of normal, or local or systemic disease. The term macule would be used to clinically describe the following conditions: oral melanotic macule, ephelis, amalgam tattoo, and focal argyrosis. Conditions that appear as macules are discussed in detail under Pigmented Lesions (Figs. 46.1–48.8).

**Patch (Figs. 4.3 and 4.4)** A patch is a circumscribed area that is larger than the macule and differentiated from the surrounding epidermis by color, texture, or both. Like the macule, the patch is neither elevated nor depressed. Focal argyrosis, lichen planus, mucous patch of secondary syphilis, and snuff dipper's patch represent patch-like lesions that may be seen intraorally. Conditions that appear as patches are discussed in detail under White Lesions (Figs. 37.1–39.8), Pigmented Lesions (Figs. 46-1–48.8), and Sexually Transmissible Diseases (Figs. 60.1–62.8).

**Erosion (Figs. 4.5 and 4.6)** Erosion is a clinical term that describes a soft tissue lesion in which the epithelium above the basal cell layer is denuded. Erosions are moist and slightly depressed and often result from a broken vesicle or trauma. Healing rarely results in scarring. Pemphigus and erosive lichen planus are diseases that produce mucocutaneous erosions. Conditions that appear as erosions are discussed in detail under Vesiculobullous Lesions (Figs. 52.1–56.8).

**Ulcer (Figs. 4.7 and 4.8)** An ulcer is an uncovered wound of cutaneous or mucosal tissue that exhibits gradual tissue disintegration and necrosis. Ulcers extend deeper than erosions, from beyond the basal layer of the epithelium and into the dermis. Scarring may follow healing of an ulcer. Ulcers may result from aphthous stomatitis or infection by such viruses as herpes simplex, variola (smallpox), and varicella-zoster (chickenpox and shingles). Ulcers are usually painful and often require topical drug therapy for effective management. Conditions that appear as ulcers are discussed in detail under Vesiculobullous Lesions (Figs. 52.1–56.8).

# Diagnostic and Descriptive Terminology

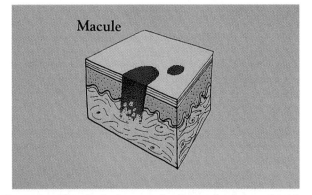

Figure 4.1. Macule. A circumscribed, nonraised area of epidermis altered in color from its surroundings.

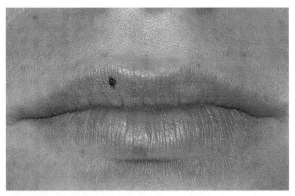

Figure 4.2. Oral melanotic macule on the lip.

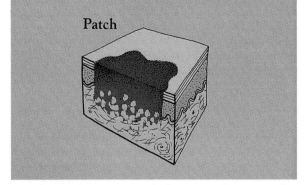

Figure 4.3. Patch. A circumscribed pigmented or textured area larger than the macule.

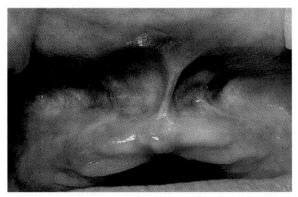

Figure 4.4. Patch: focal argyrosis caused by leaching of silver points from root canal–treated teeth that were previously extracted.

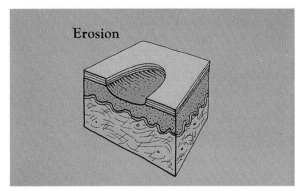

Figure 4.5. Erosion. A denudation of epithelium above the basal cell layer.

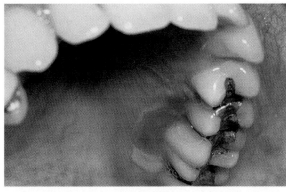

Figure 4.6. Erosion: erosive lichen planus of the palatal gingiva.

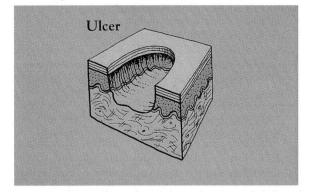

Figure 4.7. Ulcer. A loss of epithelium that extends below the basal cell layer.

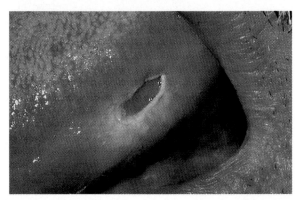

Figure 4.8. Traumatic ulcer of the lateral border of the tongue.

# Diagnostic and Descriptive Terminology

**Wheal (Figs. 5.1 and 5.2)** A wheal is an edematous papule or plaque that results from acute extravasation of serum into the upper dermis. Wheals are generally pale red, pruritic, and of short duration. By definition they are only slightly raised; they often occur in persons with allergies. The wheal develops as a result of histamine release from mast cells or activation of the complement cascade. Wheals may be seen after insect bites, an allergic reaction to food, or mechanical irritation (such as that occurring in patients with dermatographia). Conditions that appear as wheals are discussed in detail under Allergic Reactions and Vesiculobullous Lesions (Figs. 54.1–54.8).

**Scar (Figs. 5.3 and 5.4)** A scar is a permanent mark or cicatrix remaining after a wound heals. These lesions are visible signs that indicate a disruption in the integrity of the epidermis and dermis and healing of epithelium with collagen connective tissue. Scars are infrequently found in the oral cavity but may be of any shape or size. The color of an intraoral scar is usually lighter than that of the adjacent mucosa. A scar is more dense than the adjacent epithelium. Periapical surgery, burns, or intraoral trauma may result in a scar. Scars are discussed in detail under White Lesions (Figs. 35.1–35.8).

**Fissure (Figs. 5.5 and 5.6)** A fissure is a normal or abnormal linear cleft in the epidermis that affects the lips and perioral tissues. The presence of a fissure can indicate a condition representing a variant of normal or disease. Diseased fissures result when pathogenic organisms infect a fissure, causing pain, ulceration, and inflammation. Fissured tongue is an example of a variation of normal, whereas angular cheilitis and exfoliative cheilitis are examples of diseased fissures.

**Sinus (Figs. 5.7 and 5.8)** A sinus is an abnormal tract or fistula that leads from a suppurative cavity, cyst, or abscess to the surface of the epidermis. An abscessed tooth often produces a sinus tract together with a clinically evident parulis, which is the terminal end of the sinus. Gutta percha points can be placed into the tract; when radiography is done, the nonvital tooth can be identified by locating the tip of the point. Actinomycosis is a condition characterized by several yellow sinus tracts.

# Diagnostic and Descriptive Terminology

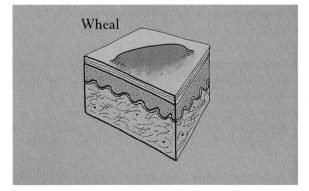

**Figure 5.1. Wheal.** A pinkish-red, edematous, serum-filled papule or plaque.

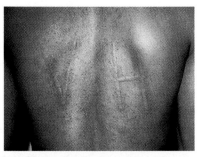

**Figure 5.2. Wheal: dermatographism.** A condition of hypersensitivity characterized by wheals produced by rubbing the skin.

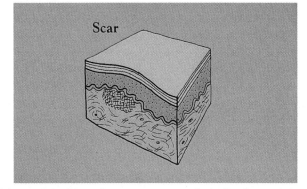

**Figure 5.3. Scar.** A permanent mark indicating previous wound healing.

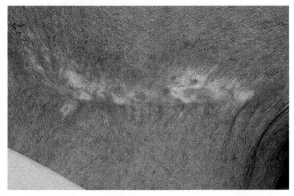

**Figure 5.4. Scar:** taut fibrotic tissue caused by a **burn**.

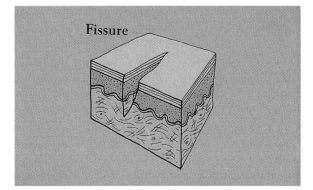

**Figure 5.5. Fissure.** A linear crack in the epidermis.

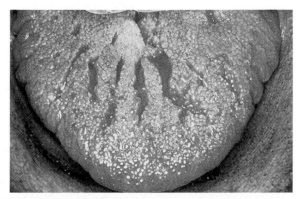

**Figure 5.6. Fissure: fissured tongue.** A variant of normal.

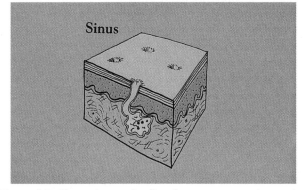

**Figure 5.7. Sinus.** A tract leading from a suppurative cavity, cyst, or abscess.

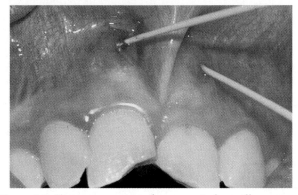

**Figure 5.8. Sinus tracts** exiting from nonvital maxillary central incisors that have been delineated by insertion of gutta percha points.

# Diagnostic and Descriptive Terminology

**Papule (Figs. 6.1 and 6.2)** A papule is a superficial, elevated, solid lesion that is less than 1 cm in diameter. Papules may be of any color and may be attached by a stalk or firm base. A papule often represents a benign or slow-growing lesion such as condyloma acuminatum, parulis, and squamous papilloma. However, basal cell carcinoma can appear as a papule. Conditions that appear as papules are discussed in the section on Papulonodules (Figs. 51.1–51.8).

**Plaque (Figs. 6.3 and 6.4)** A plaque is a flat, solid, raised area that is larger than 1 cm in diameter. Although essentially superficial, plaques may extend deeper into the dermis than papules. The edges may be sloped, and sometimes surface keratin proliferates (a condition known as lichenification). Lichen planus, leukoplakia, or melanoma may initially appear as a plaque. Lichen planus is discussed under Red and Red/White Lesions (Figs 43.1–43.8).

**Nodule (Figs. 6.5 and 6.6)** A nodule is a solid mass of tissue that has the dimension of depth. Like papules, these lesions are less than 1 cm in diameter; nodules, however, extend deeper into the dermis. The nodule can be detected by palpation. The overlying epidermis is usually nonfixed and can be easily moved over the lesion. Nodules can be asymptomatic or painful and usually are slow growing. Benign mesenchymal tumors such as the fibroma, lipoma, lipofibroma, and neuroma often appear as oral nodules. Other examples of nodules are discussed under Figs. 50.1–50.8.

**Tumor (Figs. 6.7 and 6.8)** "Tumor" is a term used to indicate a solid mass of tissue larger than 1 cm in diameter that has the dimension of depth. The term is also used to represent a neoplasm—a new, independent growth of tissue with uncontrolled and progressive multiplication of cells that have no physiologic use. Tumors may be any color and may be located in any intraoral or extraoral soft or hard tissue. Tumors are classified as benign or malignant. **Benign tumors** grow more slowly and are less aggressive than **malignant tumors**. Benign tumors often appear as raised, rounded lesions that have well-defined margins; they do not metastasize. Malignant tumors spread rapidly and often have ill-defined margins. Persistent tumors may be umbilicated or ulcerated in the center. The term tumor is often used to describe a benign tissue mass such as a neurofibroma, granular cell tumor, or pregnancy tumor. The term **carcinoma** is reserved for malignant cancers of epithelial tissue. The term **sarcoma** is reserved for a malignant neoplasm of embryonic connective tissue origin, such as osteosarcoma, a malignant neoplasm of bone.

# Diagnostic and Descriptive Terminology

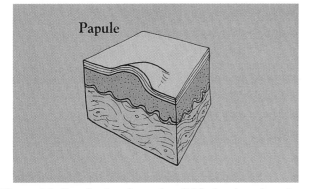

**Figure 6.1. Papule.** An elevated, solid lesion less than 1 cm in diameter.

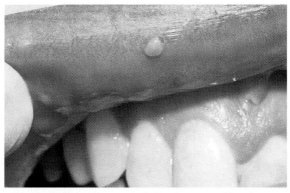

**Figure 6.2. Papule: fibroepithelial polyp** caused by chronic inflammation.

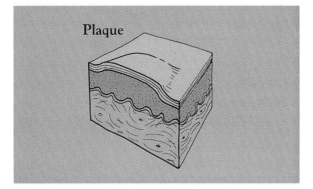

**Figure 6.3. Plaque.** A flat, raised area larger than 1 cm in diameter.

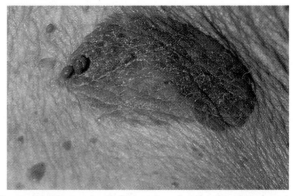

**Figure 6.4. Plaque: senile keratosis,** a benign skin discoloration that develops in elderly persons.

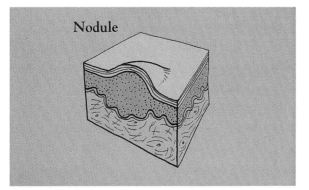

**Figure 6.5. Nodule.** A raised, solid mass that has the dimension of depth and is less than 1 cm in diameter.

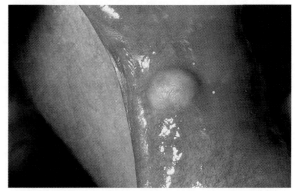

**Figure 6.6. Nodule: irritation fibroma.** Common location is the buccal mucosa near commissure.

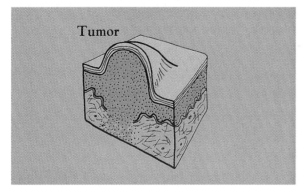

**Figure 6.7. Tumor.** A solid, raised benign or malignant mass that has the dimension of depth and is larger than 1 cm in diameter.

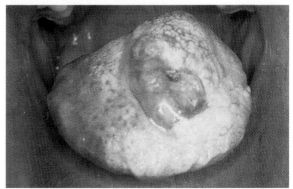

**Figure 6.8. Tumor: squamous cell carcinoma** of the tongue.

**15**

# Diagnostic and Descriptive Terminology

**Vesicle (Figs. 7.1 and 7.2)** A vesicle is a circumscribed, fluid-filled elevation in the epidermis that is less than 1 cm in diameter. The fluid of a vesicle generally consists of lymph or serum but may contain blood. The epithelial lining of a vesicle is thin and will eventually break down, thus causing an ulcer and eschar. Vesicles are common in such viral infections as herpes simplex, herpes zoster, chickenpox, and smallpox. In viral infections, the vesicle is laden with virus and is highly infectious. Conditions characterized by vesicles are discussed under Vesiculobullous Lesions (Figs. 52.1–56.8).

**Pustule (Figs. 7.3 and 7.4)** A pustule is a circumscribed elevation filled with purulent exudate resulting from an infection. Pustules are less than 1 cm in diameter and may be preceded by a vesicle or papule. They are creamy white or yellowish and are often associated with an epidermal pore. Within the mouth, a pustule is represented by a pointing abscess or parulis. Herpes zoster also produces pustules that eventually ulcerate and cause intense pain. See the discussions under Localized Gingival Lesions (Figs. 22.1–22.2), Caries Progression (Fig. 17.8), and Vesiculobullous Lesions (Figs. 53.1–53.4) for examples of diseases that produce pustules.

**Bulla (Figs. 7.5 and 7.6)** When the diameter of a vesicle exceeds 1 cm, the vesicle is termed a bulla. This condition develops from the accumulation of fluid in the epidermal-dermis junction or a split in the epidermis. Because of their size, bullae represent a more severe disease than do conditions associated with vesicles. Bullae are commonly seen in pemphigus, pemphigoid, burns, and epidermolysis bullosa. These conditions are discussed under Vesiculobullous Lesions (Figs. 56.1–56.8).

**Cyst (Figs. 7.7 and 7.8)** A cyst is an epithelially lined mass located in the dermis or subcutaneous tissue. Cysts result from entrapment of epithelium or remnants of epithelium that grow to produce a cavity. They range in diameter from a few millimeters to several centimeters. Aspiration of a cyst may or may not yield luminal fluid, depending on the nature of the cyst. Cysts that contain clear fluid appear pink to blue, whereas keratin-filled cysts often appear yellow or creamy white. Some of the many types of oral cysts are dermoid cysts, eruption cysts, implantation cysts, incisive canal cysts, lymphoepithelial cysts, mucus retention cysts, nasoalveolar cysts, and radicular cysts.

# Diagnostic and Descriptive Terminology

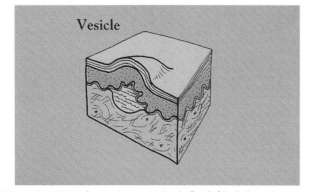

Figure 7.1. **Vesicle.** A circumscribed, fluid-filled skin elevation less than 1 cm in diameter.

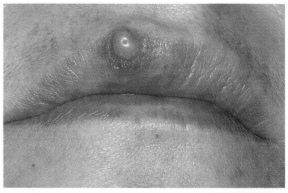

Figure 7.2. **Vesicle: recurrent herpes simplex.** Vesicular fluid is contagious.

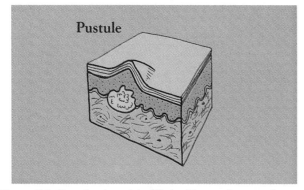

Figure 7.3. **Pustule.** A vesicle filled with purulent exudate.

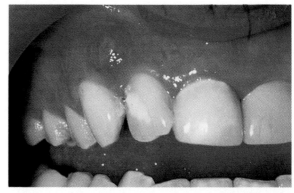

Figure 7.4. **Pustule: abscessed lateral incisor.** Drainage reduces the swelling and relieves symptoms.

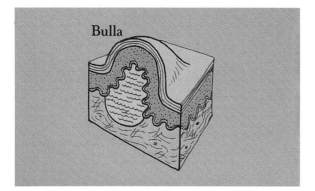

Figure 7.5. **Bulla.** A fluid-filled mucocutaneous elevation greater than 1 cm in diameter.

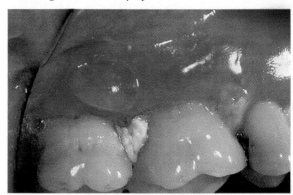

Figure 7.6. **Bulla: bullous lichen planus.** A rare manifestation of this disease.

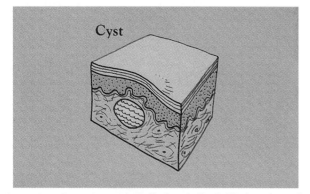

Figure 7.7. **Cyst.** An epithelially lined, fluid-filled mass in the dermis, subcutaneous tissue, or jaw bones.

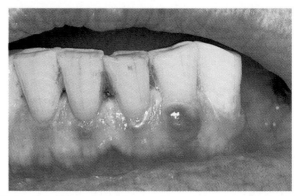

Figure 7.8. **Cyst: gingival cyst,** the peripheral variant of the developmental lateral periodontal cyst.

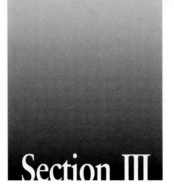

# Section III

# Oral Conditions Affecting Infants and Children

# Oral Conditions Affecting Infants and Children

**Commissural Lip Pits (Fig. 8.1)** Commissural lip pits are dimple-like invaginations of the corner of the lips. They may be unilateral or bilateral but generally occur on the vermilion portion of the lip. They are generally less than 4 mm in diameter, and exploration of the pits yields a sealed depression. Commisural lip pits represent failure of fusion of the embryonic maxillary and mandibular processes. The pits occur more frequently in males than in females, and prevalence differs between adults and children. For example, lip pits have been documented in less than 1% of children but in up to 10% of adults. These figures indicate that the invaginations may be developmental and not congenital. However, an autosomal dominant pattern of transmission has been reported in some families. No treatment is required.

**Paramedian Lip Pits (Fig. 8.2)** Paramedian lip pits are congenital depressions that occur in the mandibular lip, most often on either side of the midline. They probably develop from the lateral sulci of the embryonic mandibular arch that fail to regress during the sixth week in utero. Paramedian lip pits are more often bilateral, symmetric depressions with raised, rounded borders. However, single pits and unilateral pits have been described. Inspection reveals a sealed depression that may express mucinous saliva. Paramedian lip pits are often inherited as an autosomal dominant trait in combination with cleft lip or cleft palate. When these features occur together, the condition is called **van der Woude's syndrome**. The gene responsible for lip pits shows variable penetrance; some patients who carry the gene may have a minor or submucosal cleft palate or no cleft yet pass the full syndrome on to their children. By themselves, paramedian lip pits require no treatment unless they are of esthetic concern. The clinician should inquire about affected family members and examine them for cleft lip and palate.

**Cleft Lip (Figs. 8.3 and 8.4)** Cleft lip is the result of a disturbance of lip development in utero. The maxillary lip is most commonly affected. Cleft lip results when the medial nasal process fails to fuse with the lateral portions of the maxillary process of the first branchial arch. Fusion normally occurs during the sixth and seventh week of embryonic development.

Cleft lip occurs in about 1 in 900 births and more often in Asian and Native American persons than in white persons. The condition occurs more often in males than in females and is more severe in males than in females. About 85% of cleft lips are unilateral and non-midline; 15% are bilateral. Midline cleft lip, resulting from failure of fusion of the right and left medial nasal processes, is rare.

The severity of cleft lips varies. A small cleft that does not involve the nose is called an incomplete cleft; these sometimes appear as a small notch in the lip. A complete cleft lip involves the nasal structures and is often (45% of cases) associated with cleft palate. Cleft lip and cleft palate can be caused by abnormal patterning genes that are transmitted by autosomal dominant and recessive inheritance, as well as X-linked inheritance. Certain drugs, such as nicotine and antiepileptic agents, also appear causative.

**Cleft Palate (Figs. 8.5–8.8)** The palate develops from the primary and secondary palate. The primary palate is formed by fusion of the right and left medial nasal processes. It is a small triangular mass that encompasses bone, connective tissue, labial and palatal epithelium, and the four incisor tooth buds. The secondary palate is formed by fusion of the palatine processes (shelves) of the maxillary process. Palatal fusion is initiated during the eighth week in utero by expansion of the mandible; this permits the tongue to drop down and allows the palatal processes to grow inward. The palatal shelves merge with the primary palate, and fusion progresses posteriorly. Except for the posterior soft palate and uvula, fusion of the palate is generally completed by the twelfth week of gestation.

Disruption in palatal fusion leads to clefting. A cleft palate can involve the soft palate only; the hard palate only; the hard and soft palates; or the hard and soft palates, alveolus, and lip. Cleft palate without lip involvement occurs in about 30% of cases.

**Bifid uvula** is a minor cleft of the posterior soft palate. It occurs most commonly in Asian and Native American persons; the overall incidence is about 1 in 250 people. A **submucosal palatal cleft** may occur with bifid uvula. It develops when the muscles of the soft palate are clefted but the surface mucosa is intact. The clefted region is palpably notched. An **incomplete cleft palate** is a small break in the hard or soft palate that permits communication between the oral and nasal cavities. A **complete cleft palate** extends forward to include the incisive foramen. The triad of cleft palate, micrognathia and retrognathia of the mandible, and glossoptosis (posterior displacement of the tongue) is called **Pierre Robin's syndrome** (anomalad). This condition is characterized by respiratory difficulty.

Cleft lip and palate are often associated with cleft alveolus, missing teeth (most commonly the lateral incisor), malpositioned teeth, and occasionally supernumerary teeth. Cleft palate causes feeding and speech impairment and prominent malocclusion. Treatment involves a multidisciplinary team consisting of a pediatrician, pediatric dentist, oral and plastic surgeon, orthodontist, and speech therapist. Surgical lip closure is generally accomplished early in the infant's life, whereas cleft palate may require several surgical procedures because of growth plate considerations.

# Oral Conditions Affecting Infants and Children

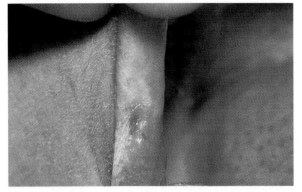

Figure 8.1. **Commissural lip pits:** blind depression at commissure of lip.

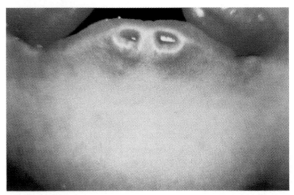

Figure 8.2. **Paramedian lip pits:** with cleft lip and palate (van der Woude's syndrome).

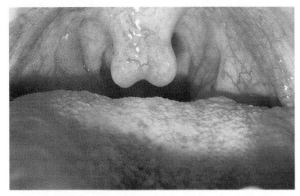

Figure 8.3. **Incomplete cleft lip:** rare midline type.

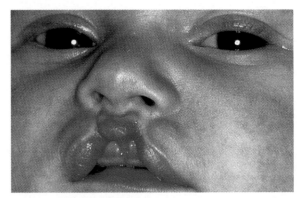

Figure 8.4. **Bilateral cleft lip.**

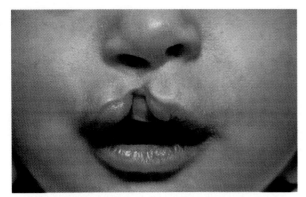

Figure 8.5. **Bifid uvula:** mild case.

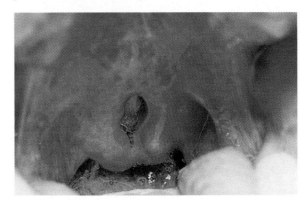

Figure 8.6. **Bifid uvula:** more severe case than that shown in Figure 8.5.

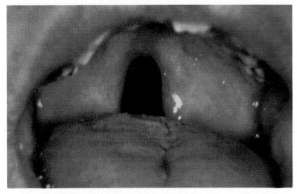

Figure 8.7. **Cleft soft palate.** If untreated, the condition causes problems with speech and swallowing.

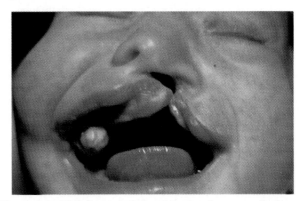

Figure 8.8. **Cleft lip and cleft palate:** involvement of primary and secondary palates.

# Oral Conditions Affecting Infants and Children

**Congenital Epulis (Fig. 9.1)** The congenital epulis of the newborn is a benign, soft tissue polypoid growth arising from the edentulous alveolar ridge. It usually occurs in the anterior maxilla and is 10 times more likely to occur in females than in males. The lesion is pink, soft, and compressible. The surface shows prominent telangiectasis and is attached to the alveolar ridge by a pedunculated stalk. Lesions can be several centimeters in diameter. The lesion is treated by excision, and recurrence is unlikely. Histologic examination shows granular cells. In one of 10 cases, multiple lesions are present.

**Melanotic Neuroectodermal Tumor of Infancy (Fig. 9.2)** The melanotic neuroectodermal tumor of infancy is a benign, rapidly growing neuroblastic neoplasm commonly located in the anterior maxilla. The tumor shows no sex predilection and begins as a small pink or red-purple nodule that resembles an eruption cyst. Radiography usually shows localized and irregular destruction of underlying alveolar bone and a primary tooth bud floating in a soft tissue mass. Urinary levels of vanyllmandelic acid are elevated in conjunction with this tumor. Treatment is conservative excision. Histologic examination often shows pigmentation. Recurrence and metastasis are rarely documented complications.

**Dental Lamina Cysts (Fig. 9.3)** Remnants of the dental lamina that do not develop into a tooth bud may degenerate to form dental lamina cysts. These cysts are classified according to clinical location. The **gingival cyst of the newborn** are tiny keratin-filled cysts. They are often multiple and whitish and usually resolve when the tooth erupts. The **palatal cysts of the newborn** can be either Epstein's pearls or Bohn's nodules. Epstein's pearls arise from epithelial inclusions that become entrapped at the median palatal raphe during fusion of opposing embryonic palatal shelves; Bohn's nodules arise from minor salivary glands. The pearls and nodules are usually small, firm, and whitish and may occur in small groups anywhere on the hard palate or at the junction of the hard and soft palates. Dental lamina cysts may be incised if they do not resolve spontaneously.

**Natal Teeth (Fig. 9.4)** Natal teeth are teeth that are present at birth or erupt within 30 days of birth. Some natal teeth have been referred to as "supernumerary" or as "predeciduous" and consist only of cornified and calcific material; the teeth are mobile and do not have roots. However, most natal teeth simply represent premature eruption of the primary teeth. The most common natal teeth are the incisors; the mandible is affected 10 times more often than the maxilla. Natal teeth have been reported to cause ulcers of the ventral tongue (Riga-Fede's disease) that result from irritation during nursing. In this case, extraction may be needed. However, a radiograph should be taken to determine whether the tooth is predeciduous or deciduous.

**Eruption Cyst (Gingival Eruption Cyst, Eruption Hematoma) (Fig. 9.5)** The eruption cyst is a soft tissue variant of the dentigerous cyst that forms around an erupting tooth crown. Children younger than 10 years of age are most commonly affected. It appears as a small, dome-shaped, translucent swelling overlying an erupting primary tooth. The cyst is lined by odontogenic epithelium and is filled with blood or serum. The presence of blood casts a blue-gray appearance to the cyst. No treatment is necessary because the erupting tooth eventually breaks the cystic membrane. Symptoms can be relieved by incising the lesion and allowing the fluid to drain.

**Congenital Lymphangioma (Fig. 9.6)** The congenital lymphangioma is a benign hamartoma of dilated lymphatic channels that may present in the mouth of infants. The tongue, alveolar ridge, and labial mucosa are common locations. There is a 2:1 predilection for males. In 1 in 20 African-American neonates, one or more alveolar lymphangiomas may be seen. The lymphangioma typically produces a swelling that is asymptomatic, compressible, and negative on diascopy. When superficial, the swelling is composed of single or multiple discrete papulonodules that may be pink to dark blue. Deep-seated tumors produce diffuse swellings with no alteration of the color of the overlying tissue. Large lymphangiomas of the neck are called cystic hygromas. Intraoral lymphangiomas may regress spontaneously, but persistent lesions should be excised.

**Thrush (Candidiasis, Moniliasis) (Fig. 9.7)** Thrush, or acute pseudomembranous candidiasis, is a fungal infection of mucosal membranes that is caused by *Candida albicans* and is primarily seen in infants. Thrush is a surface infection that produces milky-white curds on the oral mucosa. These curds are easily wiped off and leave a red, raw, painful surface. The buccal mucosa, palate, and tongue are common locations. Newborns often acquire the infection from the mother's birth canal during partuition and show clinical signs of infection within the first few weeks of life. Fever and gastrointestinal irritation may accompany the disorder. Treatment consists of topically applied antifungal agents.

**Parulis (Gum Boil) (Fig. 9.8)** The parulis is an inflammatory response to a chronic bacterial infection of a nonvital tooth draining through a sinus tract. It most commonly occurs in children when pulpal infection spreads beyond the furcal area of a posterior tooth. The parulis appears as a small, raised, fluctuant yellow-to-red boil that is located near the mucogingival junction adjacent to the affected tooth. Pressure to the area and the resulting discharge of pus are pathognomonic. Spontaneous pain is not a feature, although palpation of the lesion, tooth, or surrounding structures may elicit pain. The condition resolves when the odontogenic infection is eliminated.

# Oral Conditions Affecting Infants and Children

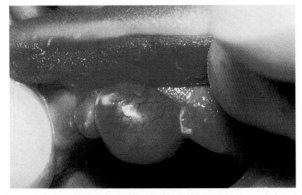

**Figure 9.1. Congenital epulis of the newborn:** pink nodule with surface telangiectasis. (Courtesy Dr Sheryl Hunter)

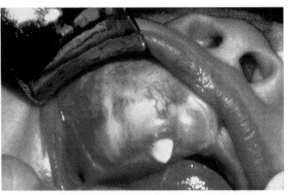

**Figure 9.2. Melanotic neuroectodermal tumor of infancy:** floating tooth in a large expanding tumor. (Courtesy Dr Chris Nortjé)

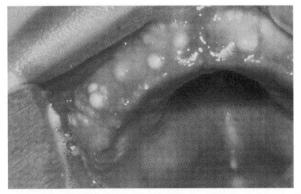

**Figure 9.3. Dental lamina cysts (Bohn's nodules)** on the maxillary alveolar ridge and **Epstein's pearl** on median palatal raphe.

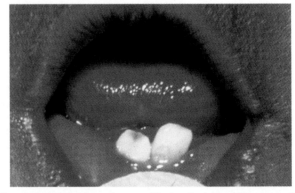

**Figure 9.4. Natal teeth:** mandibular incisors. (Courtesy Dr Ron Jorgenson)

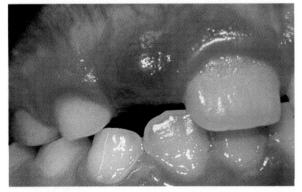

**Figure 9.5. Eruption cyst:** blue dome-shaped cyst coronal to an erupting lateral incisor. (Courtesy Dr F Garcia-Godoy)

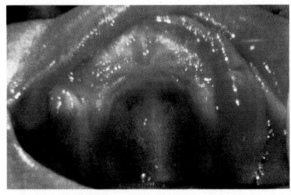

**Figure 9.6. Congenital lymphangioma.** At this location, also known as congenital alveolar lymphangioma. (Courtesy Dr Ron Jorgenson)

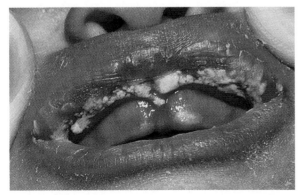

**Figure 9.7. Thrush** caused by *Candida albicans*. (Courtesy Dr Ron Jorgenson)

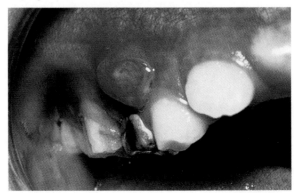

**Figure 9.8. Parulis:** nonvital primary first molar. (Courtesy Dr Al Lugo)

# Section IV

# Abnormalities by Anatomic Location

# Alterations in Tooth Morphology

**Microdontia (Figs. 10.1–10.2) and Macrodontia** Microdontia refers to teeth that are considerably smaller than normal. The condition is usually seen bilaterally and is often a familial trait. Microdontia may occur as an isolated finding, a relative condition, or in a generalized pattern. The most common form occurs as an isolated finding involving one permanent tooth, usually the maxillary lateral incisor. The term "peg lateral" is often used to describe this variant because the tooth is cone-shaped or peg-shaped. Third molars are the second most frequently affected teeth.

When microdontia occurs in a generalized pattern it may be relative to the size of the jaws. True generalized microdontia is rare and occurs when the size of the jaws is normal and the actual tooth size is small. Generalized microdontia has been associated with pituitary dwarfism and cancer therapy during the formative stage of tooth development. True microdonts should be distinguished from small overretained primary teeth and should be examined for the presence of a frequently coexisting anomaly, the dens in dente (see Fig. 10.7).

Macrodontia is the opposite of microdontia and refers to an abnormal increase in tooth size. This condition may affect one, several, or, infrequently, all teeth. It is usually a relative phenomenon. Macrodontia is often seen in incisors, in mandibular third molars, and in a developmental condition known as hemihypertrophy, in which the affected side is larger than the unaffected side. A single macrodont should be distinguished from fusion or gemination, a common finding of incisors and cuspids. True generalized macrodontia is rare and may be a result of pituitary gigantism.

**Fusion (Figs. 10.3–10.4) and Gemination (Figs. 10.5 and 10.6)** Fusion and gemination are opposite conditions that involve alterations in tooth morphology that result from a developmental disturbance during tooth formation. In fusion, the union of two tooth buds at the level of the dentin forms one tooth. This condition is often hereditary, and it affects the primary teeth more often than the permanent teeth. Incisor teeth are the most frequently involved. Clinical manifestations are an enlarged crown, often with an extra cusp; a notch at the incisal edge; and a vertical groove of variable length in the enamel. Radiography may show one large root or two roots with separate pulp canals. In rare instances, a normal tooth bud fuses with a developing supernumerary tooth and creates an appearance that greatly resembles gemination.

Gemination is the condition in which one tooth attempts to split in two. It appears as an incompletely divided or bifid tooth. The teeth most often affected are the primary mandibular incisors and permanent maxillary incisors. Heredity appears to be an important etiologic factor.

The two developmental anomalies, fusion and gemination have similar clinical and radiographic appearances and may be difficult to distinguish. Geminated teeth appear wide in the mesio-distal dimension and more commonly lack the vertical groove that delineates the two crowns. To confirm the diagnosis, the teeth should be counted. If a clinically large tooth is seen and there is no increase or decrease in the number of teeth, the condition is gemination. If an enlarged tooth is seen and a neighboring tooth is missing, fusion has occurred. Treatment is usually cosmetic; in this case, the pulp chambers should be located radiographically before crown preparation or endodontic treatment.

**Dens Invaginatus (Dens in Dente) (Fig. 10.7) and Dens Evaginatus (Leong's Tubercle) (Fig. 10.8)** About 1% of the population has dens invaginatus, a developmental anomaly in which enamel and dentin of the crown invaginate in an apical direction into the pulp chamber along the palatal or lingual aspect of the tooth. The degrees of invagination vary. The term "dens in dente," which literally means a tooth within a tooth, should be reserved for only the most severe form of this disorder, in which the disturbance extends apically into the root. Dens invaginatus is usually bilateral; the cingulum of maxillary lateral incisors is the most frequent point of invagination, followed by the maxillary central incisors, mesiodens, cuspids, and mandibular lateral incisors. Clinical examination shows a deep crevice or an accentuated lingual pit. Food can easily become impacted in the invagination and result in caries; the latter can rapidly lead to pulpal necrosis and periapical inflammation. Generally, prophylactic restorations are placed if the risk for carious involvement is high. Radiography shows longitudinal and bulb-shaped layers of enamel, dentin, and pulp centrally located within the crown of the tooth. A radiolucency involving the periapical and lateral periapical region of the maxillary lateral incisor (previously called a globulomaxillary cyst) is a sign of a pulpally involved dens invaginatus.

Dens evaginatus is less common than dens invaginatus. It is represented by a small, dome-shaped accessory cusp emanating from either the central groove of the occlusal surface or the lingual incline of the buccal cusp of a permanent posterior tooth. This condition occurs almost exclusively in mandibular premolars and thus has been termed Leong's tubercle. Asian persons exhibit Leong's tubercle more frequently than do others. The tubercle consists of enamel, dentin, and a prominent pulp chamber. Care should be taken to prevent pulp injury during tooth preparation. Pathologic exposure of the pulp may occur with attrition.

# Alterations in Tooth Morphology

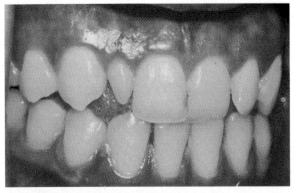

Figure 10.1. Microdontia: peg-lateral incisor.

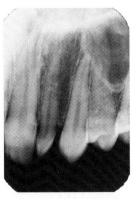

Figure 10.2. Microdontia: periapical radiograph of a peg lateral incisor.

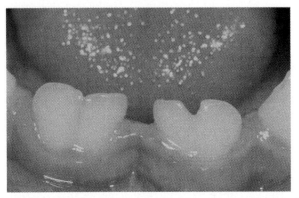

Figure 10.3. Fusion: bilateral fused primary mandibular incisors with prominent vertical grooves between crowns. (Courtesy Dr Rick Myers)

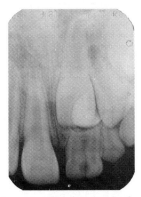

Figure 10.4. Fusion: periapical radiograph of fused primary maxillary incisors.

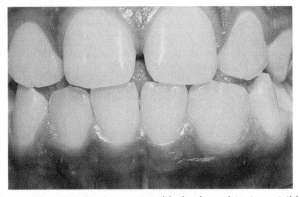

Figure 10.5. Gemination: a mandibular lateral incisor visibly enlarged in the mesial distal diameter because of gemination.

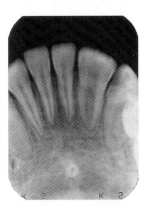

Figure 10.6. Gemination: periapical radiograph of a geminated mandibular lateral incisor.

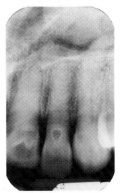

Figure 10.7. Dens invaginatus: common radiographic appearance.

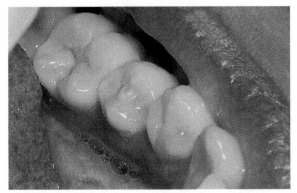

Figure 10.8. Dens evaginatus: note the tubercle on occlusal of mandibular second premolar.

# Alterations in Tooth Numbers: Hypodontia

**Hypodontia (Figs. 11.1–11.3)** Hypodontia is the congenital absence of one or a few teeth because of agenesis. Similar in meaning is the term **oligodontia**, which is used to refer to *numerous* congenitally missing teeth. The term **anodontia** is reserved for the rare condition in which no teeth develop. When missing teeth are discovered, the patient must be carefully questioned to determine the reason for hypodontia. If teeth are missing for reasons such as previous removal or lack of eruption, the use of the term hypodontia is inappropriate.

Hypodontia may involve either sex, any race, and the primary or permanent teeth; however, it is most common in the permanent dentition. About 5% of the population is affected, and a familial tendency is common. The most frequent congenitally missing teeth are the third molars, followed by the mandibular second premolars, the maxillary second premolars, and the maxillary lateral incisors. Visible space or over-retained primary teeth are often the clinical signs of a missing tooth. Counting the teeth together with radiographs confirms the condition.

Many syndromes are associated with congenitally missing teeth, including Böök's syndrome, chondroectodermal dysplasia, ectodermal dysplasia, Hajdu-Cheney's (acro-osteolysis) syndrome, incontinentia pigmenti, otodental dysplasia, and Rieger's syndrome. Radiation therapy to the head and neck in infants or children and rubella (measles) during pregnancy have been implicated in the failure of teeth to develop.

**Acquired Hypodontia (Partial and Complete Edentulism) (Fig. 11.4)** Acquired hypodontia is the loss of teeth as a result of trauma or extractions. Sporting accidents and motor vehicle accidents contribute to most traumatic cases, whereas periodontal disease, caries, and space requirements for orthodontia contribute to dental extraction. Tooth loss produces excess space that may result in drifting, tipping, rotation, and supraeruption of adjacent or opposing teeth. In particular, splaying and spacing of the anterior teeth is an indirect result of loss of a posterior tooth because of distribution of the occlusal load onto the remaining anterior teeth. The single-rooted anterior teeth are less able to handle the load and tilt anteriorly when the periodontal support is poor. Acquired hypodontia can produce alterations in occlusion that require orthodontic, periodontic, and prosthodontic therapy to restore function and esthetics. Persons missing all their teeth are completely edentulous.

**Ankylosis (Figs. 11.5 and 11.6)** Ankylosis, a term meaning fused to bone, is associated with hypodontia. It occurs when a primary molar fails to exfoliate, usually as a result of a missing permanent tooth. Ankylosis is associated with loss of the periodontal ligament and fusion of the cementum of the roots with the bone. The most commonly ankylosed tooth is the primary second molar; the permanent second premolar is the tooth that usually fails to develop and erupt. The ankylosed tooth is typically submerged several millimeters below the marginal ridges of adjacent teeth; the adjacent teeth are slightly or severely tipped toward the ankylosed tooth. The opposing maxillary tooth may be supraerupted. Percussion of the ankylosed tooth produces a dull sound. Ankylosed teeth often remain in the arch for many years but may exfoliate and create a small edentulous space. Exfoliation is often preceded by tooth mobility and pocket formation.

**Ectodermal Dysplasia (Figs. 11.7 and 11.8)** Ectodermal dysplasia is a group of more than 150 inherited diseases characterized by hypoplasia or aplasia of ectodermal structures, such as the hair, nails, skin, sebaceous glands, and teeth. In its best known **hypohidrotic form**, it demonstrates an X-linked recessive inheritance. This means that the defective gene located on the X chromosome is carried by the female and manifested in the male. Less common forms of ectodermal dysplasia have been reported in females and can be caused by autosomal dominant and autosomal recessive transmission. One in 50,000 persons are affected. These patients have fine, smooth dry skin; hypodontia; hypothrichosis (sparse hair); and hypohidrosis (partial or complete absence of sweat glands). Other signs include a depressed bridge of the nose, pronounced supraorbital ridges, periorbital hyperpigmentation, thin sparse hair and eyebrows, protuberant lips, indistinct vermilion border, and varying degrees of xerostomia. Most patients have many missing teeth, and the teeth that are present often are conical and tapered. The canine is the most commonly present tooth, whereas incisors are generally missing. When present, molars show reduced coronal diameter. Anodontia sometimes occurs. Most patients do not perspire and consequently suffer from heat intolerance. Treatment involves several health care workers, genetic counseling, and the avoidance of heat. Partial dentures, full dentures, overdentures, and implants can be fabricated and placed for functional and esthetic purposes. Patients do well with prostheses even at a young age. However, new dentures must be reconstructed periodically as the jaws grow.

# Alterations in Tooth Numbers: Hypodontia

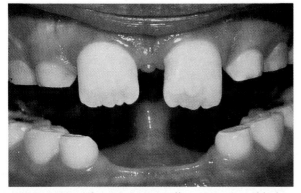

**Figure 11.1. Hypodontia:** congenitally missing mandibular incisors.

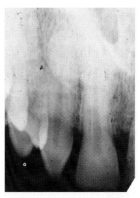

**Figure 11.2. Hypodontia:** periapical radiograph reveals a congenitally missing maxillary lateral incisor.

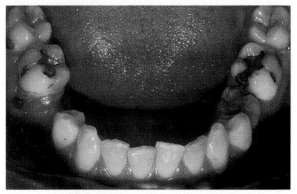

**Figure 11.3. Hypodontia:** congenitally missing maxillary lateral incisor (same patient shown in Figure 11.2).

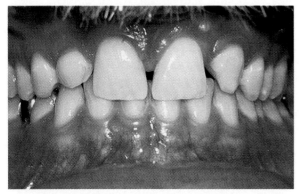

**Figure 11.4. Acquired hypodontia:** extracted mandibular central incisor for orthodontic space requirements.

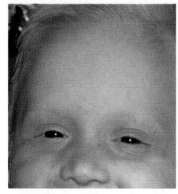

**Figure 11.5. Ankylosis** of second primary molar. Note absence of second premolar on opposite side.

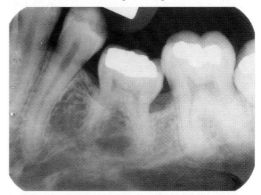

**Figure 11.6. Ankylosis:** periapical radiograph of ankylosis of second primary molar and tipped adjacent teeth.

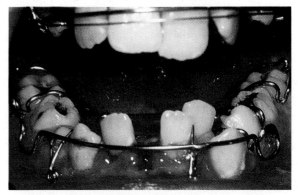

**Figure 11.7. Hypohydrotic ectodermal dysplasia:** sparse hair and eyebrows, periorbital pigmentation, and prominent supra-orbital ridges.

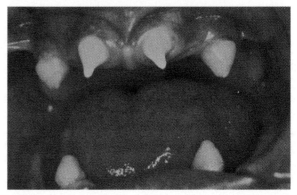

**Figure 11.8. Hypohydrotic ectodermal dysplasia:** several teeth missing, conical teeth (same patient shown in Figure 11.7).

# Alterations in Tooth Numbers: Hyperdontia

**Hyperdontia (Figs. 12.1–12.4)** Hyperdontia refers to an extra or supernumerary deciduous or permanent tooth. The condition results from focal overproliferation of the developing dental lamina. It occurs more often in the maxilla than in the mandible (a ratio of 8:1), more often in males than females (a ratio of 2:1), more often in the permanent dentition than the primary dentition (1.0% of the population compared with 0.5%), and more often unilaterally than bilaterally. The most common supernumerary tooth is the mesiodens; this tooth is located, either erupted or impacted, near the midline between the maxillary central incisors. It may be of normal size and shape but is usually a small tooth with a short root and conically shaped crown that tapers toward the incisal surface.

The second most common supernumerary tooth is the maxillary fourth molar, which can be fully developed or microdontic in size. If the fourth molar is buccal or lingual to the erupted third molar, the term "paramolar" is used. When the fourth molar is positioned behind the third molar, the term "distomolar" is used. Mandibular premolars are the third most common supernumerary tooth. They are usually malpositioned because of late eruption into the arch.

Supernumerary teeth may fail to erupt or may erupt improperly. Those impacted in the jaw have the propensity to cause dentigerous cysts. Other supernumerary teeth have been reported to erupt into the gingiva, palate, tuberosity, nasal cavity, and orbital rim. Space limitations in the arch often force the supernumerary tooth to erupt buccally or lingually. Such teeth are often nonfunctional and may cause inflammation; food impaction; interference with tooth eruption; and positional, esthetic, and masticatory problems. In general, supernumerary teeth should be extracted to permit proper growth, development, and occlusion.

One supernumerary tooth may be an isolated occurrence, but it more commonly affects several family members. Familial hyperdontia is probably related to a common defective gene that has not yet been identified. The presence of several supernumerary teeth is commonly associated with specific syndromes such as cleidocranial dysplasia and Gardner's syndrome and have occasionally been reported in Hallermann-Streiff's and orofaciodigital syndromes. These syndromes should be ruled out whenever supernumerary teeth are present.

## Cleidocranial Dysplasia (Figs. 12.5 and 12.6)

Cleidocranial dysplasia is an autosomal dominant hereditary disturbance of unknown cause. However, up to 40% of cases result from spontaneous mutation. The syndrome affects women and men equally and is usually discovered during childhood or early adolescence.

Cleidocranial dysplasia is a developmental disorder characterized by defective ossification of the clavicles and cranium together with oral and sometimes long-bone disturbances. Prominent features include delayed closure of the frontal, parietal, and occipital fontanelles of the skull; short stature; broad shoulders; prominent frontal eminences with bossing; small paranasal sinuses; an underdeveloped maxilla with a high narrow palate; and relative prognathism of the mandible. The head appears large compared with the short body, the neck appears long, and the shoulders appear narrow and drooping. The clavicles may be absent or underdeveloped, permitting hypermobility of the shoulders whereby patients can bring their shoulders together in front of the chest.

The oral changes are dramatic, particularly as seen on the panoramic radiograph, which can lead to early diagnosis of the condition. The palate is usually high, arched, narrow and sometimes clefted. There is prolonged retention of the primary dentition; numerous unerupted supernumerary teeth, especially in the premolar and molar areas; and delayed eruption of the permanent teeth. The permanent teeth are often short-rooted and lack cellular (secondary) cementum, which may be the cause of the defective eruption pattern. Treatment is complex, involving surgical exposure of unerupted teeth and orthodontic therapy to produce a functional and esthetic occlusion.

## Gardner's Syndrome (Figs. 12.7 and 12.8)

Gardner's syndrome is an autosomal dominant condition with prominent orofacial features characterized by hyperdontia, impacted supernumerary teeth, odontomas, and jaw osteomas. In addition to these features, patients have several epidermal cysts, many dermoid tumors, and many intestinal polyps. The osteomas occur most frequently in the craniofacial skeleton, especially in the mandible, mandibular angle, and paranasal sinuses; however, osteomas of the long bones are possible. Maxillofacial radiographs often demonstrate several supernumerary teeth, many odontomas, numerous round osteomas, and multiple diffuse enostoses that impart a cotton-wool appearance to the jaws. When superficial in the skin, these slow-growing tumors are clinically detectable as rock-hard nodules. The skin cysts (epidermoid, dermoid, or sebaceous) are smooth-surfaced lumps that are commonly located on the ventral and dorsal thorax. Lipomas, fibromas, leiomyomas, or desmoid tumors may accompany this disorder.

The most serious consideration of Gardner's syndrome is the presence of multiple polyps that affect the colorectal mucosa. These intestinal polyps have an extremely high potential for malignant transformation, resulting in adenocarcinoma of the colon in nearly 100% of patients by the age of 40 years. Early recognition of the orofacial manifestations necessitates prompt referral to a gastroenterologist and genetic counseling. Close annual colorectal examination is required; prophylactic colectomy is usually recommended.

# Alterations in Tooth Numbers: Hyperdontia

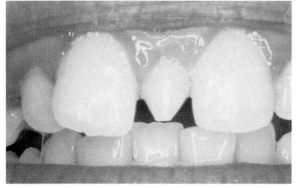

**Figure 12.1. Hyperdontia:** fully erupted mesiodens in midline between maxillary central incisors.

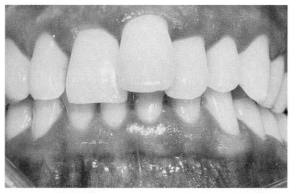

**Figure 12.2. Hyperdontia:** extra maxillary lateral incisor.

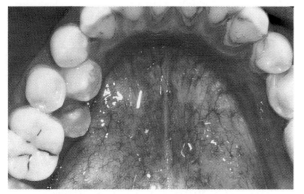

**Figure 12.3. Hyperdontia:** two erupted supernumerary mandibular premolars.

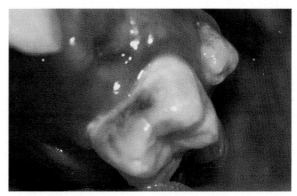

**Figure 12.4. Hyperdontia:** buccally erupted maxillary fourth molar (paramolar).

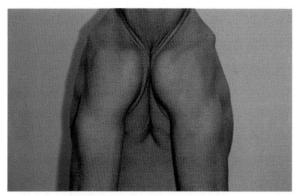

**Figure 12.5. Cleidocranial dysplasia:** absent clavicles and hypermobility of the shoulders.

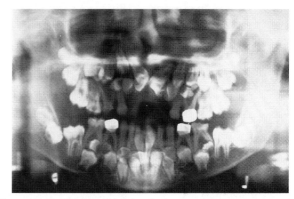

**Figure 12.6. Cleidocranial dysplasia:** many supernumerary impacted teeth and prolonged retention of primary teeth.

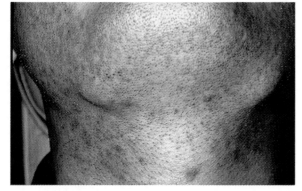

**Figure 12.7. Gardner's syndrome:** mandibular osteomas. (Courtesy Dr Geza Terezhalmy).

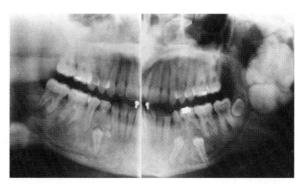

**Figure 12.8. Gardner's syndrome:** periosteal and endosteal osteomas, impacted and supernumerary teeth.

# Alterations in Tooth Structure and Color

**Enamel Hypoplasia (Figs. 13.1 and 13.2)** Enamel that is decreased in quantity is called hypoplastic. This condition results from a disturbance in enamel deposition during amelogenesis. Various interfering influences, including genetic factors (amelogenesis imperfecta), local factors (trauma), or systemic factors (fluorosis, exanthematic microbial infections in which body temperature is elevated), and nutritional deficiencies (vitamin D deficiency), may be involved. Depending on the severity of hypoplasia, enamel discolorations, surface pitting, or distinct horizontal grooves may appear. The pattern of enamel hypoplasia depends on the nature of the influencing factor, the phase of ameloblastic production at the time of the insult, and the duration of the insult. If the entire phase of amelogenesis is affected, the enamel of the entire dentition is thin and may appear "snow-capped," yellowish-brown, rough, pitted, or mottled. If the influence is systemic and lasts only a short time, only enamel then being formed is affected, producing a linear band of hypocalcification on teeth developing during this period. If the injury is local, such as with trauma from an intruded primary tooth, damage to the labial enamel surface of the permanent successor is likely. Enamel hypoplasia of a single permanent tooth that results from periapical or perifurcal inflammation of a primary tooth is referred to as a "**Turner's tooth**." Permanent premolars are often affected by diseases from nonvital primary molars.

**Amelogenesis Imperfecta (Figs. 13.3 and 13.4)** Amelogenesis imperfecta is a hereditary disorder characterized by a generalized defect in enamel formation of the primary or permanent dentition. The condition has been divided into four main types (hypoplastic, hypomature, hypocalcified, and hypomaturation-hypoplasia with taurodontism) and 11 subtypes according to clinical, histologic, radiographic, and genetic features.

The most common form, the **hypoplastic type**, is deficient in normal enamel; thus, the crowns of the teeth appear blanched, "snow-capped," yellow-brown, pitted, or grooved. Radiography usually shows a full complement of teeth, but the crowns of the teeth have either very thin enamel or completely lack enamel. The teeth resemble crown preparations, with characteristic excessive interdental spacing.

The **hypocalcified type**, like the hypomature type, has soft enamel but loses it at a much faster rate than the hypomature type. Dentin becomes exposed soon after eruption. Patients with hypocalcified amelogenesis imperfecta usually have honey-brown teeth with roughened surface texture, several unerupted teeth, and an anterior open bite.

The **hypomature type** has quantitatively normal amounts of enamel, but the enamel is soft and poorly mineralized; thus, a dental explorer under pressure will pit the enamel surface. In this type of amelogenesis imperfecta, the crowns contact interproximally but appear chalky, rough, grooved, and discolored. Fracturing of the enamel is common.

In the **hypomaturation-hypoplasia with taurodontism** type, the teeth are yellowish with opaque mottling, cervical pitting, attrition, and taurodontism. Treatment of all forms of amelogenesis imperfecta usually involves full veneer coverage for esthetic reasons (caries is not usually a problem).

**Dentinogenesis Imperfecta (Figs. 13.5 and 13.6)** Dentinogenesis imperfecta is a hereditary disorder that affects the development of dentin. Three types have been classified according to systemic involvement, clinical features, and histologic findings: Shields type I, Shields type II (hereditary opalescent dentin), and Shields type III (Brandywine type).

Shields type I is a manifestation of osteogenesis imperfecta, a systemic condition involving bone fragility, blue sclerae, joint laxity, and hearing impairment. It is caused by a defect in collagen formation. Shields type II consists of the same dentinal features as type I but has no osteogenic component. Shields type III occurs in isolated racial groups. The teeth affected by type III are opalescent (as in types I and II) but have a shell-like appearance.

Dentinogenesis imperfecta affects the primary and permanent teeth, the latter less severely. On clinical examination, the teeth look normal when they first erupt but shortly thereafter become discolored, gray-brown, or opalescent. The incisal and occlusal surfaces chip and flake away, resulting in fissuring and significant attrition. Radiography shows bulbous crowns, exaggerated cervical constrictions, short tapered roots, and progressive obliteration of the root canal. Affected teeth are more susceptible to root fractures.

**Dentin Dysplasia (Figs. 13.7 and 13.8)** Dentin dysplasia is a hereditary disorder of dentin characterized by alterations in pulp configuration—the presence of pulp stones and idiopathic radiolucencies of the root apices. The term "rootless teeth" has been used to describe this condition. The abnormality has been classified into two types: type I, radicular dentin dysplasia, and type II, coronal dentin dysplasia. Both types are autosomal dominant and may affect the primary and permanent dentition.

The distinction between types I and II is based on radiographic and histopathologic findings. In type I, the primary and permanent teeth look normal on clinical examination, but radiographs reveal defective root development with almost complete absence of root formation, as well as large pulp stones and complete pulpal obliteration of the primary teeth before tooth eruption. Loose teeth and multiple periapical radiolucencies of unknown cause are characteristic.

In type II, the pulp canals of the primary teeth are often completely obliterated, as they are with dentinogenesis imperfecta. The permanent teeth, in contrast, appear normal clinically except for narrower, thistle-shaped pulp canals that are frequently occupied by denticles. The roots may be short, blunted, and tapered and may have horizontal radiolucent lines.

# Alterations in Tooth Structure and Color

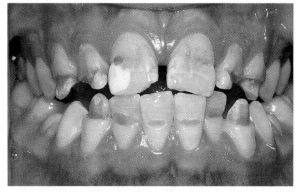

**Figure 13.1. Enamel hypoplasia** characterized by horizontal grooves, deficient enamel, brown color, and linear and pitted defects.

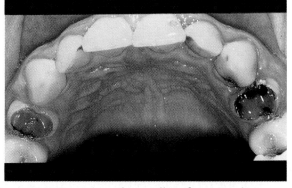

**Figure 13.2. Turner's teeth:** maxillary first premolars.

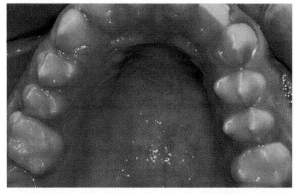

**Figure 13.3. Amelogenesis imperfecta hypoplastic type.** Teeth resemble crown preparations; yellow color resulting from dentin exposure.

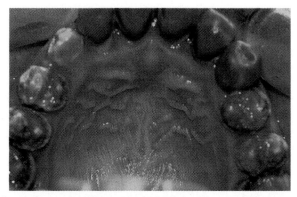

**Figure 13.4. Amelogenesis imperfecta, hypocalcified type:** brown, rough, and chipped teeth.

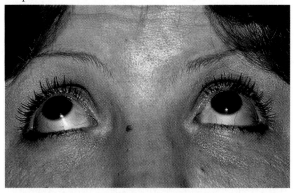

**Figure 13.5. Dentiogenesis imperfecta Shields type I:** osteogenesis imperfecta and blue sclerae. (Courtesy Dr Jerald Katz)

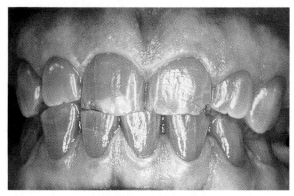

**Figure 13.6. Dentinogenesis imperfecta Shields type II:** opalescent, cracked, and chipped teeth. (Courtesy Dr Charles Morris)

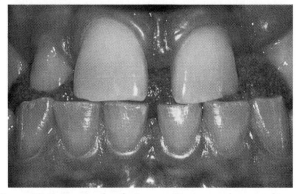

**Figure 13.7. Dentin dysplasia type II:** tan opalescence hue of mandibular incisors.

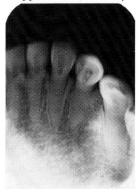

**Figure 13.8. Dentin dysplasia type II:** thistle-tube-shaped pulp chambers and pulp calcifications (same patient shown in Figure 13.7).

# Alterations in Tooth Color

**Intrinsic Staining (Figs. 14.1–14.4)** A change in tooth color from the usual whitish appearance indicates a genetic or acquired abnormality. Genetic processes that alter tooth color include amelogeneis and dentinogenesis imperfecta and dentin dysplasia. Acquired alterations in tooth color result from intrinsic or extrinsic processes. Intrinsically stained teeth are caused by loss of tooth vitality, intake of drugs (such as tetracycline) and chemicals (such as excess fluoride), and certain disease states (hepatitis, biliary disease, erythroblastosis fetalis, and porphyria) that occur during periods of tooth development. Extrinsic processes that stain teeth result from adherence of dark substances to the external tooth surface (see Extrinsic Staining).

**Nonvital Teeth (Figs. 14.1 and 14.2)** A nonvital tooth can be discolored (yellow-brown to brown-gray) because of loss of pulpal fluids and the darkening of dentin. These teeth often have concurrent signs of caries, restorations, fractured incisal edges, or vertical fracture lines. A large amalgam restoration may contribute to the gray-blue hue seen.

Nonvital teeth can also darken from the extravasation of pulpal blood into the dentin as the result of trauma or the accumulation of blood in the teeth at the time of nonvitality. This situation usually produces a pink to purple tooth in which the neck of the crown is more discolored than the incisal edge. A pink, discolored nonvital tooth has been called the "**pink tooth of Mummery.**" Lepromatous leprosy has also been reported to cause rupture of pulpal blood vessels and pink teeth.

**Tetracycline Staining (Fig. 14.3)** The tetracyclines are a group of bacteriostatic antibiotics that inhibit protein synthesis of certain bacteria. The drug is used to treat skin and periodontal infections as well as chlamydial, certain rickettsial, and penicillin-resistant gonococcal infections. Embryos, infants, and children who receive tetracyclines are prone to develop varying degrees of permanent discoloration. This is more likely to occur during long-term use and repeated short-term courses and is directly related to the total quantity of drug absorbed during embryogenesis and tooth development. Presence of tetracycline in the bloodstream promotes deposition of the drug in the developing enamel and dentin of teeth and bones in the form of tetracycline-calcium-orthophosphate. This complex causes teeth to become discolored when they erupt and are exposed to sunlight (that is, ultraviolet light). The discoloration is generalized and band-like if the drug was administered in courses; prolonged use produces a more homogeneous appearance. The discoloration appears light yellow with oxytetracycline (Terramycin); yellow with tetracycline (Achromycin); or green to dark gray with the synthetic tetracycline, minocycline. Chlortetracycline (Aureomycin), which is no longer available in oral form, was best known for its ability to produce gray-brown staining. Doxycycline and oxytetracycline appear to be the least discoloring. The diagnosis can be confirmed by using an ultraviolet light, which will make the teeth fluoresce. Adults receiving long-term tetracycline therapy have been reported to acquire tetracycline staining. Accordingly, alternate antibiotics should be selected in children younger than age 8 years, and long-term tetracycline treatment should be avoided in adults if possible.

**Fluorosis (Fig. 14.4)** Fluoride is a caries-preventive chemical that has its greatest benefit when used at the appropriate concentration. Research has shown that the optimal fluoride concentration in the drinking water is between 0.7 and 1 part per million (ppm). At this level, fluoride is incorporated into the enamel matrix and adds hardness and caries resistance. At levels of 1.2 ppm and 4 ppm there is a increased risk for mild to severe fluorosis, respectively.

Fluorosis is a disturbance of the developing enamel that is caused by excess levels of fluoride in the blood and plasma. Blood levels are directly related to the level of fluoride ingested in water; excess levels can be acquired from drinking well water (endemic fluorosis) or from excessive treatment with and ingestion of fluoride. At elevated fluoride levels, ameloblasts are affected during the apposition of enamel and produce deficient organic matrix. At high levels, interference of the calcification process occurs. Mild fluorosis produces isolated, lusterless, whitish-opaque spots in the enamel. The occurrence of these spots near the incisal edge have been called "snow-capped." Moderate fluorosis is characterized by more generalized yellow to brown spots, whereas severe fluorosis has many symmetrically and bilaterally affected teeth with mottled and pitted enamel and brown and white spots. In the severe form, the morphology of the crown can be grossly altered.

**Extrinsic Staining (Figs. 14.5–14.8)** Extrinsic stains result from the adherence of colored material or bacteria to the enamel of teeth. Most extrinsic stains tend to localize in the gingival third of the tooth above the gingival collar, where bacteria accumulate and absorb the stain. Chromogenic bacteria can produce green to brown stains in this region; these stains result from the interaction of bacteria with ferric sulfide and iron in the saliva and gingival crevicular fluid. Colored fluids, such as coffee, tea, and chlorhexidine, and inhaled tobacco smoke can cause brown to black stains. These stains appear darkest in the gingival third of the tooth and develop as a result of frequent oral contact and enhanced contact by bacterial absorption. Amalgam restorations that leak into dentin produce blue-gray to black stains. This is most often apparent in the facial aspect of maxillary premolars that have a large class II restoration or a central incisor that has a lingually placed amalgam restoration. Along the gingival margin, the stain should be distinguished from calculus and caries. Calculus adheres to the external surface of the tooth and appears greenish-black when subgingival or tan when supragingival. Like stains, caries can be dark; unlike stains, caries causes loss of tooth structure.

# Alterations in Tooth Color

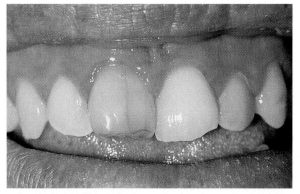

**Figure 14.1. Intrinsic staining.** Traumatic insult resulting in nonvitality shown by yellow-brown color, broken incisal edge, and vertical fracture line.

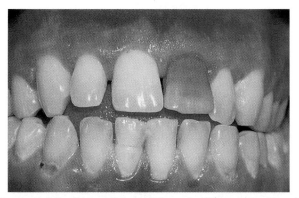

**Figure 14.2. Intrinsic staining: pink tooth of Mummery.** Nonvitality characterized by red-purple color caused by extravasated blood.

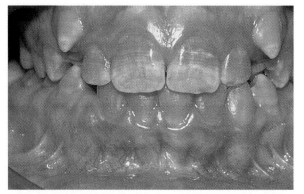

**Figure 14.3. Intrinsic staining: tetracycline staining.** Brown-gray, band-like appearance.

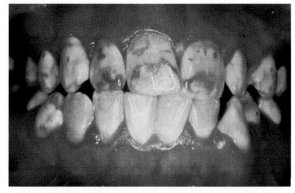

**Figure 14.4. Intrinsic staining: fluorosis.** Characterized by generalized brown mottling and focal white spotting.

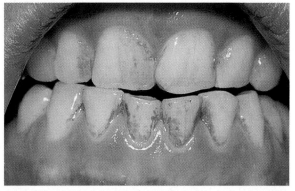

**Figure 14.5. Extrinsic staining: chlorhexidine staining.** Regions of plaque accumulation with greatest stain.

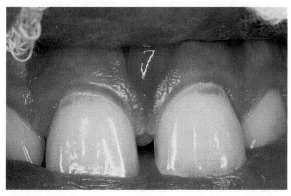

**Figure 14.6. Extrinsic staining caused by marijuana use.**

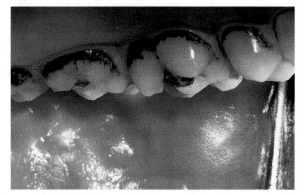

**Figure 14.7. Extrinsic staining caused by tobacco and coffee.**

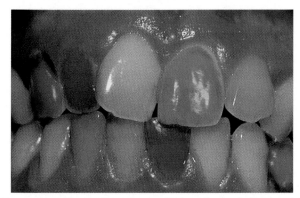

**Figure 14.8. Extrinsic stain:** applied with the holiday spirit (Courtesy Dr David Molina).

# Acquired Defects of Teeth: Noncarious Loss of Tooth Structure

**Attrition (Fig. 15.1)** Attrition, considered a physiologic process, is the wearing down and loss of occlusal and incisal tooth structure because of chronic tooth-to-tooth frictional contact. Although the condition occurs most frequently in older adults, the primary teeth of young children may also be affected. Attrition is usually a generalized condition accelerated by bruxism and abnormal use of selective teeth. Flattening of the incisal and occlusal surfaces and wear facets are common findings. Close examination reveals a smooth and highly polished tooth surface that is broad and angled, loss of the superior interproximal space, the outline of the dentin-enamel junction, and a receded pulp chamber. Pulp exposure is rare, however, because the deposition of secondary dentin and pulpal recession occur concurrently with attrition. Affected teeth are generally not sensitive to hot, cold, or the explorer tine. Restoration of worn teeth may be challenging because of acquired changes in vertical dimension.

**Abrasion (Figs. 15.2–15.5)** Abrasion is the pathologic loss of tooth structure caused by abnormal and repetitive mechanical wear. Various agents can cause abrasion, but the most common form is "**toothbrush abrasion,**" which results from abrasive toothpastes being brushed against the teeth too frequently, with improper technique, and with too much vigor. Toothbrush abrasion produces a rounded, saucer-shaped, or V-shaped notch in the cervical portion of the facial aspect of several adjacent teeth. The abraded area is usually shiny or polished and yellow (because of exposed dentin). The dentin is typically firm and noncarious, little plaque accumulation is present, and the marginal gingiva is not inflamed. Premolars opposite to the dominant hand are most often affected. Abraded teeth demonstrate dentinal sensitivity to hot, cold, or the explorer tine and are more susceptible to pulp exposure and tooth fracture.

Abrasive notching of the teeth also can be created by clasps of partial dentures, pins or nails habitually held with the teeth, or a pipe stem persistently clamped between the teeth. Inappropriate use of toothpicks and dental floss can also abrade the interproximal regions of teeth. Porcelain restorations placed in occlusion against nonrestored teeth usually result in abrasion of the incisal and occlusal surfaces of the teeth in the opposite arch. When the porcelain teeth are maxillary incisors, the mandibular incisors are abraded at an upward and backward angle. Exposure to abrasive substances in the diet; chewing tobacco; powder cocaine; and long-term inhalation of sand, quartz, or silica can also promote abrasion. Abrasion caused by chewing tobacco frequently occurs on the side of the mouth in which the tobacco is most often placed. Cocaine addiction can cause localized abrasion of the maxillary anterior teeth when the drug is chronically rubbed against the gingiva and teeth.

Abrasion is a slow and chronic process, requiring many years before giving rise to signs. Restoration of normal tooth contour may be unsuccessful if the patient is not made aware of the causative factors.

**Abfraction (Stress-Induced Cervical Lesions) (Fig. 15.4)** Abfraction means "to break away" and is a term used in dentistry to define the pathologic loss of tooth structure at, or under, the cemento-enamel junction caused by abnormal biomechanical loading. Abfraction appears as a sharp, wedge-shaped, or V-shaped defect of enamel and dentin along the cervical region of the facial aspect of a tooth. Defects occur as a result of eccentric occlusal loading, which creates tensile and compressive forces, flexure and shearing stresses, and disruption of the chemical bond between enamel and dentin. Invariably, the periodontal support around these teeth is excellent, occlusal wear facets are present, and abrasive and erosive factors are nonidentifiable. Adults older than age 35 years are most often affected. One tooth in a quadrant is typically involved, particularly mandibular premolars. Abfraction may be associated with multiple lesions and with concurrent abrasion and attrition.

**Erosion (Figs. 15.6–15.8)** Erosion refers to the loss of tooth structure caused by such chemicals as dietary, gastric, or environmental acids that are placed in prolonged contact with the teeth. The condition is exacerbated by xerostomia and drugs that produce xerostomia, because loss of saliva reduces the buffering capacity of the oral cavity. The most commonly affected tooth surfaces are the labial and buccal surfaces.

The pattern of tooth erosion often indicates the causative agent or a particular habit. For example, sucking on lemons (citric acid) produces characteristic changes of the facial surfaces of the maxillary incisors. Horizontal ridges are initially apparent, followed by smooth, cupped-out, yellowish depressions. Eventually the incisal edges thin and fracture. A similar erosive pattern may be seen in dedicated swimmers whose anterior teeth are chronically exposed to chlorinated swimming pools.

Erosion limited to the lingual surfaces of the maxillary teeth (**perimolysis,** also known as perimylolysis) indicates chronic regurgitation caused by bulimia, anorexia, pregnancy, hiatal hernia, gastroesophageal reflux, or alcohol abuse. The occlusal margins of several existing amalgams are often raised above the eroded and adjacent enamel. Sensitivity of the exposed area is an early symptom. Excessive consumption of sweetened beverages and carbonic acid-containing beverages may accelerate the condition. Fluoride treatments for early erosions and restorations that cover exposed dentin for more extensive lesions are the treatment of choice. Elimination of the causative habit or behavior modification is required for success.

# Acquired Defects of Teeth: Noncarious Loss of Tooth Structure

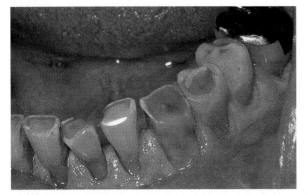

Figure 15.1. **Attrition:** exposed, smooth yellowish dentin and large wear facets on masticatory surfaces. Abrasion also apparent along cervical regions.

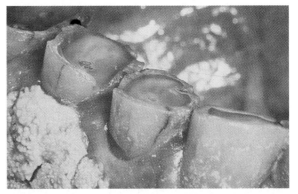

Figure 15.2. **Attrition and abrasion** of teeth and leukoplakia caused by 40-year history of use of chewing tobacco.

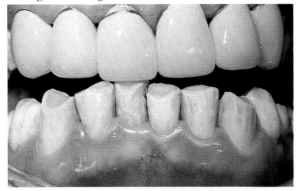

Figure 15.3. **Abrasion:** angled wear pattern on mandibular incisors and canines from chronic friction against porcelain.

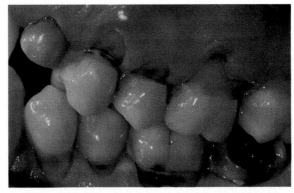

Figure 15.4. **Toothbrush abrasion and abfraction** along cervical margins of teeth.

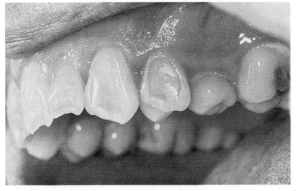

Figure 15.5. **Abrasion** caused by rubbing of powder cocaine on alveolar mucosa, attached gingiva, and teeth.

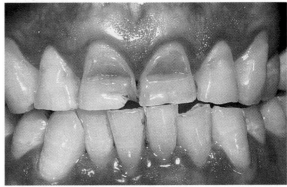

Figure 15.6. **Erosion:** notchlike depressions of enamel caused by lemon sucking and dissolution of citric acid.

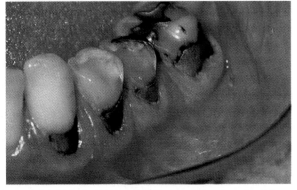

Figure 15.7. **Erosion caused by** frequent intake of acidic carbonated beverages in combination with xerostomia.

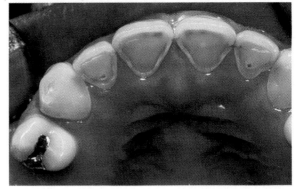

Figure 15.8. **Erosion** affecting lingual surfaces of maxillary incisors (**perimolysis**) caused by chronic vomiting in bulimic patient.

# Acquired Defects of Teeth: Carious Loss of Tooth Structure

**Caries (Figs. 16.1–16.8)** Dental caries is one of the most common bacterial infections affecting humans. Caries is characterized by demineralization and destruction of the organic matrix of teeth and results from an interaction of bacterial plaque, diet components, altered host responses, and time. Electrochemical changes produced by acid generation and calcium and phosphate ion flow out of the tooth appear to be causative. The primary pathogen, *Streptococcus mutans*, together with *Actinomyces viscosus*, *Lactobacillus* species, and *Streptococcus sanguis* are involved in tooth adherence and the production of lactic acid needed for enamel dissolution.

Caries begins as an enamel decalcification that appears as a chalky white spot or fissure. The initial lesion is termed "incipient." Maturation of caries causes destruction of the enamel and lateral spread along the dentin-enamel junction, through the dentin, and eventually toward the pulp. The classic clinical features of a carious lesion are 1) color change (chalky white, brown, or black discoloration), 2) loss of hard tissue (cavitation), and 3) stickiness to the explorer tine. The color change is caused by decalcification of enamel, exposure of dentin, or demineralization of dentin. The dental explorer tip is used to determine whether the lesion is decalcified (smooth to the explorer tip), incipient (small "catch" with the explorer tine), or carious (soft and sticky to the explorer tip). Although stain is sometimes confused with caries, it only meets one of the three criteria. Stains are not associated with loss of tooth structure or stickiness to the explorer tine.

The classic symptoms of caries are sensitivity to sweets, hot, and cold. These symptoms are generally absent with incipient lesions. Larger lesions permit ingress of fluids into exposed dentinal tubules. The hydrostatic changes are sensed by pulpal nerves that transmit the changes to the trigeminal sensory complex and result in the perception of pain.

There are two types of caries, which are classified according to location: fissural and smooth surface. **Fissural caries** is the most common form. It occurs most often in deep fissures in the chewing surfaces of the posterior teeth. **Smooth surface caries** usually occurs at places that are protected from plaque removal, such as just below the interproximal contact, at the gingival margin, and along the root surface. Caries is subdivided into six classes according to their anatomic location. Class I caries is fissural; the remaining five classes are smooth surface caries.

**Class I Caries (Fig. 16.1)** Class I caries is characterized by decay that affects the occlusal surface of a posterior tooth. The disease arises when bacteria invade a deep occlusal groove or fissure, remain sheltered for many months, and then produce acid and enamel dissolution. Destruction of enamel and dentin permits the carious groove to enlarge, darken, and become soft. Small class I caries is the size of the sharp tip of a lead pencil. Larger lesions can encompass the entire occlusal surface, leaving only a shell of facial or lingual enamel.

**Class II Caries (Figs. 16.2 and 16.4)** Class II caries is characterized by decay that affects the interproximal surface of a posterior tooth. These lesions are often difficult to identify clinically and require an astute eye; a clean, dry tooth surface; and a bitewing radiograph. One feature that may help in the detection of class II caries is decalcification (chalkiness or translucency) along the marginal ridge that is caused by hollowing of the subjacent dentin. The caries can occasionally be seen from the lingual or buccal aspect of the interproximal contact. Class II caries is most easily recognized on bitewing radiographs. The carious lesion appears as a triangular radiolucency in the enamel just below the contact point; the base of the triangle parallels the external aspect of the tooth, and the tip of the triangle points inward toward the dentin. As the lesion reaches dentin, the demineralization spreads along the dentino-enamel junction and spreads toward the pulp.

**Class III Caries (Figs. 16.3 and 16.5)** Class III caries is characterized by decay that affects an interproximal surface of an anterior tooth. Like class II interproximal caries, class III caries begins just below the contact point. Invasion results in triangular destruction of enamel and lateral spread into dentin. Interproximal caries (classes II and III) are common in persons who seldom floss their teeth and have a frequent intake of liquid sugar, such as carbonated beverages. Class III caries is also prominent in Asian and Native American persons who have prominent marginal ridges (shovel-shaped incisors).

**Class IV Caries (Fig. 16.6)** Class IV caries results when class III caries does not receive dental treatment and the dentin that supports the incisal line angle is undermined. Involvement of the incisal line angle defines a class IV carious lesion.

**Class V Caries (Fig. 16.7)** Class V caries is characterized by decay along the gingival margin of a posterior or anterior tooth. Early signs of class V caries are chalky, white decalcification lines running parallel to the gingiva. Any plaque covering the lesion must be removed for adequate detection of the caries. With time, the lesions enlarge mesially and distally faster than they do gingival-incisally, thereby producing an oval defect. As Class V caries reaches interproximal regions, spread toward the contact point occurs and the lesion becomes L-shaped. Patients with class V caries usually consume large amounts of sugary carbonated drinks, sip on such drinks for several hours during the day, or are xerostomic.

**Class VI Caries (Fig. 16.8)** Class VI caries is characterized by decay of the incisal edge or cusp tip. This type of caries is seldom seen but is more common in persons who frequently chew sugary gums or consume sticky candy bars. Patients with low salivary flow are also predisposed to this type of caries.

# Acquired Defects of Teeth: Carious Loss of Tooth Structure

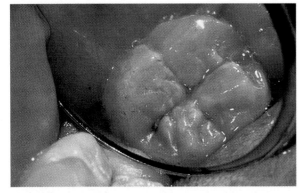

Figure 16.1. **Class I caries** in a mandibular molar; the occlusal decay exhibits the features of color change, cavitation, and softness to the explorer tine.

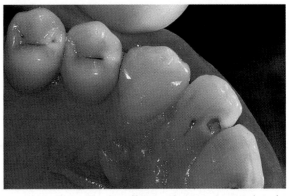

Figure 16.2. **Class II caries** affecting the interproximal surfaces of the premolars. Pinpoint mesial occlusal decay of second premolar and class III lesion in the lateral incisor.

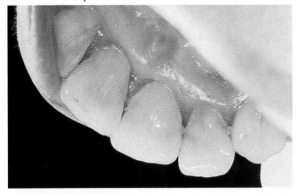

Figure 16.3. **Class III caries:** interproximal decay of incisors that appears as a brownish triangle just below the contact point.

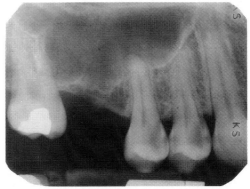

Figure 16.4. **Class II caries:** radiographic evidence of interproximal decay in same patient shown in Figure 16.2.

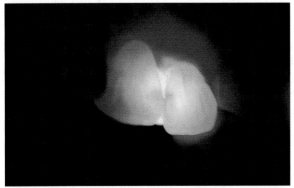

Figure 16.5. **Class III caries** evident by transillumination (same patient as shown in Figure 16.3).

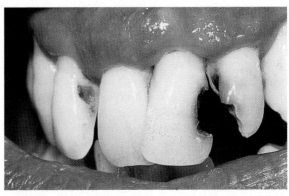

Figure 16.6. **Class III caries** at the distal of the central incisor and **class IV caries** in the mesial of the lateral incisor.

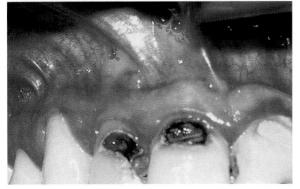

Figure 16.7. **Class V caries** along the gingival margin of the incisors.

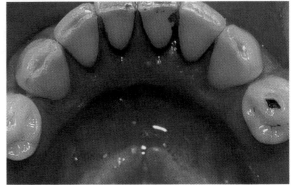

Figure 16.8. **Class VI caries:** decay of the cusp tip of the first premolar.

# Acquired Defects of Teeth: Carious Loss of Tooth Structure

**Progression and Classification of Caries (Figs. 17.1–17.8)** The invasion of caries may be a slow or fast process and may involve the pulp before the patient is aware of the carious lesion. In most cases, it takes several years for caries to reach the pulp. Some caries are particularly aggressive or have a unique cause. These caries have received descriptive definitions. For example, **rampant caries** are a type of caries that develop at an extremely rapid pace in some children and young adults. **Radiation, or amputation caries** are another form of caries that occur in patients receiving radiotherapy who lack the protective action of saliva. These caries appear along the gingival margin of teeth and can weaken teeth so severely that the crown fractures. **Root caries** has an appearance similar to that of radiation caries but is not associated with a history of radiation therapy; rather, affected patients usually have a history of xerostomia or drug-induced xerostomia. Root caries progresses more slowly than radiation caries because xerostomia is less severe. **Nursing bottle caries** results from prolonged contact of teeth with sugar-containing liquids in infants.

If caries is left untreated, the bacterial infection can progress through tooth dentin and produce pulpal inflammation. The initial stage of pulpal involvement is **reversible pulpitis,** which is characterized by pulpal hyperemia and tooth sensitivity to hot and cold that dissipates when the temperature source is removed. Persistent pulpal inflammation produces irreversible changes, or **irreversible pulpitis,** in which the patient experiences spontaneous and persistent pain in the tooth after removal of the temperature source. Death of pulpal tissue from bacterial infection or interruption of the blood supply to the pulp produces a nonvital pulp and periapical changes.

Prevention is the best way to reduce the incidence of caries. Clinical examinations should be provided twice a year to minimize the sequela of caries. Bitewing radiographs should be taken at six-month intervals in children if clinical caries are detected or the patient has a high risk for caries. Adults at high risk should receive bitewing radiography annually. Plastic sealants should be placed over deep fissures of posterior teeth in caries-susceptible children and adolescents. Remineralization products such as fluoride are advocated to prevent caries. Pulp vitality should be tested when a carious lesion has invaded to, or beyond 50% of the space between the dentino-enamel junction and pulp margin.

**Pulp Polyp (Fig. 17.2)** The pulp polyp is an inflammatory and hyperplastic response of a wide open pulp chamber to a chronic bacterial infection. Extensively carious primary molars and 6-year molars of young children are most frequently affected. Upon clinical examination, the soft, red, nonpainful, pedunculated mass is seen projecting up from the pulp chamber beyond the broken-down occlusal surface of the tooth. Although the tooth is initially vital, the condition eventually erodes and results in nonvitality. Treatment is extraction or endodontic therapy.

**Periapical Inflammation (Apical Periodontitis) (Figs. 17.4–17.6)** Periapical inflammation or apical periodontitis are clinical terms used to describe the radiographic changes and clinical findings associated with inflammation that involves the periodontal ligament at the periapex of the tooth. The condition is most commonly associated with a nonvital tooth but may occur in vital teeth from occlusal traumatism or constant and repetitive pressure placed on a tooth. Radiography shows a widening of the apical periodontal ligament space. The condition may be symptomatic or asymptomatic, acute or chronic. Chronic periapical inflammation has chronic inflammatory cells at the periapex and often shows greater periradicular destruction of alveolar bone than acute periapical inflammation. In contrast, acute periapical inflammation is usually symptomatic. Chronic periapical inflammation can stimulate epithelium at the apex of a nonvital tooth to form a **periapical cyst,** or cause a **periapical granuloma** (an accumulation of granulation tissue, lymphocytes, plasma cells, histiocytes, and polymorphonuclear leukocytes). These two entities are distinguished by their histologic appearance.

**Periapical Abscess (Figs. 17.7 and 17.8)** Periapical abscess is the acute phase of an infection that spreads from a nonvital tooth through the alveolar bone into the adjacent soft tissue. The abscess is composed of polymorphonuclear leukocytes and necrotic debris. Clinical examination shows a red or reddish-yellow, swollen nodule that is warm and fluctuant to the touch. The affected tooth is tender to percussion and responds abnormally or not at all to heat, cold, and electric pulp testing. Abscesses can be drained by opening into the pulp chamber or incising the soft tissue swelling. An alternate treatment is extraction, which provides an avenue for drainage. Antibiotics are used when the abscess is large and spreading, lymphadenopathy and fever are present, and drainage is not established. Penicillin VK is the antibiotic of choice. If the infection is unresponsive to penicillin, a bacterial culture and sensitivity should be obtained. Antibiotics are generally not needed if the affected tooth is extracted and adequate drainage is established.

# Acquired Defects of Teeth: Carious Loss of Tooth Structure

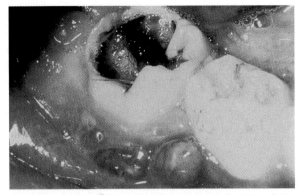

Figure 17.1. **Extensive caries** of the occlusal, facial, and distal surfaces of the mandibular first molar. Infection has resulted in a parulis.

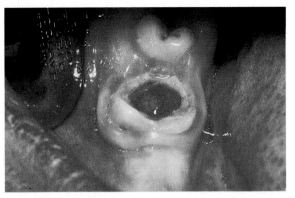

Figure 17.2. **Pulp polyp:** reddish, exuberant mass projecting from the pulp chamber of a nonvital tooth with chronic hyperplastic pulpitis.

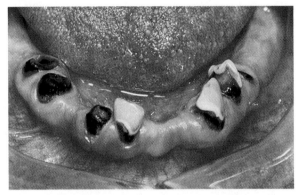

Figure 17.3. **Rampant caries** associated with xerostomia.

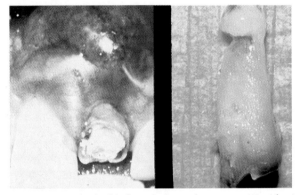

Figure 17.4. **Periapical inflammation:** abscess associated with fractured mandibular incisor. **Granuloma** apparent at the apex of the extracted tooth.

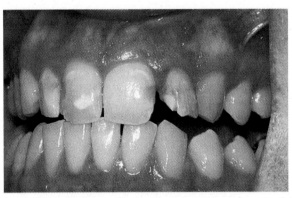

Figure 17.5. **Periapical inflammation** draining at the site of the parulis near the periapex of the nonvital maxillary lateral incisor.

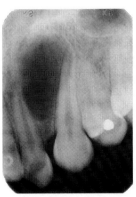

Figure 17.6. **Periapical inflammation:** radiograph showing the nonvital maxillary incisor with periapical radiolucency (same patient shown in Figure 17.5).

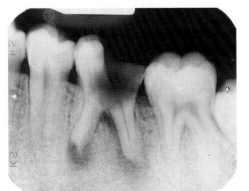

Figure 17.7. **Caries and chronic periapical inflammation** of the mandibular first molar.

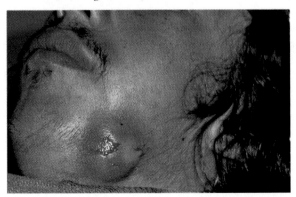

Figure 17.8. **Abscess** draining through the mandible on to the soft tissues of the face (same patient shown in Figure 17.7).

# Periodontal Diseases: Plaque, Calculus, and Regressive Changes

**Plaque (Fig. 18.1–18.2)** Plaque is bacteria and matrix that adheres to the outer tooth surface. The development of plaque is a well characterized, stepwise process. The first step is the attachment of the **acquired pellicle**, a thin film of salivary proteins. Within a few days, Gram-positive facultative cocci overlay the pellicle and colonize the tooth surface. Additional bacterial types such as *Veillonella* species, a Gram-negative anaerobe; *Actinomyces* species, a Gram-positive rod; and *Capnocytophaga* species, a Gram-negative rod enter the region and colonize plaque. *Prevotella intermedia* and filamentous *Fusobacterium* species colonize plaque between the first week and third weeks as an anaerobic environment becomes established. If the plaque grows undisturbed, late colonization with *Porphyromonas gingivalis*, motile rods, and *Treponema* species (spirochetes) occurs during and after the third week. The exact composition of the microbial population within plaque varies according to site, available substrate, salivary components (adhesins and secretory immunoglobulin), duration, and the patient's oral hygiene practices.

Plaque is white and soft and is composed of bacteria and an extracellular, sticky matrix called "glucan." Secreted by streptococci, glucans promote adherence of the bacteria to the pellicle.

**Supragingival plaque** is bacteria that adheres above the gingiva; **subgingival plaque** is bacteria below the gingiva. Growth in supragingival plaque mass results from nutrients obtained from ingested simple carbohydrates (glucose), lactic acid, and other plaque components. Instead of glucose, subgingival (plaque) bacteria preferentially use metabolized peptides and amino acids that are obtained from tissue breakdown products, the gingival crevicular fluid, and interbacterial feeding. Inflamed gingival tissues produce more gingival crevicular fluid, which favors the proliferation of subgingival bacterial replication. Subgingival bacterial populations prefer an anaerobic environment, whereas supragingival bacterial populations prefer a low-oxygen environment. The latter are called facultative anaerobes. Long-standing plaque is mostly composed of Gram-negative anaerobes.

Persistent microbial plaque can lead to caries, gingivitis, calculus formation, gingival recession, and periodontitis.

**Calculus (Figs. 18.3–18.5)** Calculus (lay term, tartar) consists primarily of mineralized, dead bacteria with a small amount of mineralized salivary proteins. Its chemical components are mostly calcium phosphate, calcium carbonate, and magnesium phosphate. Calculus is hard, like bone and other mineralized substances, and firmly adheres to the tooth. Above the gingival margin, calculus is called **supragingival calculus**. It appears yellow or tan and is usually located near large salivary sources in patients who do not mechanically remove plaque regularly. Supragingival calculus accumulates preferentially along the lingual of the mandibular incisors adjacent to the duct for the sublingual and subman-

dibular glands, and along the buccal of maxillary molars adjacent to Stenson's duct of the parotid gland. It darkens in color with age and increases in size. A **calculus bridge** is an extensive matrix of calculus that extends across several tooth surfaces. A calculus bridge is often associated with gingival recession and periodontal disease. Removal of the bridge may reveal several mobile teeth. Patients should be advised of this possibility prior to debridement.

**Subgingival calculus** forms below the gingival collar and is not usually visible unless gingival recession has occurred. This type of calculus is most often detected with a periodontal probe or explorer as a rough mass projecting from the cementum. Subgingival calculus is usually brown, black, or green because of its chronic exposure to gingival crevicular fluid, blood, and blood breakdown products. It is frequently associated with the development of a pyogenic granuloma, an epulis-like lesion on the gingiva.

**Gingival Recession (Figs. 18.6 and 18.7)** In health, the gingival margin normally extends about 1 mm above the cementoenamel junction. Gingival recession is the apical shift of gingiva below the cementoenamel junction toward the root. By definition, recession results in exposure of cementum. It usually occurs in persons older than age 30 on the facial aspect of teeth; it occurs less frequently on the lingual and rarely in the interproximal regions. Recession may be localized or generalized and often progresses during periods of inflammation that are combined with bad habits (improper toothbrushing technique, fingernail injuries), prominently located teeth and thin gingiva. Localized causes include excessive occlusal loading, temporary crowns, plaque and calculus, inadequate bands of attached gingiva, high muscle attachments, frenal pull, bony fenestrations, and dehiscences. Gingival recession begins as a small oval defect but may progress to expose the entire root. A variant form is narrow clefting. Surgical grafting procedures that provide root coverage should be offered if patients report hypersensitivity from exposed root surfaces, if esthetics are a concern, the condition is progressive, or root caries develop.

**Dehiscence and Fenestration (Fig. 18.8)** A dehiscence is loss of alveolar bone on the facial (rarely lingual) aspect of a tooth that leaves a characteristic oval, root-exposed defect from the cementoenamel junction apically. The defect may be 1 or 2 mm long or may extend the full length of the root. The three features of dehiscence are gingival recession, alveolar bone loss, and root exposure.

A fenestration is a "window" of bone loss on the facial or lingual aspect of a tooth that places the exposed root surface directly in contact with gingiva or alveolar mucosa. It can be distinguished from the dehiscence in that the fenestration is bordered by alveolar bone along its coronal aspect.

# Periodontal Diseases: Plaque, Calculus, and Regressive Changes

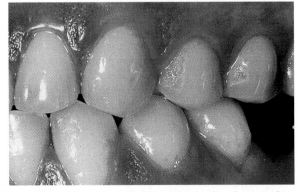

Figure 18.1. **Plaque** along the interproximal and gingival margin, stained pink-red by disclosing solution.

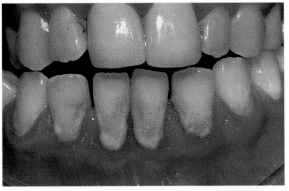

Figure 18.2. **Plaque:** heavier deposits along facial gingival margins of mandibular incisors.

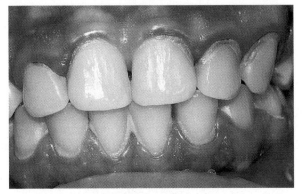

Figure 18.3. **Calculus:** early formation at interproximal of mandibular incisors.

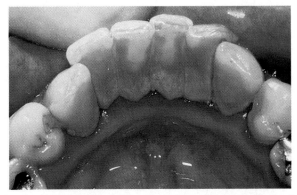

Figure 18.4. **Calculus bridge** along lingual of mandibular incisors.

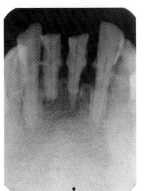

Figure 18.5. **Calculus:** periapical radiograph showing bony destruction associated with plaque-derived calculus.

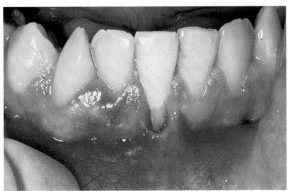

Figure 18.6. **Gingival recession:** 4-mm oval defect during active inflammatory phase.

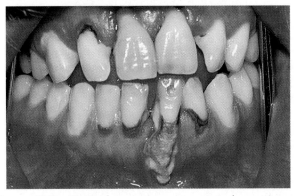

Figure 18.7. **Gingival recession:** extensive destruction of attached gingiva of central incisors beyond the mucogingival junction and brown calculus on roots.

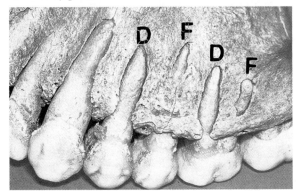

Figure 18.8. **Fenestration and dehiscence:** fenestration (F) on second premolar and distobuccal root first molar; dehiscence (D) of canine, first premolar, and mesiobuccal root of first molar.

# Gingivitis

**Gingivitis (Figs. 19.1–19.4)** Inflammation of the gingiva, or gingivitis, is a bacterial infection that can occur at any age but most frequently arises during adolescence. It is a disease that requires the presence and maturation of bacterial plaque.

Gingivitis is diagnosed by bleeding and by changes in the color, contour, and consistency of the gingiva. Features include red swollen marginal gingiva; loss of stippling; red-purple, bulbous interdental papillae; and increased fluid flow from the gingival crevice (gingival crevicular fluid). Gingival bleeding and pain are induced by toothbrushing and slight probing.

Gingivitis has no gender or racial predilection and can be classified according to distribution, duration, cause, and severity. The distribution may be general, local, marginal, or papillary; the duration may be acute or chronic. An abbreviated list of the many types of gingivitis based on cause includes actinomycotic, diabetic, hormonal, leukemic, plasma cell, psoriasiform, scorbutic, and necrotizing. Severe cases of gingivitis destroy gingival tissues.

Treatment of gingivitis consists of frequent and regular removal of supragingival and subgingival plaque. Intervals of debridement should be based on the level of plaque accumulation and gingival alterations that develop between evaluation periods.

**Gingivitis Caused by Mouth Breathing (Figs. 19.3 and 19.4)** Chronic mouth breathing is characterized by nasal obstruction, a high narrow palatal vault, snoring, xerostomia, a sore throat upon wakening, and a characteristic form of gingivitis. Soft tissue changes are limited to the anterior labial gingiva of the maxilla and, sometimes, the mandible. These changes may be an incidental finding or noticed in conjunction with caries limited to the incisors. Plaque accumulation at the gingival margin and multiple anterior restorations often serve as a diagnostic clue. Early changes consist of diffuse redness of the labial, marginal, and interdental gingiva. The interproximal papillae become red, bulbous, and hemorrhagic. Progression results in inflammatory changes of the entire attached gingiva and bleeding upon probing. Improved oral hygiene reduces these signs but does not resolve the condition. Protective dressings (i.e. emollients) placed on the affected gingiva promote healing. However, definitive treatment should address the reestablishment of a patent nasal airway.

**Acute Necrotizing Ulcerative Gingivitis (Fig. 19.5)** Acute necrotizing ulcerative gingivitis (ANUG) is a type of gingivitis that is linked to specific bacterial species and stress. The condition is also known as Vincent's infection, or "trench mouth." This multifactorial disease has a bacterial population high in fusiform bacillae and spirochetes that are evident in smears viewed by dark-field microscopy. The condition is characterized by fever, lymphadenopathy, malaise, fiery red gingiva, extreme oral pain, hypersalivation, and an unmistakable fetor oris. The interdental papillae are punched out, ulcerated, and covered with a grayish pseudomembrane. The condition is common in persons between the ages of 15 and 25 years, particularly students and military recruits enduring times of increased stress and reduced host resistance, and in HIV-infected patients. In rare instances, the infection can extend to other oral mucosal surfaces or can recur if mismanaged. Treatment of ANUG requires irrigation, gentle debridement, antibiotics (if constitutional symptoms are present), and stress reduction. Partial loss of the interdental papillae can be expected despite normal healing.

**Actinomycotic Gingivitis (Fig. 19.6)** Actinomycotic gingivitis is a rare form of marginal gingivitis that presents with redness, intense burning pain, and lack of a response to normal therapeutic regimens. Biopsy of tissue reveals the non–acid-fast, filamentous fungal organism. Gingivectomy or long-term antimicrobial therapy provides effective treatment.

**Hormonal Gingivitis (Pregnancy Gingivitis) (Fig. 19.7)** Hormonal gingivitis is an hyperplastic reaction to microbial plaque that generally affects women during puberty, pregnancy, or menopause. Elevated estrogen or progesterone levels resulting from hormonal shifts and use of birth control pills have been implicated. These hormones enhance tissue vascularity, which permits an exaggerated inflammatory reaction to plaque. Hormonal gingivitis produces fiery red, swollen, and tender marginal gingiva and compressible and swollen interdental papillae. Severity is related to microbial accumulation and poor oral hygiene. This is often the case with the gravid female because toothbrushing may precipitate nausea. Hormonal gingivitis is usually transitory and responds to meticulous home care, oral prophylaxis, and a decrease in hormone levels. Persistence results in fibrosis and pinker, firmer, and lumpy tissues. Gingivectomy is needed to reduce fibrotic gingivae.

**Diabetic Gingivitis (Fig. 19.8)** Diabetes mellitus is a common disease, affecting approximately 1–3% of the U.S. population. It is a progressive metabolic disorder characterized by hyperglycemia, glucosuria, polyuria, polydipsia, pruritis, and weight loss. Poor control of blood glucose levels is related to lack of production or use of insulin. Complications of diabetes include many vascular-related problems, risk for infection, dry mouth, burning tongue, and persistent gingivitis. The severity of diabetic gingivitis is disease dependent. In the patient with uncontrolled diabetes, peculiar proliferations of exuberant tissue arise from the marginal and attached gingiva. The well-demarcated swellings are soft, red, irregular, and hemorrhagic. The surface of the hyperplastic tissue is bulbous or papulonodular. The gingivitis is difficult to manage when blood glucose levels remain elevated. Successful treatment requires meticulous home care and control of the blood glucose level with diet, hypoglycemic agents, or insulin.

# Gingivitis

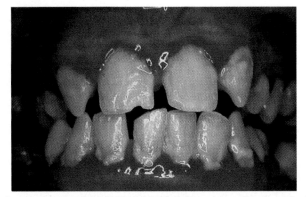

Figure 19.1. Marginal gingivitis: bright red, swollen marginal gingiva. Plaque-induced pain and bleeding reduces willingness to brush.

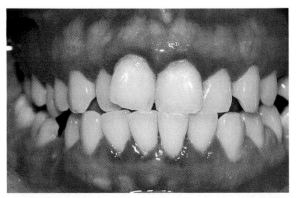

Figure 19.2. Gingivitis: early inflammatory changes along the labial marginal gingiva caused by mouth breathing.

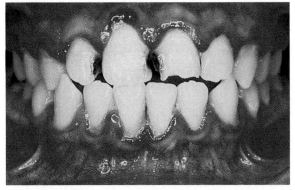

Figure 19.3. Gingivitis caused by mouth breathing. More severe gingival inflammation and caries. (Courtesy Dr Charles Morris)

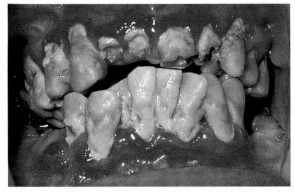

Figure 19.4. Chronic gingivitis extending onto the attached gingiva. (Courtesy Dr Tom McDavid)

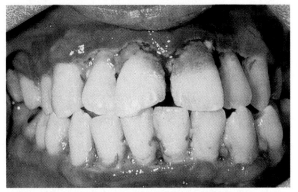

Figure 19.5. Acute necrotizing ulcerative gingivitis: punched-out necrotic papillae. (Courtesy Dr Bill Baker)

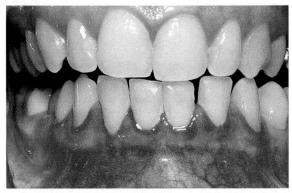

Figure 19.6. Actinomycotic gingivitis: unresponsive to local measures; confirmed by biopsy.

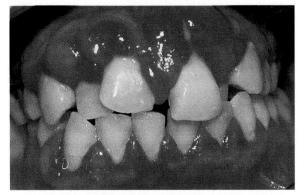

Figure 19.7. Hormonal gingivitis (pregnancy): chronic hyperplastic stage; swollen and fiery red interdental papillae.

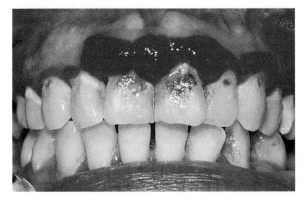

Figure 19.8. Diabetic gingivitis: papulonodular and fiery-red hyperplastic gingiva in a diabetic patient. (Courtesy Dr Margot Van Dis)

# Periodontitis

**Periodontitis (Figs. 20.1–20.8)** Peridontitis is inflammation of the periodontium caused by persistent microbial plaque. It is characterized by progressive loss of epithelial attachment and destruction of the periodontal ligament and alveolar bone. It is preceded by gingivitis and a maturation of bacterial plaque toward anaerobic species. The most common form is **adult periodontitis**. It can be localized or generalized, and it appears to progress episodically. During periods of exacerbation there is advancing loss of epithelial attachment, increased periodontal pocket depth, increased gingival crevicular fluid, loss of alveolar bone and the connective tissue attachment and gingival bleeding. Disease activity can be assessed by monitoring these findings clinically and radiographically and by analyzing the content of the gingival crevicular fluid, which contains inflammatory mediators. Periodontitis usually results in mobile teeth, shifting of teeth and loss of teeth. Nonvitality and periodontal abscess are two less common outcomes.

Adult periodontitis is divided into three types (mild, moderate, and advanced) based on severity. Other types of periodontitis are classified according to early-onset periodontitis (**prepubertal periodontitis** and **juvenile periodontitis**), clinical characteristics (**rapidly progressing periodontitis** and **necrotizing ulcerative periodontitis** [formerly, HIV periodontitis]), and responsiveness to therapy (**refractory periodontitis**). The predominant species associated with adult periodontitis are *Actinobaccillus actinomycetemcomitans* (25–30%), *Actinomyces naeslundii, Bacteriodes forsythus, Campylobacter rectus, Eikenella corrodens, Eubacterium* species, *Fusobacterium nucleatum, Peptostreptococcus micros, Prevotella intermedia, Porphyromonas gingivalis, Selenomonas sputigena, Streptococcus intermedius*, and *Treponema* species. Certain bacterial species are detected more often with specific types of periodontitis; and certain systemic diseases, such as blood dyscrasias, endocrine disorders, and Ehlers-Danlos syndrome, are associated with periodontal disease. Smoking also increases the risk. Treatment depends on the causal factors but generally involves the removal of plaque, calculus and diseased cementum by scaling, curettage, and root planing. Topical antibiotics, short-course therapy with systemic antibiotics (tetracycline and metronidazole), and periodontal surgery have proven successful. Control of systemic factors and implementation of good oral hygiene practices are also required to reverse periodontitis.

## Mild (Early) Adult Periodontitis (Figs. 20.1 and 20.2)

Mild adult periodontitis is microscopically characterized by minor breakdown of pocket epithelium, migration of neutrophils, increasing population of plasma cells, apical migration of junctional epithelium, minor destruction of the connective tissue attachment, and localized resorption of alveolar bone. This stage is defined by 3 mm **of epithelial attachment loss or less**, periodontal pocket depths of 3–5 mm, class I furcation involvement, and alveolar crestal bone loss of 2 mm or less. Pocket depth is determined using a periodontal probe. The **class I furcation** is limited destruction of bone between the superior aspect of the roots immediately below the tooth crown that is detectable by 1-mm entry of an explorer or probe. Alveolar bone loss is determined by vertical periapical bitewing radiographs or subtraction radiography. Although the latter technique is the most accurate and reproducible, the former is generally used because of cost.

## Moderate Adult Periodontitis (Figs. 20.3–20.5)

Moderate adult periodontitis is the second stage of adult periodontitis. Microscopic examination shows ulceration of the pocket epithelium, infiltrating populations of plasma cells and T cells, significant migration of junctional epithelium, and significant destruction of the connective tissue attachment and alveolar bone. Moderate adult periodontitis is defined by 4–5 mm **of epithelial attachment loss**, periodontal pocket depths of 4–6 mm, alveolar bone loss that is 3–5 mm, gingival exudate, and bleeding. **Horizontal bone loss, vertical bone loss, osseous defects (moats, craters), mobile teeth, and class II furcation involvement** are additional radiographic and clinical features of the disease. The class II furcation is a 2- to 4-mm defect of cortical and alveolar bone located superiorly between the roots.

## Advanced Adult Periodontitis (Figs. 20.6 and 20.8)

Advanced adult periodontitis is characterized microscopically by major destruction of the pocket epithelium, connective tissue attachment and alveolar bone, and large populations of plasma cells and T cells. Advanced adult periodontitis is defined by at least 6 mm **of epithelial attachment loss**. Typically, periodontal pocket depths exceed 6 mm; alveolar bone loss is more than 5 mm; and gingival recession, significant tooth mobility, and **class III fucation involvement** (a through-and-through bony defect) are seen.

## Periodontal Abscess (Fig. 20.7)

A periodontal abscess is a fluctuant swelling of the gingiva resulting from pathogenic bacteria that are occluded in the gingival crevice. The condition is evidenced clinically by a rapidly progressing, smooth-surfaced, red-purple papule or nodule emanating from the attached gingiva. Other characteristics are increased mobility of the periodontally involved tooth, purulence, tissue necrosis, and loss of stippling of the free marginal groove. Patients often report well-localized, dull, and continuous pain, especially if the purulent exudate has no avenue for escape. Pain intensifies when pressure is applied to the tooth or the overlying soft tissue. Diagnostic evaluation using a periodontal probe may initially produce discomfort but is often therapeutic for a short time because it may drain the abscess. Fever, malaise, lymphadenopathy and an unpleasant taste may accompany the condition. The pulp of a tooth associated with a periodontal abscess usually tests vital. Treatment should be directed toward removal of necrotic material, adequate drainage, localized periodontal therapy, and improved plaque control measures.

# Periodontitis

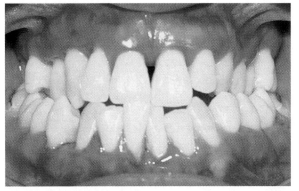

Figure 20.1. Mild periodontitis: loss of attachment evident by gingival recession and blunting of interdental papillae; inflammation evident by bleeding of premolar periodontal pocket.

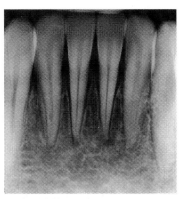

Figure 20.2. Mild periodontitis: radiographic features showing crestal loss of alveolar bone.

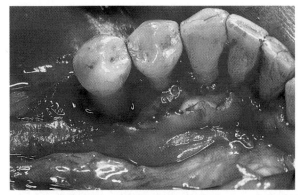

Figure 20.3. Moderate periodontitis: 4-mm moat defect surrounding second premolar evident during periodontal surgery.

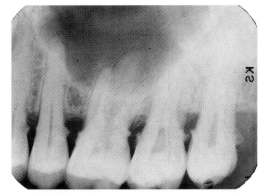

Figure 20.4. Moderate periodontitis: interproximal calculus and horizontal bone loss in the posterior quadrant.

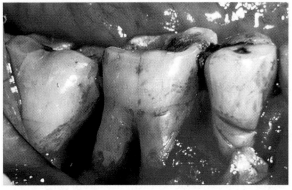

Figure 20.5. Class II furcation: a sign of moderate periodontitis. This defect was 3 mm deep.

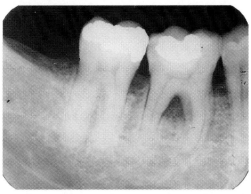

Figure 20.6. Furcation involvement: radiographic evidence of a class III furcation consistent with advanced periodontitis.

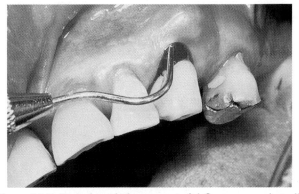

Figure 20.7. Periodontal abscess: painful fluctuant, red swelling. Periodontal probe depth was 12 mm.

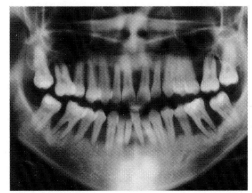

Figure 20.8. Advanced periodontitis: panoramic film shows generalized horizontal alveolar bone loss greater than 6 mm.

# Localized Gingival Lesions

**Pyogenic Granuloma (Figs. 21.1 and 21.2)** Pyogenic granuloma (a misnomer because the condition is neither pus-filled nor a granuloma) is a form of inflammatory hyperplasia rich in neocapillaries and immature fibrous connective tissue. The growth is an exaggerated response to irritation and appears bright red, fleshy, and soft. The surface is glossy and ulcerated. The base is polypoid or pedunculated. Although the condition is usually asymptomatic, minor manipulation induces bleeding because of the thinned epithelium and highly vascular tissue. Maturation of the lesion results in increased fibrosis, decreased vascularity, and pinker color.

Pyogenic granulomas develop in patients who have poor oral hygiene or a chronic oral irritant such as overhanging restorations and calculus. Females are more susceptible to the condition because of hormonal imbalances that occur during puberty, pregnancy, or menopause; in such cases, the granulomas are called hormonal or pregnancy tumors. About 1% of pregnant women develop this lesion.

Pyogenic granulomas most frequently arise from the interdental papilla and can enlarge from the labial and lingual aspects to several centimeters. Other sites of development include the tongue, lips, buccal mucosa, and edentulous ridge. Treatment is surgical excision that, in the gravid female, should be delayed until after partuition. Recurrence is possible, if excision and local debridement are incomplete or plaque control is inadequate.

**Peripheral Giant Cell Granuloma (Figs. 21.3 and 21.4)** The peripheral giant cell granuloma is a reactive epulis-like growth that develops exclusively on the gingiva. It is generally associated with a history of trauma or irritation and is thought to originate from the mucoperiosteum or periodontal ligament. Therefore, the peripheral giant cell granuloma demonstrates a restricted area of development—the dentulous or edentulous ridge. The mandibular gingiva anterior to the molars is particularly affected, especially in women between the ages of 40 and 60. Histologic examination shows multinucleated giant cells and numerous fibroblasts.

The peripheral giant cell granuloma is a well-defined, firm swelling that seldom ulcerates. The base is sessile, the surface is smooth or slightly granular, and the color is pink to dark red-purple. The nodule is usually a few millimeters to 1 cm in diameter, although rapid enlargement may produce a large growth that encroaches on adjacent teeth. The lesion is generally asymptomatic; however, because of its aggressive nature, the underlying alveolar bone is often involved, producing a pathognomonic superficial "peripheral-cuff" radiolucency. Treatment is surgical excision that includes the base of the lesion and curettage of the underlying bone. Incomplete removal may result in recurrence. On histologic examination, this lesion cannot be distinguished from the central giant cell granuloma and the brown tumor of hyperparathyroidism.

**Peripheral Ossifying Fibroma (Figs. 21.5 and 21.6)** The peripheral ossifying fibroma is a reactive growth that is especially prone to occur in the anterior region of the maxilla of young females in the second decade of life. The cause of the peripheral ossifying fibroma is uncertain, but inflammatory hyperplasia of superficial periodontal ligament origin has been suggested. The condition arises exclusively from the gingiva, usually the interdental papillae. When calcifications are present, they may consist of bone, cementum, or dystrophic calcification. Peripheral ossifying fibroma is unrelated to the central ossifying fibroma. The salient clinical features of this solitary swelling are firmness, red or pink color, possible ulceration, and sessile attachment. An important diagnostic clue is the condition's marked tendency to cause displacement of adjacent teeth. The chief sign is often an asymptomatic, slow-growing round or nodular swelling. Immature lesions are soft and bleed easily, whereas older lesions become firm and fibrotic. Radiographs may reveal central radiopaque foci and mild resorption of the crest of the ridge at its base. Treatment is excision. The recurrence rate is about 15%.

**Irritation Fibroma** The irritation fibroma is a common benign oral lesion that occasionally develops on gingival tissues. It is more typically seen on moveable mucosa and is discussed in Section VI (Figs. 50.1 and 50.2).

**Peripheral Odontogenic Fibroma (Fig. 21.7)** The peripheral odontogenic fibroma is clinically similar to the irritation fibroma but is characterized by its unique location and tissue of origin. In most cases, the peripheral odontogenic fibroma is found as a circumscribed swelling in the region of the interdental papilla, generally located anterior to the molar teeth. A cup-like erosion of the underlying alveolar bone may be seen radiographically. It probably arises from cellular components of the periodontal ligament. Microscopic examination shows clusters of odontogenic epithelium among dense collagenous tissue.

**Desmoplastic Fibroma (Fig. 21.8)** The desmoplastic fibroma is a rare tumor composed of fibroblasts and abundant collagen that most frequently affects the metaphyseal regions of the long bones of the arms and legs. The fourth most commonly affected site is the mandible. Most cases occur in adults younger than age 30; the posterior jaw is the most common intraoral location. These tumors begin as painless firm swellings within bone that appear unilocular radiographically. Erosion of the cortical bone results in root resorption and a pink, firm soft tissue mass of the alveolar ridge or gingiva. The tumor is locally aggressive and recurs in about 30% of patients who receive surgical treatment. Resection is recommended for recurrent lesions.

# Localized Gingival Lesions

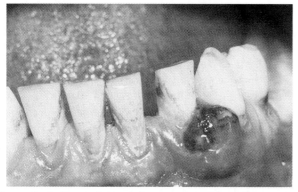

Figure 21.1. **Pyogenic granuloma** arising from the interdental papilla.

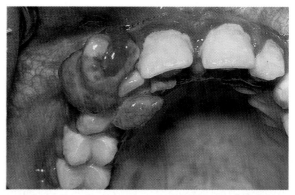

Figure 21.2. **Pregnancy tumor:** 3 days after partuition.

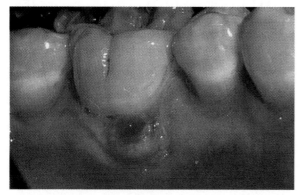

Figure 21.3. **Peripheral giant cell granuloma** arising from marginal gingiva. (Courtesy Dr Ed Heslop)

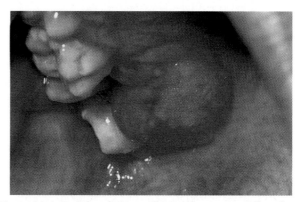

Figure 21.4. **Peripheral giant cell granuloma:** a rapidly enlarging lesion. (Courtesy Dr James Cottone and Dr Steve Bricker)

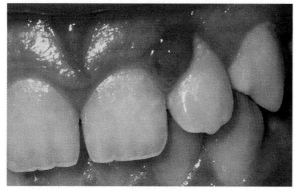

Figure 21.5. **Peripheral ossifying fibroma:** typical location in a teenaged female (Courtesy Dr James Cottone)

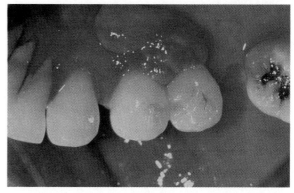

Figure 21.6. **Peripheral ossifying fibroma:** older lesion becoming pink and firm to palpation. (Courtesy Dr Pete Benson)

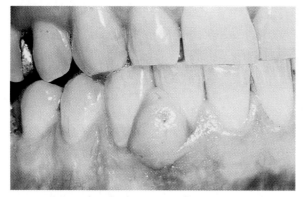

Figure 21.7. **Peripheral odontogenic fibroma:** pink with interdental location.

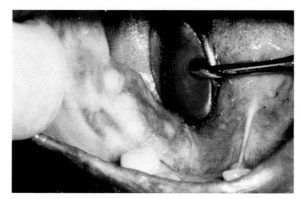

Figure 21.8. **Desmoplastic fibroma:** aggressive firm lesion on lingual aspect of posterior gingiva.

# Localized Gingival Lesions

**Parulis (Gumboil) (Figs. 22.1 and 22.2)** The parulis, or gumboil—the latter term being reserved for children—is a localized area of inflammatory hyperplasia that occurs at the end point of a draining dental sinus tract. It appears as a soft, solitary reddish papule, located apical and facial to a chronically abscessed tooth, usually on or near the labial mucogingival junction. Occasionally the parulis is slightly yellow in the center and emits a purulent yellowish exudate upon palpation. Acute swelling and pain may accompany the condition if the sinus tract is obstructed.

To locate the nonvital tooth from which the parulis arises, a sterile gutta-percha point may be inserted into the sinus tract. Periapical radiographs are then taken to demonstrate the proximity of the gutta-percha point to the apex of the offending tooth. After the nonvital tooth is diagnosed, the treatment of choice is root canal therapy. Shortly thereafter, the parulis usually regresses. If the problematic tooth is left untreated, the parulis may persist for years. A persistent lesion may mature into a pink-colored fibroma.

**Pericoronitis (Operculitis) (Figs. 22.3 and 22.4)** Pericoronitis is inflammation of the soft tissue surrounding the crown of a partially erupted or impacted tooth. Pericoronitis may develop at any age but most frequently occurs in children and young adults whose teeth are erupting. Generally, it is associated with an erupting mandibular third molar that is in good alignment but is limited in its eruption by insufficient space. Radiographs of the region reveal a flame-shaped radiolucency in the alveolar bone distal to the tooth, with the cortical outline either absent or distinctly thickened because of infection or deposition of reactive bone.

Pericoronitis develops from bacterial contamination beneath the operculum, resulting in gingival swelling, redness, and halitosis. Pain varies and may be extreme, but the discomfort usually resembles that of gingivitis, a periodontal abscess, or tonsillitis. Regional lymphadenopathy, malaise, and low-grade fever are common. If edema or cellulitis extends to involve the masseter muscle, trismus often accompanies the condition. Pericoronitis is frequently complicated by pain induced by trauma from the opposing tooth during closure.

Pericoronitis is best managed by entering the follicular space, flushing the purulent material from the gingival sulcus with saline solution, and eliminating any occlusal trauma. Definitive treatment is usually extraction of the involved tooth. Antibiotic coverage is recommended when constitutional symptoms are present and the spread of infection is likely. Recurrences and chronicity are likely if the condition is managed only with antibiotics.

**Periodontal Abscess** The periodontal abscess produces a localized gingival swelling. An example is seen in Figure 20.8.

**Epulis Fissuratum (Irritation Hyperplasia) (Figs. 22.5 and 22.6)** The epulis fissuratum is a reactive inflammatory fibrous hyperplasia caused by a chronic irritant, usually the flange area of an old, poorly fitting complete or partial denture. The overextended denture margin initially produces an ulcer that heals incompletely because of repeated trauma. Hyperplastic healing results in a pink-red, fleshy exuberance of mature granulation tissue. The hyperplastic lesion, located where the denture flange rests, is found mostly in older women. It is nonpainful, grows slowly on either side of the denture flange, and causes the patient little concern.

The epulis fissuratum in the early stages consists of a single fold of smooth soft tissue. As the swelling grows, a central cleft or several clefts become apparent, the boundaries of which may drape over the denture flange. The mucolabial fold of the anterior region of the maxilla is the most common location, followed by the mandibular alveolar ridge and the mandibular lingual sulcus. Adjustment of the denture or construction of a new denture may reduce the trauma and inflammation but will not cause the underlying fibrous tissue to regress. Likewise, surgical excision without alteration of the dentures promotes recurrence. Successful treatment usually requires surgical removal of the redundant tissue, microscopic examination of the excised tissue, and correction or reconstruction of the denture.

**Gingival Carcinoma (Figs. 22.7 and 22.8)** The gingiva accounts for approximately 5–10% of all cases of oral squamous cell carcinoma. Generally, at the time of diagnosis the disease is advanced because of its asymptomatic nature, posterior location, and delay of examination.

The appearance of gingival carcinoma varies. It usually appears as a reddish mass with focal white areas proliferating from the gingiva but may mimic benign inflammatory gingival conditions, erythroplakia, leukoplakia, or a simple ulceration. Carcinoma should be suspected when close examination reveals a pebbly surface, many small blood vessels in the overlying epithelium, and surface ulceration. Etiologic factors include tobacco use, alcoholism, and poor oral hygiene. Elderly men are especially susceptible, and the condition seems to have a slight predilection for the alveolar ridge of the posterior mandible. Completely dentulous persons rarely have this disease.

Gingival carcinoma may extend onto the floor of the mouth or mucobuccal fold, or it may invade the underlying bone. Radiographs may reveal a "cupping out" of the alveolar crest. Metastasis to regional lymph nodes occurs frequently. Metastatic nodes are firm, rubbery, matted, nonmovable, and nonpainful. Treatment consists of surgery and radiotherapy.

# Localized Gingival Lesions

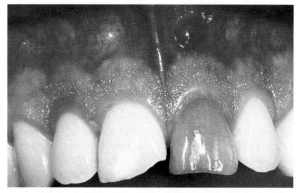

Figure 22.1. **Parulis:** reddish papule associated with the discolored nonvital maxillary central incisor.

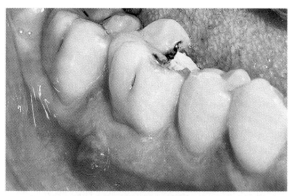

Figure 22.2. **Parulis:** more pinkish papule at mucogingival junction adjacent to a nonvital first molar.

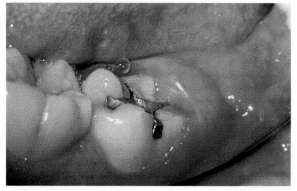

Figure 22.3. **Pericoronitis** surrounding a partially erupted mandibular molar.

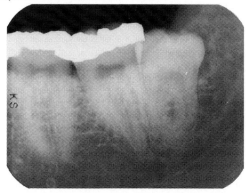

Figure 22.4. **Pericoronitis** has produced a flame-shaped radiolucency and reactive sclerotic margin because of underlying osteitis.

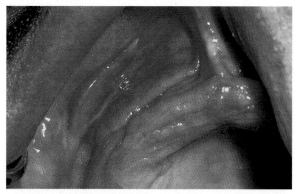

Figure 22.5. **Epulis fissuratum:** reddish hyperplastic folds caused by irritating denture flange.

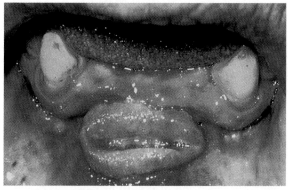

Figure 22.6. **Epulis fissuratum** where the partial denture flange rests.

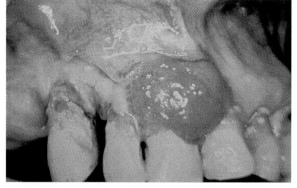

Figure 22.7. **Gingival carcinoma** in a patient with poor oral hygiene and advanced age. (Courtesy Dr Jack Sherman)

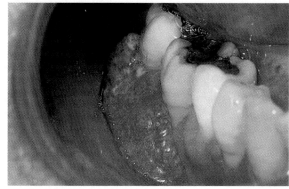

Figure 22.8. **Gingival carcinoma:** squamous cell type with reddish, granular, and telangiectatic surface. (Courtesy Dr Tom Aufdemorte)

# Generalized Gingival Enlargements

**Primary Herpetic Gingivostomatitis (Fig. 23.1)**
Herpes simplex virus is a DNA virus with a propensity to infect human epithelium. The initial infection is subclinical (not readily visible) or prominent depending on the amount of initial inoculum, location, integrity of the epithelium, and the host response. Herpetic gingivostomatitis is the prominent finding of primary oral infection. Replication of the virus in gingival epithelium causes generalized swelling, redness, and pain of the marginal gingiva. The interdental papillae become bulbous and bleed easily about 4 days after infection. Several vesicles and ulcers also develop. Antiviral agents are recommended early during the herpetic infection. Antibiotics are occasionally needed when patients become septic and their temperature is persistently elevated above 101 ° F. Healing normally takes about 14 to 21 days. Recurrent herpes simplex virus infections develop in 30–40% of infected patients (see Figs. 52.1–52.6 for more information).

**Fibromatosis Gingivae (Fig. 23.2)** Fibromatosis gingivae is a rare progressive fibrous enlargement of the gingiva that is usually inherited as an autosomal dominant trait. The condition begins with tooth eruption and becomes more prominent with age. The enlargement is usually generalized and noninflammatory, affecting the buccal and lingual surfaces of one or both jaws. The free, interproximal, and marginal gingiva are enlarged, uniformly pink, firm, nonhemorrhagic, and often nodular.

There are two varieties of fibromatosis gingivae: generalized and localized. The generalized type is nodular and diffuse, exhibiting several coalesced areas of globular gingival overgrowths that encroach on and eventually cover the crowns of the teeth. In the occasionally seen localized variety, solitary overgrowths are limited to the palatal vault of the maxillary tuberosity or the lingual gingiva of the mandibular arch. These gingival overgrowths appear smooth, firm, and symmetrically round. The localized involvement may be unilateral or bilateral, and the term "focal gingival fibromatosis" has been suggested for this variant.

Fibromatosis gingivae may interfere with tooth eruption, mastication, and oral hygiene. In severe cases, noneruption of the primary or permanent teeth may be the chief symptom. Regression is not a feature of this disease, even with effective oral hygiene measures. Gingivectomy, with either a blade or a carbon dioxide laser, is the treatment of choice. Continued growth may require several operations. The condition may be accompanied by acromegalic facial features, hypertrichosis, mental deficits, deafness, and seizures.

**Drug-Induced Gingival Hyperplasia (Figs. 23.3–23.6)** Gingival enlargement is an adverse effect associated with use of some prescription drugs. It occurs in 25–50% of patients taking phenytoin (Dilantin) and cyclosporine (Sandimmune). Phenytoin is taken for its antiepileptic properties; cyclosporine is taken because it inhibits T-cell proliferation and prevents transplant rejection. Gingival hyperplasia also occurs in 1–10% of patients who take calcium channel blocker drugs (such as nifedipine [Procardia], diltiazem [Cardizem], verapamil [Calan], felodipine [Plendil]), sodium valproate (Depakene), and estrogen (in birth control pills and Premarin). Although the mechanism of drug-induced gingival hyperplasia remains unknown, many of these drugs affect calcium ion flux in gingival fibroblasts that may alter normal homeostasis and collagenase activity. Estrogen may work separately by increasing the blood supply and inflammatory mediators to the gingiva.

Drug-induced gingival hyperplasia can occur at any age and in either sex. Although the enlargement results from a hyperplastic response, an inflammatory component induced by dental bacterial plaque often coexists and tends to exacerbate the condition. The gingival enlargement is usually generalized and begins at the interdental papillae. It appears most exaggerated on the labial aspects of the anterior teeth. The overgrowths form soft red lumpy nodules that bleed easily. Progressive growth results in fibrotic changes: the interdental tissue becomes enlarged, pink, firm, and resilient to palpation. With time the condition can completely engulf the crowns of the teeth; this aggravates home care, limits mastication, and compromises esthetics. Treatment may involve changing drug therapy or minimizing the overgrowth with meticulous and frequent plaque control measures. The gingival swelling may completely regress by discontinuing drug use. However, excess fibrotic tissue unresponsive to changes in drug therapy must be surgically removed.

**Gingival Edema of Hypothyroidism (Figs. 23.7 and 23.8)** Hypothyroidism is a relatively common disorder in which clinical manifestations depend on the age at onset, duration, and severity of the thyroid insufficiency. When the patient is deficient in hormone at an early age, cretinism results. This disease is characterized by short stature, mental retardation, disproportionate head-to-body size, delayed tooth eruption, mandibular micrognathism, and swollen lips and tongue. Regardless of the age of onset, hypothyroid patients have coarse, dry, yellowish skin; intolerance to cold; and lethargy. Swelling is the classic feature and is most prominent in the face, particularly around the eyes.

Within the mouth, macroglossia and macrocheilia are common and may cause an altered speech pattern. The gingiva appears uniformly enlarged, pale pink, and compressible. Swelling occurs in all directions on both the facial and lingual sides of the dental arches. When secondary inflammation is present, the tissues become red and boggy and have a tendency to bleed easily. Treatment for the gingival condition depends on the degree of thyroid deficiency. Patients with marginal deficiency require only strict oral hygiene measures, whereas frank cases require supplemental thyroid therapy to achieve resolution of the systemic and oral condition.

# Generalized Gingival Enlargements

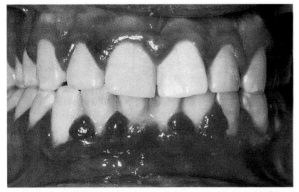

Figure 23.1. Primary herpetic gingivostomatitis: interdental papillae red, swollen, and painful.

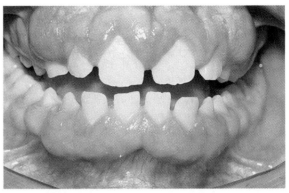

Figure 23.2. Fibromatosis gingivae: generalized type. (Courtesy Dr Kenneth Abramovitch)

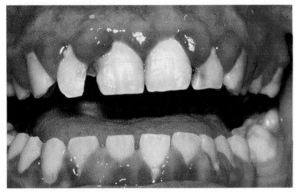

Figure 23.3. Dilantin-induced gingival hyperplasia: inflamed, hyperplastic interdental papillae (Courtesy Dr James Cottone)

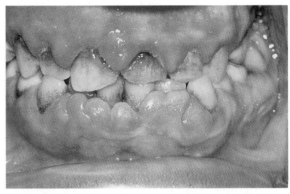

Figure 23.4. Dilantin-induced gingival hyperplasia: generalized fibrous appearance.

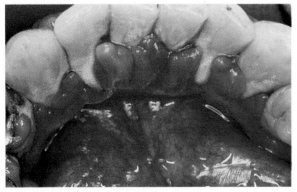

Figure 23.5. Nifedipine-induced gingival hyperplasia. Patient was taking Procardia.

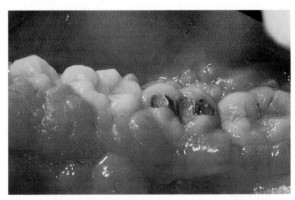

Figure 23.6. Cyclosporine-induced gingival hyperplasia: severely affected lingual gingiva.

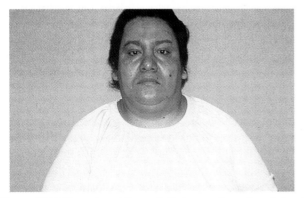

Figure 23.7. Hypothyroidism. Called myxedema in adults, it produces gingival edema and yellowish, thick, coarse skin.

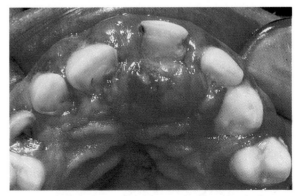

Figure 23.8. Hypothyroidism: generalized gingival edema and inflammation in same patient shown in Figure 23.7.

# Spontaneous Gingival Bleeding

**Leukemic Gingivitis (Figs. 24.1 and 24.2)** Leukemia, a malignant condition characterized by overproduction of leukocytes, is classified according to cell morphology (monocytic, myelogenous, or lymphoblastic) and the clinical course of the disease (acute or chronic). Oral manifestations are more frequently encountered in acute leukemia of the monocytic and myelogenous subtypes. Oral features occur early in the course of the disease because of neoplastic proliferation of one blood cell type, which reduces the normal production of the other hematopoietic cells.

Consistent signs of acute leukemia are cervical lymphadenopathy, malaise, anemic pallor, leukopenia-induced ulcerations, and gingival changes. Leukemic gingival tissues are usually red, tender, and spongy and tend to peel away from the teeth. With progression of the disease, the swollen gingiva becomes purple and shiny. Stippling of the tissue is lost and spontaneous bleeding from the gingival sulcus eventually occurs. The edematous tissue is most prominent interdentally and results from leukemic infiltration of leukocytes. In certain patients the neoplastic cells may invade pulpal and osseous tissue, inducing vague symptoms of pain without corresponding radiographic evidence of pathosis. Purpuric features, such as petechial lesions and ecchymoses on pale mucosal membranes, together with gingival hemorrhage, occur frequently. Systemic control of leukemia often involves intensive radiotherapy, chemotherapy, blood transfusions, and bone marrow transplantation. Difficulty may be encountered in maintaining optimal oral health because of the chemotherapy-induced oral ulcerations. Meticulous oral hygiene combined with antimicrobial rinses is recommended to reduce the inflammatory and ulcerative sequelae of chemotherapy.

**Agranulocytosis (Neutropenia) and Cyclic Neutropenia (Figs. 24.3 and 24.4)** Agranulocytosis (also known as neutropenia) is a disease characterized by a decrease in the number of circulating polymorphonuclear neutrophils. In most instances, the condition is recognized by its clinical symptoms, which consist of chronic infections and an almost complete absence of neutrophils in laboratory blood tests. Antimetabolic, antibiotic, and cytotoxic drugs are the etiologic agents involved in more than half of all cases. In rare instances the condition may be congenital. An uncontrollable infection in the neutropenic patient can result in bacterial pneumonia, sepsis, or death.

A distinct form of agranulocytosis is cyclic neutropenia, which is characterized by a periodic diminution of circulating polymorphonuclear neutrophils that occurs about every 3 weeks and lasts for about 5 days. The condition is idiopathic and usually begins in childhood. It is sometimes accompanied by arthritis, pharyngitis, fever, headache, and lymphadenopathy. A history of repeated infections of the ear and upper respiratory tract is common.

Oral manifestations include inflammatory gingival changes and mucosal ulcerations. The ulcerations are usually large, oval, and persistent. They vary in size and location; they are sometimes found on the attached gingiva and other times on the tongue and buccal mucosa. The gingivitis is periodic and ulcerative. At stages that correspond to elevated levels of polymorphonuclear neutrophils, minimal inflammation is evident. In contrast, when the polymorphonuclear neutrophil count decreases precipitously, generalized inflammatory hyperplasia and erythema occur. If left untreated, the condition is exacerbated by the presence of local factors such as plaque and calculus, which result in alveolar bone loss, tooth mobility, and early exfoliation of teeth.

The periodic appearance and spontaneous regression of signs and symptoms should cause the clinician to suspect cyclic neutropenia. Daily measurement of the leukocyte count is required to diagnose this condition. Curative treatment is unavailable. Management is therefore palliative and consists of antibiotic and antimicrobial therapy and repeated oral prophylaxis.

**Thrombocytopathic and Thrombocytopenic Purpura (Figs. 24.5–24.8)** Platelets play an integral role in maintaining hemostasis by providing the primary hemostatic plug and by activating the intrinsic system of coagulation. A decrease in the number of circulating platelets (thrombocytopenia) may be idiopathic or may be the result of decreased platelet production in the bone marrow, increased peripheral destruction, or increased splenic sequestration. Decreased function of circulating platelets (thrombocytopathia) is often related to hereditary syndromes or acquired states such as drug-induced bone marrow suppression, liver disease, or dysproteinemic states like uremia.

The normal platelet count is 150,000–400,000 cells/mm$^3$. Vascular-related clinical manifestations of platelet disorders usually do not develop until the count decreases to less than 100,000 cells/mm$^3$. These features include petechiae, ecchymoses, epistaxis, hematuria, hypermenorrhea, and gastrointestinal bleeding resulting in melena. Spontaneous gingival bleeding is a frequent, early, and dramatic occurrence. Blood profusely oozes from the gingival sulcus, either spontaneously or after minor trauma such as toothbrushing. The fluid then turns into purplish-black globs of clotted blood that adhere to the oral structures. Clotted blood is sometimes swallowed, which results in nausea. Mild traumas, particularly at the occlusal line of the buccal mucosa and tongue, are sites of extensive hemorrhage. Multifocal red petechial spots on the soft palate are another frequent clinical sign of bleeding disorders. Measurement of the platelet count, clot retraction time, tourniquet test, and template bleeding time should be done to diagnose a platelet disorder. Platelet transfusions may be necessary if local measures do not control oral bleeding.

# Spontaneous Gingival Bleeding

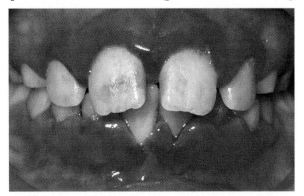

Figure 24.1. Leukemic gingivitis (acute myelogenous leukemia): swollen, shiny, and bleeding gingiva. (Courtesy Dr Monique Michaud)

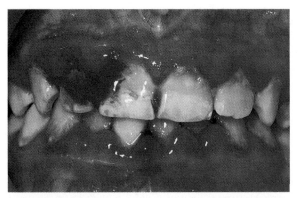

Figure 24.2. Leukemic gingivitis (acute lymphocytic leukemia): gingival enlargement and spontaneous bleeding. (Courtesy Dr Monique Michaud)

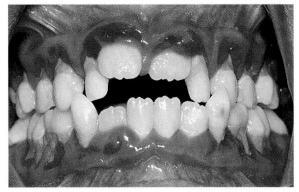

Figure 24.3. Cyclic neutropenia associated with gingival erythema and epithelial erosion.

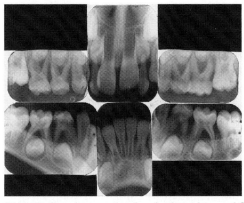

Figure 24.4. Cyclic neutropenia: alveolar bone loss and floating teeth (same patient shown in Figure 24.3).

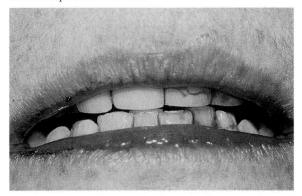

Figure 24.5. Thrombocytopathia: hemorrhagic crusts on lips of a 57- year-old woman with cirrhosis and clotting-factor deficiency. (Courtesy Dr Roger Rao)

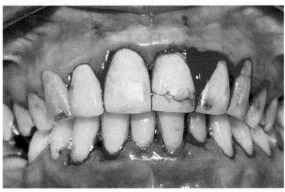

Figure 24.6. Thrombocytopenia: spontaneous gingival bleeding in same patient shown in Figure 24.5. (Courtesy Dr Roger Rao)

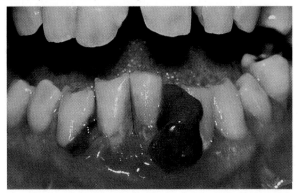

Figure 24.7. Thrombocytopenia: platelet count was 26,000 cells/mm³; gingival bleeding and the resultant blood clot. (Courtesy Dr Larry Skoczylas)

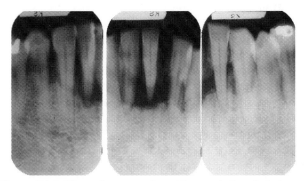

Figure 24.8. Thrombocytopenia evidence of chronic irritants contributing to the bleeding in patient shown in Figure 24.7.

# Conditions Peculiar to the Tongue

**Scalloped Tongue (Crenated Tongue) (Figs. 25.1 and 25.2)** A scalloped tongue is a common entity characterized by indentations on the lateral margins of the tongue. The condition is usually bilateral but may be unilateral or isolated to a region where the tongue is held in close contact with the teeth. Abnormal pressure of the teeth on the tongue imprints the characteristic pattern, which appears as depressed ovals that are circumscribed by a raised white scalloped border. Causes of scalloped tongue include situations that cause abnormal tongue pressure, such as frictional movement of the tongue against teeth and diastemata, tongue thrusting, tongue sucking, clenching, bruxing, or an enlarged tongue. A prominent linea alba on the buccal mucosa is a frequent coexisting finding caused by the negative intraoral pressure associated with tongue sucking in persons who clench or brux their teeth. A crenated tongue may be seen in association with temporomandibular joint disorders, such systemic conditions as acromegaly and amyloidosis, and such genetic disorders as Down's syndrome, as well as in normal patients. The condition is harmless and asymptomatic. Treatment is often aimed at habit elimination.

**Macroglossia (Figs. 25.3 and 25.4)** Macroglossia involves an abnormally enlarged tongue. For assessment of tongue size, the tongue should be completely relaxed. The normal height of the dorsum of the tongue should be even with the occlusal plane of the mandibular teeth; the lateral borders of the tongue should be in contact with, but not overlapping, the lingual cusps of the mandibular teeth. A tongue that extends beyond these dimensions is said to be enlarged.

Macroglossia is either congenital or acquired. Congenital macroglossia can be caused by idiopathic muscular hypertrophy, muscular hemihypertrophy, benign tumors, hamartomas, or cysts. Idiopathic muscular hypertrophy is often associated with a mental deficiency or may be a component of a syndrome such as Beckwith-Wiedemann's syndrome. Acquired macroglossia may be the result of passive enlargement of the tongue when mandibular teeth are lost. In this case, the enlargement may be localized or diffuse, depending on the size of the edentulous area. Systemic disease, such as acromegaly, cretinism, and amyloidosis, or malignant neoplasms, which can occlude lymphatic drainage and produce a swollen tongue, can cause macroglossia. Indicators of an enlarged tongue are speech difficulties, displaced teeth, malocclusion, or a scalloped tongue. The affected region of the tongue often demonstrates enlarged fungiform papillae. If the enlarged tongue is hindering function, elimination of the primary cause or surgical correction may be necessary.

**Hairy Tongue (Lingua Villosa, Coated Tongue) (Figs. 25.5 and 25.6)** Hairy tongue is an abnormal elongation of the filiform papillae that gives the dorsum of the tongue a hairlike appearance. The cause of the hypertrophic response of the filiform papillae is poorly understood but seems to be related to either increased keratin deposition or delayed shedding of the cornified layer. Patients who do not cleanse their tongues are most commonly affected. Cancer therapy, infection with *Candida albicans,* irradiation, poor oral hygiene, change in oral pH, smoking, and the use of antibiotics have also been associated with this condition.

Hairy tongue may be white, yellow, brown, or black, hence the names white coated tongue and yellow, brown, or black hairy tongue. The color of the lesion is a result of intrinsic factors (chromogenic organisms) combined with extrinsic factors (food and tobacco stains). Hairy tongue occurs more frequently in males, primarily in persons older than age 30 years, and the prevalence seems to increase with age. The lesion begins near the foramen cecum on the dorsal surface of the tongue and spreads laterally and anteriorly. The affected filiform papillae discolor, progressively elongate, and may reach a length of several millimeters. Generally, hairy tongue is only of cosmetic concern and the tongue remains asymptomatic. Vigorous brushing with abrasive pastes and topical antifungal agents leads to resolution. In refractory cases, an underlying endocrinopathy such as diabetes mellitus should be sought.

**Hairy Leukoplakia (Figs. 25.7 and 25.8)** Hairy leukoplakia is a significant leukoplakic-like finding that indicates immunosuppression. The lesion is seen almost exclusively in patient's infected with HIV or persons with immunosuppression resulting from drugs taken for organ transplantation or systemic disease. The white lesion is primarily located on the lateral borders of the tongue but may extend to cover the dorsal and ventral surfaces. A viral origin is likely because Epstein-Barr virus has been identified within the affected epithelial cells. Hairy leukoplakia is so named because hair-like peeling of the parakeratotic surface layer is evident histologically. *Candida albicans* is frequently associated with this lesion.

Hairy leukoplakia produces white vertical raised folds on the lateral border of the tongue. The lesion initially has alternating faint white folds and adjacent normal pink troughs that produce a characteristic vertical white-banded washboard appearance. The bands eventually coalesce to form discrete white plaques or extensive thick white corrugated patches. Large lesions are usually asymptomatic, have poorly demarcated borders, and do not rub off. A bilateral occurrence is common, but unilateral lesions are possible. Hairy leukoplakia has been documented on the palate and buccal mucosa. Antiviral agents that block replication of Epstein-Barr virus are useful in reducing the size of the lesions.

# Conditions Peculiar to the Tongue

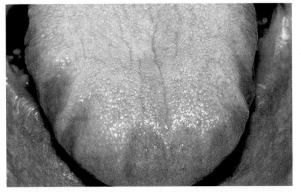

Figure 25.1. **Scalloped tongue** caused by abnormal tongue pressure against the teeth during clenching or bruxing.

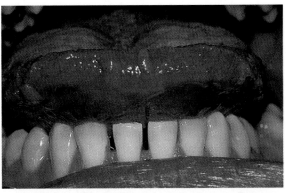

Figure 25.2. **Scalloped tongue** associated with negative oral pressure caused by tongue sucking.

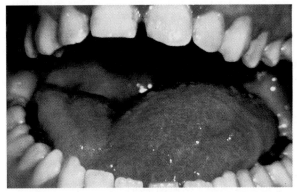

Figure 25.3. **Macroglossia:** unilateral enlargement of the tongue caused by congenital orofacial hemihypertrophy.

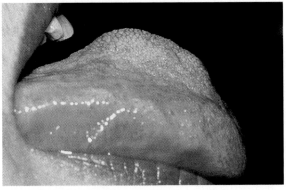

Figure 25.4. **Macroglossia** caused by a hemangioma. (Courtesy Dr Kenneth Abramovitch)

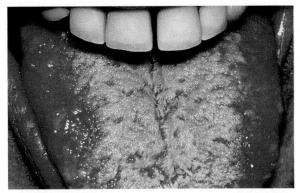

Figure 25.5. **White hairy tongue** in a patient with stomatitis medicamentosa.

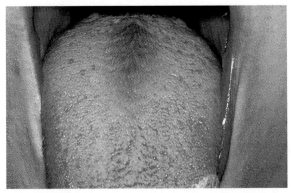

Figure 25.6. **Brown hairy tongue:** hypertrophic filiform papillae in a person who smokes.

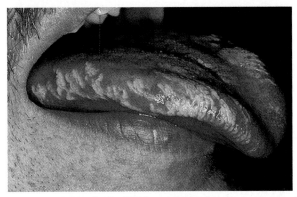

Figure 25.7. **Hairy leukoplakia:** typical white corrugations in a patient with the acquired immune deficiency syndrome. (Courtesy Dr Sol Silverman)

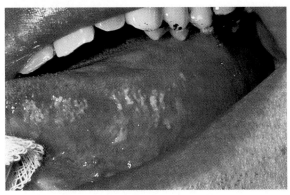

Figure 25.8. **Hairy leukoplakia** in a person who just received dental treatment. (Courtesy Dr Michaell Huber)

# Conditions Peculiar to the Tongue

**Geographic Tongue (Benign Migratory Glossitis, Erythema Migrans, Wandering Rash) (Figs. 26.1–26.6)** Geographic tongue is a benign inflammatory condition associated with desquamation of superficial keratin and the filiform papillae. The cause is unknown, but emotional stress, nutritional deficiencies, and heredity have been suggested. The condition is usually restricted to the dorsal and lateral borders of the anterior two thirds of the tongue, affecting only the filiform papillae and leaving the fungiform papillae intact.

Geographic tongue manifests in three patterns: 1) patchy areas of desquamated filiform papillae; 2) patchy areas of desquamated filiform papillae delineated by raised, white, circinate lines; and 3) patchy areas of desquamated filiform papillae, with or without white circinate lines, bordered by an erythematous band of inflammation. Admixtures of these patterns may be present in the same patient, and continuously changing patterns and migration from site to site are usual. Symptoms are uncommon in the first and second patterns, but presence of the red inflammatory band is often associated with reports of pain.

Geographic tongue is common, affecting approximately 1–2% of the population. Females and young to middle-aged adults are most frequently affected. The condition may appear suddenly and persist for months or years. Spontaneous remissions and recurrences have been observed. Geographic tongue is occasionally seen in association with a mucosal counterpart, areata erythema migrans (migratory mucositis, geographic stomatitis, ectopic geographic tongue), and fissured tongue. Erythema migrans produces red annular patches of the labial and buccal mucosa and soft palate. When asymptomatic it requires no treatment. However, mild burning is common and generally responds to topical anesthetics or topical steroids. This lesion histologically resembles psoriasis, but it is generally accepted that these conditions are distinct (although they may sometimes coexist).

**Anemia (Fig. 26.7)** Anemia is a condition of impaired oxygen delivery to bodily tissues that results from a deficiency in erythrocytes, hemoglobin, or total blood volume. Underlying causes of anemia include increased destruction of erythrocytes caused by hemolysis, increased blood loss caused by hemorrhage, or a decreased production of erythrocytes caused by a nutritional deficiency state or bone marrow suppression. Anemia is not a final diagnosis, but a sign of an underlying disease; thus, the cause of anemia must always be sought. Iron deficiency is the most common type of anemia, frequently affecting middle-aged women and young teenagers. Deficiencies in vitamin $B_{12}$ and folic acid also cause anemia and produce oral signs of the condition.

Anemia produces characteristic changes in the appearance of oral mucosal membranes. These manifestations, although suggestive of anemia, are not helpful in distinguishing the type of anemia causing the features seen. Analysis of erythrocyte morphology is recommended for a more accurate diagnosis.

Intraoral manifestations of anemia are most prominent on the tongue. The dorsum of the tongue initially appears pale, with flattening of the filiform papillae. Continued atrophy of the papillae results in a surface that is devoid of papillae and appears smooth, dry, and glazed. This condition is commonly called "bald tongue." In the final stage, a beefy or fiery red tongue is seen, sometimes with concurrent oral aphthae.

Anemic patients may report a sore, painful tongue (glossodynia) or burning tongue (glossopyrosis). The lips may be thinned and taut, and the width of the mouth may develop a narrowed appearance. Other clinical signs associated with anemia include angular cheilitis, aphthous ulceration, dysphagia, mucosal erythema and erosions, pallor, shortness of breath, fatigue, dizziness, and a bounding pulse. Patients with a vitamin $B_{12}$ deficiency may report weight loss, weakness, neurologic disturbances such as numbness and tingling of the extremities, and difficulty in walking. Therapy should be directed toward correcting the underlying cause. Improvement after therapy is reflected by changes in the oral appearance.

**Xerostomia (Fig. 26.8)** Saliva keeps the oral cavity moist and aids in mastication, deglutition, digestion, speech, and immunologic neutralization. When impaired salivary function causes a dry mouth, the condition is called xerostomia. Manifestations of decreased salivary flow can be subtle with no symptoms or severe with myriad symptoms. Xerostomia may result from advancing age, anemia, avitaminosis, dehydration, diabetes, emotional stress, mechanical blockage, surgery, collagen vascular disease, ectodermal dysplasia, mumps, Mikulicz's disease, multiple sclerosis, Sjögren's syndrome, acquired immunodeficiency syndrome, and head and neck irradiation. Many therapeutic drugs, primarily antidepressant agents, antihistamines, antihypertensive and cardiac agents, decongestants, ganglionic blocking agents, and tranquilizers also produce xerostomia.

Mild cases of xerostomia are relatively free of symptoms, and the mucosa appears normal. In moderate cases the tongue is dry, pale, red, and atrophic and its dorsal surface is wrinkled or smooth. In severe cases the tongue may be devoid of papillae, fissured, and inflamed. The mucosa appears dry, shiny, and sticky, and the lips appear cracked and fissured. Stagnant, rope-like accumulations of saliva on the tongue along with burning tongue (glossopyrosis) and alterations in taste are usually present. Progression of xerostomia can result in halitosis, candidiasis, multiple carious lesions evident at the cervical margin, and difficulty with speech, mastication, and retention of prosthodontic appliances. Chronic xerostomia requires long-term multiphasic support, including such items as emollients, artificial saliva, pilocarpine, fluoride treatment, oral hygiene instructions, antifungal agents, and nutritional counseling.

# Conditions Peculiar to the Tongue

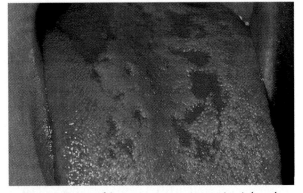

**Figure 26.1. Geographic tongue:** asymptomatic pink-red areas denuded of filiform papillae.

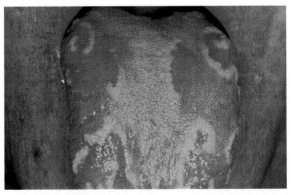

**Figure 26.2. Geographic tongue:** asymptomatic pink denudations of filiform papillae bordered by white circinate lines. (Courtesy Dr Bill Baker)

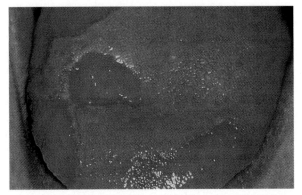

**Figure 26.3. Geographic tongue:** symptomatic denuded areas bordered by a red band of inflammation.

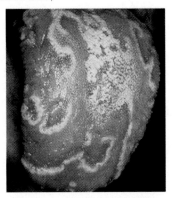

**Figure 26.4. Geographic tongue:** symptomatic denuded areas bordered by a white circinate line and red inflammatory band.

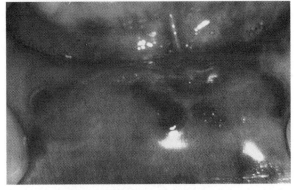

**Figure 26.5. Erythema migrans:** symptomatic involvement of the labial mucosa.

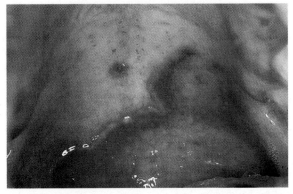

**Figure 26.6. Erythema migrans:** annular pattern on the hard and soft palate.

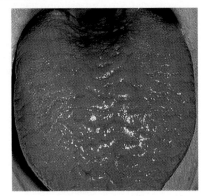

**Figure 26.7. Anemia:** smooth, bald, burning tongue caused by iron deficiency.

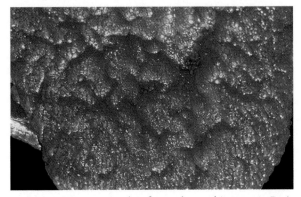

**Figure 26.8. Xerostomia:** dry, fissured atrophic tongue. Patient was receiving neuroleptic medication. (Courtesy Dr Pete Benson)

# Conditions Peculiar to the Tongue

**Median Rhomboid Glossitis (Central Papillary Atrophy of the Tongue) (Figs. 27.1–27.4)** Median rhomboid glossitis was once thought to be a developmental defect of incomplete descent of the tuberculum impar. This theory has fallen into disfavor; it is now accepted that median rhomboid glossitis is a permanent result of a *Candida albicans* infection in conjunction with other factors (possibly smoking or a change in oral pH). Median rhomboid glossitis frequently affects middle-aged men and rarely affects children. Blacks and whites are affected equally. The prevalence of this condition is often higher in patients with diabetes, immune-suppressed patients, and patients who recently completed a course of broad-spectrum antibiotics.

Median rhomboid glossitis is a smooth, denuded, beefy red patch devoid of filiform papillae. With time the lesion becomes granular, lobular, and indurated. The most common location is the midline of the dorsum of the tongue, just anterior to the circumvallate papillae. The size and shape of the lesion vary, but the lesion frequently appears as a well-demarcated 1- to 2.5-cm oval or rhomboid with irregular but rounded borders. The condition is generally asymptomatic. An erythematous palatal candidal lesion is sometimes observed directly over the lesion of the tongue. In this case, the condition is termed chronic multifocal candidiasis.

Median rhomboid glossitis is easily recognized by its clinical appearance, characteristic location, and asymptomatic nature. Early recognition and treatment with antimonilial agents usually lead to resolution. End-stage median rhomboid glossitis is usually asymptomatic but refractory to antifungal treatment. The rare possibility of anaplastic transformation exists.

**Granular Cell Tumor (Figs. 27.5 and 27.6)** The granular cell tumor is a rare benign soft-tissue tumor composed of oval cells that have an extremely granular cytoplasm. This tumor may occur in many cutaneous, mucosal, and visceral sites, but about 50% of all cases occur in the dorsal-lateral surface of the tongue. Theories of histogenesis have been controversial. Most investigators believe that the tumor is actually a benign proliferation of neurogenic cells.

The granular cell tumor can occur at any age and in any race, but it has a slight predilection for females. Usually the lesion consists of an asymptomatic, solitary, dome-shaped submucosal nodule covered clinically by normal, yellow, or white tissue. The surface may be ulcerated when it has been traumatized. The granular cell tumor is often sessile, well circumscribed, and firm to compression. Growth is very slow and painless; some tumors become several centimeters in size. Larger lesions may demonstrate a slightly depressed central area. In rare cases, these lesions are found on the ventral surface of the tongue or buccal mucosa. Approximately 10% of affected patients experience multiple lesions.

The granular cell tumor is characterized by pseudoepitheliomatous hyperplasia and granular cells that may histologically resemble epidermoid carcinoma or the congenital epulis of the newborn. Conservative local excision is the preferred treatment. These lesions do not tend to recur.

**Lingual Thyroid (Fig. 27.7)** Lingual thyroid is an uncommon nodule of thyroid tissue found just posterior to the foramen cecum on the posterior third of the tongue. It occurs when embryonic tissue from the thyroid gland fails to migrate to the anterolateral surface of the trachea. Persistent thyroid tissue occurs much more frequently in women than in men (the ratio is 4:1) and may appear at any age. If the remnant tissue becomes cystic the condition becomes a thyroglossal duct cyst.

The lingual thyroid is a raised asymptomatic mass that is usually about 2 cm in diameter. Increased surface vascularity is a prominent feature. Hemorrhage, dysphagia, dysphonia, symptoms of hypothyroidism, and (rarely) pain can be associated with the condition. Clinicians can differentiate the lesion from similar lesions by confirming its distinctive location posterior to the circumvallate papillae and by using uptake studies of radioactive iodine. Biopsy should be deferred until it is ascertained that the rest of the thyroid gland is present and functioning. In more than 50% of patients with ectopic thyroid, the lingual thyroid is the only active thyroid tissue present.

**Cyst of Blandin-Nuhn (Lingual Mucus-Retention Phenomenon) (Fig. 27.8)** The glands of Blandin-Nuhn are the accessory salivary glands on the ventral surface of the tongue and are composed of mixed serous and mucous elements. When trauma of the ventral tongue induces extravasation of saliva into the surrounding tissues, a relatively small painless swelling develops, which is termed the cyst of Blandin-Nuhn. This infrequent accessory salivary gland mucocele is located near the tip of the ventral surface of the tongue. The borders are raised and well demarcated, the mucosal surface appears pink-red, and the lesion is soft and fluctuant. When superficial, the cyst has balloon-like features and a pedunculated base. Deeper lesions have sessile bases. Although usually induced by trauma, the cyst of Blandin-Nuhn may be congenital. The congenital variant may represent a true epithelial-lined salivary duct cyst. These cysts rarely exceed 1 cm in diameter. Treatment is excisional biopsy, and recurrence is rare.

# Conditions Peculiar to the Tongue

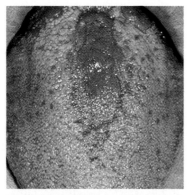

Figure 27.1. Median rhomboid glossitis: typical presentation.

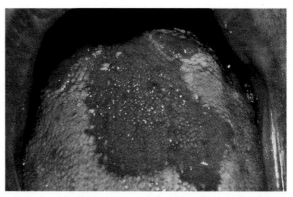

Figure 27.2. Median rhomboid glossitis: smooth denuded patch with irregular borders. (Courtesy Dr Linda Otis)

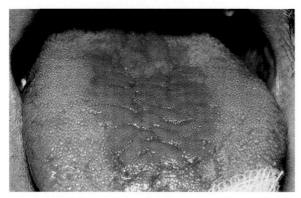

Figure 27.3. Median rhomboid glossitis in a patient with thalassemia.

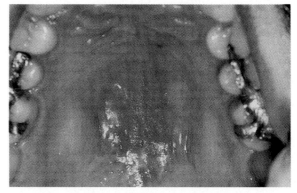

Figure 27.4. Chronic multifocal candidiasis: same patient shown in Figure 27.3 with candidal inflammation of palate in area contacting tongue.

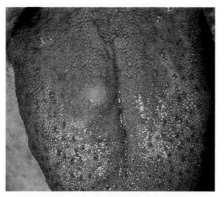

Figure 27.5. Granular cell tumor appearing as a pink tongue nodule (Courtesy Dr Jerry Cioffi)

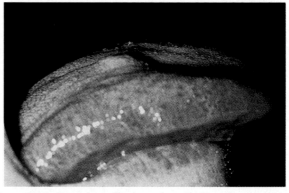

Figure 27.6. Granular cell tumor: lateral view of same patient shown in Figure 27.5. (Courtesy Dr Jerry Cioffi)

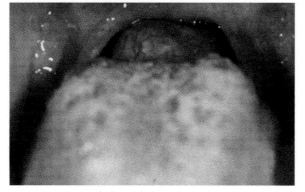

Figure 27.7. Lingual thyroid: large vascular mass in midline of base of tongue. (Courtesy Dr Tom Aufdemorte)

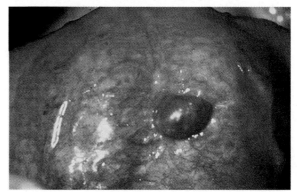

Figure 27.8. Cyst of Blandin-Nuhn: a mucocele variant in an 8-year-old boy. (Courtesy Dr James Cottone)

# Conditions Peculiar to the Lip

**Actinic Cheilosis (Actinic Cheilitis) (Figs. 28.1 and 28.2)** Actinic cheilosis is a clinical lesion of the lower lip caused by excessive solar radiation damage. Older, fair-skinned men with outdoor occupations are typically affected. In early stages, the lower lip is mildly keratotic with a subtle blending of the vermilion border with the adjacent skin. With increased exposure to the sun, focal white zones that have distinct or diffuse borders become apparent. The lip slowly becomes firm, scaly, slightly swollen, fissured, and everted. Ulceration with encrustation is typical of the chronic condition. The ulcers may be caused by loss of elasticity, or they may be an early sign of carcinomatous transformation. Histologic features include atrophic thinning of the epithelium, subepithelial basophilic degeneration of collagen, and increased elastin fibers. Biopsy is recommended to rule out similar sun-related diseases such as epithelial dysplasia, carcinoma in situ, basal cell carcinoma, squamous cell carcinoma, malignant melanoma, keratoacanthoma, cheilitis glandularis, and herpes labialis.

Actinic cheilosis is considered a precancerous condition. Clinicians should warn the patient of the likelihood of disease progression without the use of sunscreen protective agents. Dysplastic changes should be treated surgically or by topical application of 5-fluorouracil.

**Candidal Cheilitis (Figs. 28.3 and 28.4)** Candidal cheilitis is an inflammatory condition of the lips associated with *Candida albicans* and a lip-licking habit. It is believed that the candidal organisms obtain access to the surface layers of the labial epithelium after mucosal breakdown, which is caused by repeated wetting and drying of the labial tissues. Desquamation and fissuring of surface epithelium results, and a fine whitish scale consisting of dried salivary mucous may be seen. In children, the affected perilabial skin appears red, atrophic, and fissured. Chapped, dry, itchy, burning lips and the inability to eat hot spicy foods are frequent symptoms. Chronic infection is characterized by painful vertical fissures that ulcerate and are slow to heal. A hypersensitivity reaction to ingredients contained in lip balms or lipsticks may mimic the condition. In candidal cheilitis the lip-licking habit perpetuates the condition. Although nystatin ointment is helpful, ultimate resolution requires elimination of the habit. In persistent cases, an underlying systemic problem such as diabetes mellitus or HIV infection should be ruled out.

**Angular Cheilitis (Perleche) (Figs. 28.5 and 28.6)** Angular cheilitis is a painful condition consisting of radiating erythematous fissures at the corners of the mouth. The condition is most commonly seen after the age of 50 years and is usually encountered in females and denture wearers. The cause is believed to be associated with a mixed infection of *Candida albicans* and *Staphylococcus aureus*.

Angular cheilitis results from repeated pooling of saliva and carriage of pathogens from the mouth to the region. The mucocutaneous tissue at the corners of the mouth initially become soft, red, and ulcerated. With time the erythematous fissures become deep and extend several centimeters from the commissure onto the perilabial skin or ulcerate and involve the labial and buccal mucosa. The ulcers frequently develop crusts that split and reulcerate during normal oral function. Small yellow-brown granulomatous nodules may eventually appear. Bleeding is infrequent.

Angular cheilitis is chronic and usually bilateral and is often associated with denture stomatitis or glossitis. Predisposing conditions include anemia, poor oral hygiene, frequent use of broad-spectrum antibiotics, decreased vertical dimension, high sucrose intake, dry mouth, flaccid perioral folds, and vitamin B deficiency. Treatment should include preventive measures (such as elimination of traumatic factors, meticulous oral hygiene, reestablishment of the correct vertical dimension and salivary flow) combined with topical antifungal and antibiotic therapy. Vitamin supplementation may also prove beneficial.

**Exfoliative Cheilitis (Figs. 28.7 and 28.8)** Exfoliative cheilitis is a persistent condition affecting the lips that is characterized by fissuring, desquamation, and the formation of hemorrhagic crusts. *Candida albicans,* oral sepsis, stress, and habitual lip licking and biting are etiologic agents. An association with psychological and thyroid disorders has been reported. This condition usually begins as a single fissure near the midline of the lower lip and spreads to produce multiple fissures. The fissures may ultimately develop a yellow-white scale or ulcerate and form hemorrhagic crusts over the entire lip. The condition is often bothersome and unsightly; the lower lip is more adversely affected than the upper lip. When the condition is symptomatic, burning is the usual chief symptom. Exfoliative cheilitis has a predisposition for teenage girls and young women, and stress has been reported to cause acute exacerbations. Because the cause of the condition appears to be multifactorial, exfoliative cheilitis is difficult to manage and may persist for many years. Treatment is best rendered through the elimination of predisposing systemic or psychological factors together with topical application of antifungal ointments.

# Conditions Peculiar to the Lip

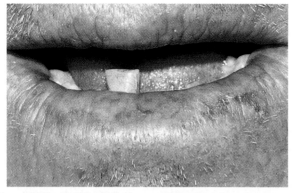

Figure 28.1. **Actinic cheilosis caused by** chronic sun exposure. Lower lip shows loss of cutaneous border and thickening and blanching of the vermilion.

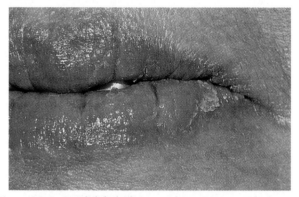

Figure 28.2. **Actinic cheilosis:** the lip is everted, focally thickened, and fissured with keratotic crusts.

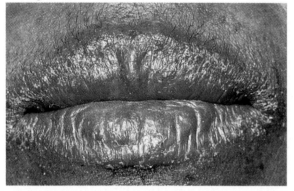

Figure 28.3. **Candidal cheilitis:** burning, red lips with whitish scale representing dried mucin. (Courtesy Dr Curt Lundeen)

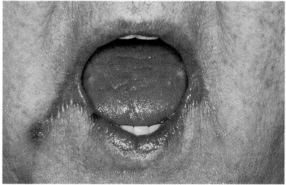

Figure 28.4. **Candidal cheilitis:** recalcitrant case with desquamation and fissuring in a patient with undiagnosed diabetes.

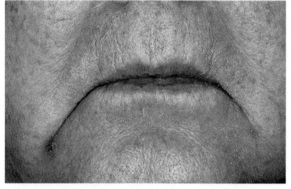

Figure 28.5. **Angular cheilitis** in an older edentulous man with flaccid perioral folds and loss of vertical dimension.

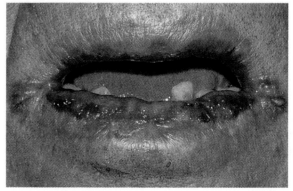

Figure 28.6. **Angular cheilitis:** same patient shown in Figure 28.5 with coexisting introral chronic atrophic candidiasis and xerostomia.

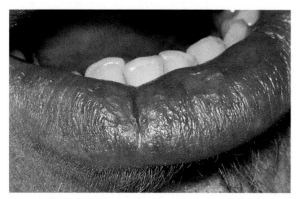

Figure 28.7. **Exfoliative cheilitis:** early lesion consisting of a single fissure.

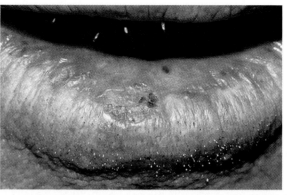

Figure 28.8. **Exfoliative cheilitis:** severe case in a psychiatric patient with yellowish-red hemorrhagic crusts and fissuring.

# Nodules of the Lip

**Mucocele (Mucus Extravasation Phenomena) (Figs. 29.1 and 29.2)** The mucocele results from retention of mucous secretions in subepithelial tissue when a salivary gland duct is severed. Most mucoceles are associated with traumatized accessory salivary gland ducts of the mandibular labial mucosa. They lack an epithelial lining and are usually surrounded by granulomatous tissue. The ranula is a variant mucocele of the floor of the mouth caused by trauma to a sublingual gland duct and rarely Wharton's duct of the submandibular gland. Mucoceles are distinguished from the rare salivary duct cyst (mucous retention cyst), which is a true cyst with an epithelial lining.

The mucocele constitutes the most common nodular swelling of the lower lip. These swellings are asymptomatic, soft, fluctuant, bluish-gray, and usually less than 1 cm in diameter. Enlargement coincident with meals may be an occasional finding. The most common location is the lower lip midway between the midline and commissure, but other locations include the buccal mucosa, palate, floor of the mouth, and ventral tongue. Children and young adults are most frequently affected. Trauma is the etiologic agent.

Superficial mucoceles often regress spontaneously, whereas deep-seated mucoceles tend to persist and exacerbate with repeated trauma. Persistent mucoceles are treated by surgical excision. Recurrence is possible if the involved accessory salivary glands are not removed or if other ducts are severed during the procedure.

**Accessory Salivary Gland Tumor (Figs. 29.3 and 29.4)** Nodular swellings of the upper lip are infrequent and are usually caused by benign neoplasia of the minor salivary glands, such as the canalicular adenoma and pleomorphic adenoma. Benign accessory salivary gland tumors constitute approximately 10% of all salivary gland tumors and are characterized by encapsulation, slow growth, and long duration (several months). Persons older than age 30 years are more commonly affected. Clinical examination shows the pleomorphic adenoma to be a pink to purple dome-shaped or multinodular lesion that protrudes from the inner aspect of the lip or vestibule. It is usually semisolid, freely movable, painless, and especially firm on palpation. The border is well circumscribed. Although it has unlimited potential for growth, the tumor generally remains less than 2 cm in diameter. Fluctuance and surface ulceration are not usual clinical features.

Malignant salivary gland tumors, such as mucoepidermoid carcinoma and adenocarcinoma, are rare in the upper lip and may be distinguished from benign neoplasia by their rapid and aggressive growth, short duration, and tendency to ulcerate and cause neurologic symptoms. Treatment of salivary gland neoplasia consists of surgical excision. If the excision is incomplete, recurrences are possible.

**Nasolabial Cyst (Nasoalveolar Cyst) (Figs. 29.5 and 29.6)** The nasolabial cyst is a developmental cyst of soft tissue located in the cuspid-lateral incisor region of the upper lip. The cause is uncertain, and two theories have been suggested. The most accepted theory is that epithelial remnants become entrapped during the embryologic fusion of the lateral nasal, globular, and maxillary processes. A more recent theory suggests that the tissue originates from the nasolacrimal duct. Proliferation and cystic degeneration of the entrapped tissue usually do not become clinically evident until after age 30 years, even though the tissue has been entrapped since birth. The condition has a slight female predilection.

The nasolabial cyst is a palpable soft tissue mass under the upper lip that may cause elevation of the ala of the nose, as well as dilatation of the nostril and alteration of the nasolabial fold. The intraoral cyst may be tense or fluctuant, depending on size. Aspiration yields a yellowish or straw-colored fluid. The cyst is most often unilateral and is generally not in contact with the adjacent bone; thus, the maxillary teeth remain vital. Infrequently, if the nasolabial cyst applies pressure to the adjacent bone, local resorption of osseous structures can result. Treatment is simple excision.

**Implantation Cyst (Epithelial Inclusion Cyst) (Fig. 29.7)** An implantation cyst is an unusual cyst arising from a foreign-body reaction to surface epithelium that is implanted within epidermal structures after traumatic laceration. The cyst can occur intraorally or extraorally, at any age, and in any race or sex. Within the mouth, the lesion appears as a firm, dome-shaped, freely movable nodule located at the site of impetus, which is often the lip. Implantation cysts are usually small, solitary, and asymptomatic. Growth appears to remain constant, and the overlying mucosa appears smooth and pink. A history of trauma should lead the clinician to suspect this lesion. Surgical excision and histopathologic examination are recommended.

**Mesenchymal Tumors (Fig. 29.8)** A variety of mesenchymal tumors, such as fibroma, lipofibroma, and neuroma, can cause nodular swellings of the lip. The example shown here is a neurofibroma. Neurofibromas may be solitary or found in conjunction with von Recklinghausen's disease. When solitary, the neurofibroma is usually an asymptomatic, sessile, smooth-surfaced nodule of the buccal mucosa, gingiva, palate, or lips. Histologic examination of the tumor shows connective tissue and nerve fibrils. The discovery of a solitary neurofibroma requires close examination for multiple neurofibromatosis because the latter condition is associated with a marked tendency toward malignant transformation.

# Nodules of the Lip

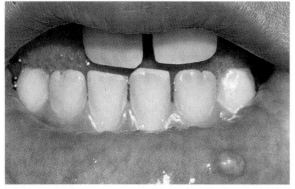

Figure 29.1. **Mucocele:** a small bluish superficial lesion of the lower lip.

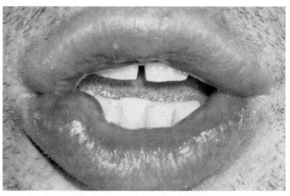

Figure 29.2. **Mucocele:** large dome-shaped surface associated with a deep-seated lesion that appeared after trauma.

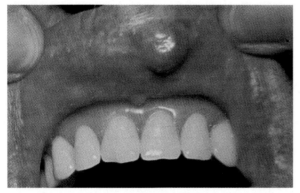

Figure 29.3. **Pleomorphic adenoma:** a firm bluish nodule.

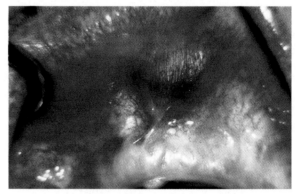

Figure 29.4. **Canalicular adenoma:** a purplish nodule in the maxillary labial mucosa.

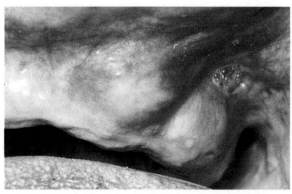

Figure 29.5. **Nasolabial cyst:** a fluctuant nodule on palpation.

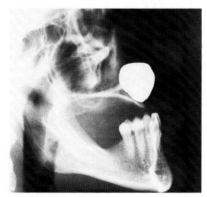

Figure 29.6. **Nasolabial cyst** injected with contrast medium. (Courtesy Dr Chris Nortjé)

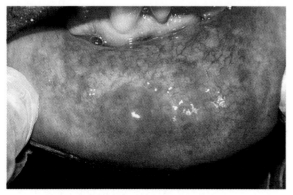

Figure 29.7. **Implantation cyst:** trauma from an automobile accident that occurred 4 years previously.

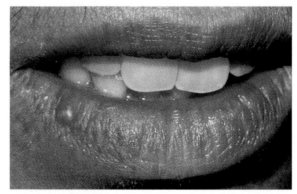

Figure 29.8. **Neurofibroma** of the lower lip with sessile base and normal coloration. (Courtesy Dr John McDowell)

# Swellings of the Lip

**Angioedema (Angioneurotic Edema) (Figs. 30.1 and 30.2)** Angioedema is a hypersensitivity reaction characterized by the accumulation of fluid within the facial tissues that results in soft, swollen areas under the skin. It occurs in hereditary and acquired forms and may be generalized or localized. Most cases of angioedema are acquired and result from IgE-mediated mast cell degranulation and release of histamine because of antigenic stimuli introduced systematically (such as through food consumption) or by contact, infection, or stress. Histamine mediates capillary permeability and the leakage of plasma into the soft tissues. Swelling develops within minutes or gradually over a few hours and is of transient duration. When swelling affects the lips it is usually uniform and diffuse but may be asymmetrical. The vermilion border appears stretched, everted, pliable, and less distinct; the surface epithelium remains normal in color or is slightly red. Swellings of the tongue, floor of the mouth, eyelids, face, and extremities may accompany the condition. Acquired angioedema is usually recurrent and self-limiting and poses little threat to the patient. Symptoms are limited to burning or itching. Management involves prescription of antihistamines, identification and withdrawal of allergenic stimuli. and stress reduction.

Angiotensin-converting enzyme drugs that are used for treating hypertension can cause angioedema in association with increased bradykinin levels. Infections and autoimmune disease can also induce angioedema by triggering capillary permeability via the formation of antigen-antibody complexes or by elevating numbers of eosinophils.

There are two types of the rare hereditary form of angioedema (type I and type II). Both are autosomal dominant. They occur in association with activation of the complement pathway. Pharyngeal and laryngeal involvement are usual and may be life threatening. Hereditary angioedema responds poorly to epinephrine, corticosteroids, and antihistamines. Management involves avoidance of violent physical activity; androgenic drugs, such as danocrine (Danazol) help to prevent attacks.

**Cheilitis Glandularis (Fig. 30.3)** Cheilitis glandularis is a chronic inflammatory disorder of the accessory labial salivary glands that most frequently affects older men. The lower lip is particularly affected and is characterized by diffuse enlargement and eversion of the lip. Although the cause remains poorly understood, the condition is associated with chronic exposure to the sun and wind and, less frequently, with smoking, poor oral hygiene, bacterial infection, and congenital predisposition.

Clinical manifestations of cheilitis glandularis include a symmetrically enlarged, everted, and firm lower lip. With time, the inflamed labial accessory salivary glands become dilated and appear as multiple small red spots. From these ductal openings a viscous, yellowish, mucopurulent exudate is secreted that makes the lip sticky. Progression of the condition causes the lip to appear atrophic, dry, fissured, and scaly and to become painful. Distinction of the vermilion border is eventually lost, and secondary infection of a deep labial fissure often results in fistulation and scarring. Emollients and sunscreens afford protection; severe cases require vermilionectomy, which produces an excellent esthetic result. These patients are at an increased risk for malignant transformation to squamous cell carcinoma.

**Orofacial Granulomatosis (Cheilitis Granulomatosa) (Figs. 30.4–30.6)** Orofacial granulomatosis is a noncaseating granulomatous condition resulting in nonpainful symmetric enlargement of orofacial tissues. The condition has two clinical variants: cheilitis granulomatosa, which usually involves only the lips, and Melkersson-Rosenthal syndrome, which has the features of unilateral facial paralysis, fissured pebbly tongue, and persistent labiofacial swelling. The cause of orofacial granulomatosis is unknown, and there is no gender predilection. The labial swelling, develops slowly at a young age. Both lips may be firm and swollen, but symmetric enlargement of the lower lip is more common. The diffuse enlargement is asymptomatic and does not affect the color of the lip, but discrete nodules can often be palpated. The tongue, buccal mucosa, gingiva, palatal mucosa, and face have also been associated with this condition. Steroids and surgery have been used with limited success. Select patients have responded to elimination of odontogenic infection and management of systemic disorders. Spontaneous regression is possible.

**Trauma (Fig. 30.7)** Trauma to the lips often results in edema that is fluctuant, irregular, and exquisitely painful. The trauma may originate from an external source or may be self-induced. External trauma may damage the soft tissue of the lip, resulting in laceration or hemorrhage. Tooth fracture may accompany the condition.

Traumatic enlargement of the lip is often a problem of children and mentally handicapped patients who inadvertently chew their lip while under local anesthesia. The best management for this type of lip injury is to limit the traumatic influence, apply ice compresses, and treat any lacerations or hemorrhage as soon as possible.

**Cellulitis (Fig. 30.8)** Cellulitis means "inflammation of cellular tissue." This degenerative process is caused by a bacterial infection in which localization of purulent material has yet to occur. When of dental origin, cellulitis typically produces grossly edematous facial tissue that is warm and painful to touch and is extremely hard to palpation. A firm, diffusely swollen lip may be the first sign of cellulitis of odontogenic origin. A nonvital tooth is usually the root of the problem. Failure of host defense mechanisms to control the infection can result in an abscess or spread of infection. Treatment involves extirpation of necrotic pulpal tissue, drainage, culture, antibiotic sensitivity testing, and antibiotic therapy. Injection of local anesthetic into the inflammatory region should be avoided to minimize spread of the infection.

# Swellings of the Lip

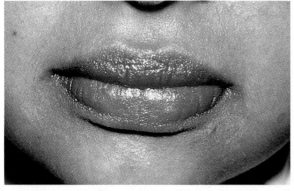

Figure 30.1. **Angioedema**: upper and lower lips are swollen and everted. (Courtesy Dr Linda Otis)

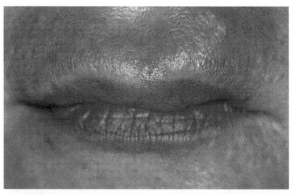

Figure 30.2. **Angioedema**: nonsymmetrical involvement of the upper lip with intense itching.

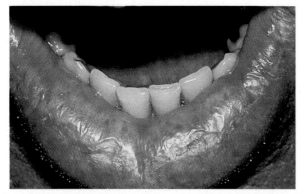

Figure 30.3. **Cheilitis glandularis**: enlarged, everted lower lip with discrete red spots.

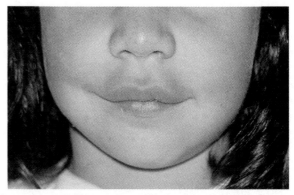

Figure 30.4. **Melkersson-Rosenthal syndrome**: cheilitis granulomatosa and facial paralysis.

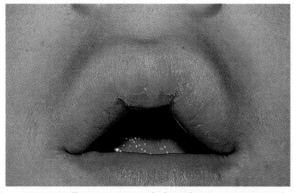

Figure 30.5. **Melkersson-Rosenthal syndrome**: symmetrical enlargement of the upper lip in same patient shown in Figure 30.4.

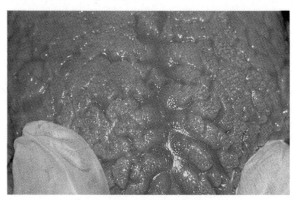

Figure 30.6. **Melkersson-Rosenthal syndrome**: fissured, pebbly tongue in same patient shown in Figure 30.4.

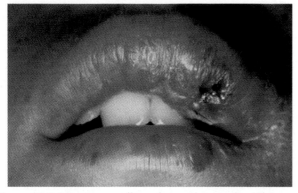

Figure 30.7. **Trauma**: swollen, ulcerated upper lip. The cause was a skateboard fall.

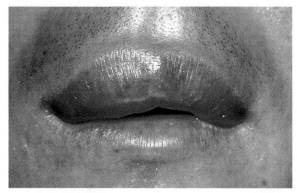

Figure 30.8. **Cellulitis** associated with an abscessed central incisor. (Courtesy Dr Geza Terezhalmy)

# Swellings of the Floor of the Mouth

**Dermoid Cyst (Figs. 31.1 and 31.2)** The dermoid cyst is a developmental cyst classified as a cystic form of teratoma. The cyst may occur anywhere on the skin but has a propensity for the floor of the mouth. Although a few appear very early in life, most occur in adults younger than age 35 years. There is no sex predilection.

When the dermoid cyst arises above the mylohyoid muscle, it appears as a painless midline, dome-shaped mass arising in the floor of the mouth. The overlying mucosa is a natural pink, the tongue is slightly elevated, and palpation yields a dough-like consistency. Patients may report difficulties in eating and speaking. The cyst grows slowly, but diameters in excess of 5 cm may be seen. Dermoid cysts may appear below the floor of mouth if the original site of development is inferior to the mylohyoid muscle. In this instance a submental swelling is noted. The lesion is histologically distinguished from an epidermoid cyst by the presence of adnexal structures in the fibrous wall such as sebaceous glands, sweat glands, and hair follicles. The lumen contains semi-solid keratin and sebum, which accounts for the doughy consistency and makes aspiration difficult. Surgical enucleation is the preferred treatment.

**Ranula (Mucocele of the Sublingual Gland) (Figs. 31.3 and 31.4)** Ranula refers to large mucoceles of the floor of the mouth. Like other mucoceles, a ranula is caused by pooling of saliva within the tissues after trauma to a salivary gland duct. A ranula is usually much larger than a mucocele. Most ranulas involve one of the major excretory ducts of the sublingual gland (ducts of Bartholin), the submandibular gland (Wharton's duct), or severed ducts of accessory salivary glands in the floor of the mouth. No sex predilection is apparent, and persons younger than age 40 years are most commonly affected.

There are two types of ranulae: the more common superficial ranula that appears as a soft compressible swelling rising up from the floor of the mouth and the dissecting or plunging ranula that penetrates below the mylohyoid muscle to produce a submental swelling. The superficial ranula is characteristically translucent or has a bluish cast; it is unilateral, dome-shaped, and fluctuant. As the asymptomatic lesion enlarges, the mucosa becomes stretched, thinned, and tense. Unlike with a dermoid cyst, digital pressure does not cause the lesion to pit, but rupture causes the escape of mucous fluid. The entire floor of the mouth may be filled by the swelling, which elevates the tongue and hinders movement. This impairs mastication, deglutition, and speech.

A ranula should be differentiated from other floor-of-the-mouth swellings such as dermoid cysts and mucoepidermoid carcinoma of the submandibular gland shown by sialography. Treatment is excision or marsupialization (Partsch operation), which consists of excising the overlying mucosa and suturing the remaining cystic lining to the floor of the mouth along the margins of the incision. Incision and drainage are not the treatment of choice because they lead to reaccumulation of fluid as healing occurs. Recurrences are common in cases involving a plunging ranula or superficial ranula that is ill-managed. Removal of the affected major salivary gland is the indicated treatment for recurrent and plunging ranulas.

**Salivary Calculi (Figs. 31.5 and 31.6)** Sialoliths (salivary calculi or stones) are accretions of calcium complexes within a salivary gland or duct that may obstruct salivary flow and cause floor-of-the-mouth swelling. They are usually round or oval and smooth or rough surfaced. Concentric laminations of different densities are often seen. Stones occur most frequently after age 25 years, twice as often in males as in females, and usually in the submandibular gland. The ascending course of the excretory duct, along with high mucous content and alkaline pH of the saliva, are significant factors in stone formation.

Obstruction of salivary flow by a calculus in Wharton's duct results in a floor-of-the-mouth swelling that is firm, tender, and painful. Acute symptoms often recur at meal time. Swelling may extend along the course of the excretory duct and last for hours or days, depending on the blockage. The overlying mucosa usually remains pink. Secondary infection results in pus emanating from the ductal opening or in redness of the swollen floor of the mouth. Another sequela of calculus formation is the development of salivary duct cyst (mucus-retention cyst) that represents ductal dilatation caused by increased intraductal pressure. Management of calculi involves appropriate occlusal radiography, sialography (if no infection is present), and surgical removal of the sialolith. Localized cellulitis and fever require the use of antibiotics before invasive procedures.

**Mucocele (Mucus-Retention Phenomenon) (Figs. 31.7 and 31.8)** The mucocele is a soft fluctuant lesion involving the retention of mucus in subepithelial tissue, usually as a result of trauma to a salivary gland duct. These clear or bluish swellings may occur on the lip, floor of the mouth, ventral tongue, palate, or buccal mucosa. They are usually asymptomatic and less than 1 cm in diameter. The base of the mucus-retention phenomenon is commonly sessile, although pedunculated bases are possible. Children and young adults are most frequently affected. Superficial lesions may heal spontaneously, whereas persistent lesions should be excised and examined microscopically. If the condition is managed properly, recurrences are rare.

# Swellings of the Floor of the Mouth

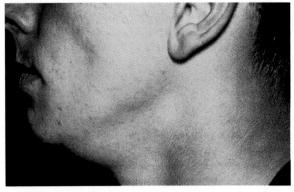

**Figure 31.1. Dermoid cyst** located below the mylohyoid muscle producing a firm double chin.

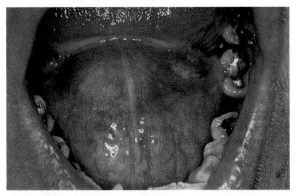

**Figure 31.2. Dermoid cyst** located above the mylohyoid muscle as a soft tissue swelling in the floor of the mouth.

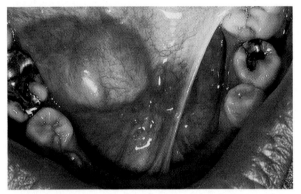

**Figure 31.3. Ranula:** typical size, color, and translucent appearance in the floor of the mouth.

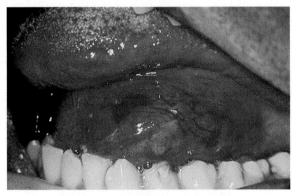

**Figure 31.4. Ranula:** rare large lesion; tongue elevation impairs eating and speaking. (Courtesy Dr Charles Morris)

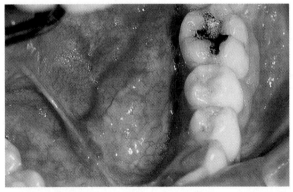

**Figure 31.5. Sialolith** producing floor-of-the-mouth swelling and salivary duct cyst.

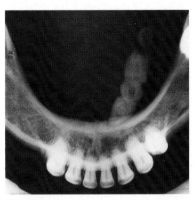

**Figure 31.6. Sialoliths:** concentric laminations of several calculi that obstruct salivary flow in Wharton's duct.

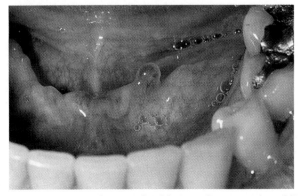

**Figure 31.7. Mucocele:** superficial lesion adjacent to the sublingual caruncle.

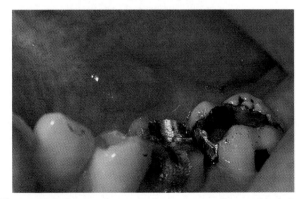

**Figure 31.8. Mucocele:** severed accessory salivary gland duct during crown preparation that was done 1 week previously.

# Swellings of the Palate

**Palatal Torus (Torus Palatinus) (Figs. 32.1 and 32.2)** A palatal torus is a form of bony exostosis that is located in the midline of the hard palate adjacent to either the bicuspid or molar teeth and affects approximately 20% of the adult population. The condition is frequently inherited, and several family members can be affected. The incidence of palatal tori is higher in women than men. After puberty there is a tendency for slow growth in all dimensions.

Tori vary greatly in size and shape. The flat torus sits on a broad base, and the surface is smooth and only slightly convex. The spindle torus is an enlarged, narrow bony ridge along the midline of the hard palate. The lobular torus sits on a single base and is divided into lobules by one or several grooves. The nodular torus represents two or more adjacent tori, each on its own separate base. The covering mucosa is pale pink, thin, and delicate; the boundary of the lesion can blend with the palatal vault or end abruptly.

The palatal torus is frequently asymptomatic unless traumatized, and some patients insist they were unaware of the torus until the traumatic episode. The resultant ulcer should always be observed until resolution. If healing does not occur, chronic irritants should be identified and eliminated. Palatal tori should be removed if they interfere with mastication, phonetics, playing a musical instrument, or the construction of prosthetic appliances.

**Nasopalatine Duct Cyst (Incisive Canal Cyst) (Figs. 32.3 and 32.4)** The nasopalatine duct cyst is a developmental cyst that arises from entrapped squamous or respiratory epithelial remnants of the nasopalatine duct within the incisive canal . It is the most common nonodontogenic cyst in the oral cavity. It may occur at any age and anywhere along the course of the incisive canal; generally, however, the cyst is confined to the palatal bone between the maxillary central incisors at the height of the incisive canal.

The nasopalatine duct cyst is usually asymptomatic and is discovered as an incidental finding during routine examination. Symptomatic cysts are usually bacterially infected. Infrequently, the cyst arises entirely in the soft tissue of the incisive papilla, where it appears as a small, superficial, fluctuant swelling. A well-developed incisive canal cyst may swell the entire anterior third of the hard palate.

The radiographic features of the nasopalatine duct cyst are characteristic: The cyst appears as a well-delineated, midline, symmetrically oval or heart-shaped radiolucency located between the roots of vital maxillary central incisors. The sclerotic margin is contiguous with the incisive canal and may vary greatly in size. Root divergence and root resorption of the central incisors are occasional findings associated with large lesions. A similar cyst that is located more posteriorly in the palate has been called the median palatal cyst. Current beliefs are that the incisive canal cyst and the median palatal cyst represent the same entity found in slightly different locations. Both conditions are treated by surgical enucleation.

**Periapical Abscess (Figs. 32.5 and 32.6)** A periapical abscess is a fluctuant soft-tissue swelling consisting of purulent material that results from bacterial infection of the pulp. It appears adjacent to a diseased tooth, which is often tender to percussion, mobile, and slightly "high" in occlusion. Regional lymphadenopathy, fever, malaise, and trismus are common accompanying features. Careful examination of the teeth and their supporting tissues along with diagnostic testing reveals the offending nonvital tooth. Radiography often shows an oval periapical radiolucency.

Any abscessed maxillary tooth may produce a swelling of the palate. Generally, the swelling is red-purple, soft, tender, and lateral to the midline if a maxillary posterior tooth is involved. In contrast, an abscessed maxillary incisor may cause a midline swelling in the anterior third of the palate. Aspiration or incision produces a creamy yellow or yellow-green purulent discharge. Immediate drainage, endodontic therapy, or extraction is indicated to prevent spread of the infection. Antibiotics, analgesics, and antipyretic agents may also be needed.

**Periodontal Abscess** The differential diagnosis for a unilateral palatal swelling should include periodontal abscess. This entity is discussed under Periodontitis (see Figs. 20.7 and 20.8).

**Lymphoid Hyperplasia (Benign Lymphoid Hyperplasia) (Figs. 32.7 and 32.8)** Lymphoid hyperplasia is a rare, benign, reactive process that involves proliferation of the lymphoid tissue of the oropharynx (enlarged tonsils), tongue, floor of the mouth, and soft palate in response to some antigenic stimuli that usually was inhaled or ingested. Authorities dispute whether the proliferation is a reaction to regional or generalized stimuli, and the exact factor is seldom identified. Persons older than age 30 years are most often affected.

Clinical examination shows that the exuberant lesion arises at the posterior extent of the hard palate and grows slowly, either unilaterally or bilaterally. The enlargement may reach 3 cm in diameter, but patients rarely report pain. The surface of the mature lesion is pink to purple, nonulcerated, and dome-shaped or lumpy. The mass is usually soft but on occasion may be firm to palpation. Biopsy is recommended if the lesion interferes with oral function or if it persists for more that 2 weeks. Generally no treatment is required if the condition is asymptomatic. Lymphoid hyperplasia may clinically resemble palatal lymphoma, benign lymphoepithelial lesion, and Sjögren's syndrome, whereas histologic features often mimic those of nodular lymphoma. Fortunately, benign lymphoid hyperplasia usually regresses spontaneously.

70

# Swellings of the Palate

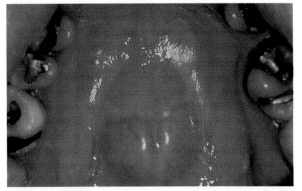

**Figure 32.1. Torus palatinus:** a flat torus with a mild central groove and slight lobulation.

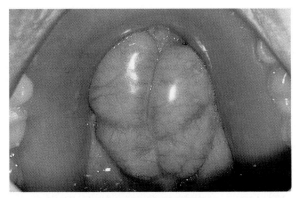

**Figure 32.2. Torus palatinus:** a lobulated torus with a denture worn around it.

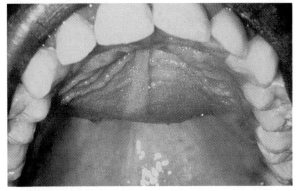

**Figure 32.3. Nasopalatine duct cyst** involving the anterior third of the palate. (Courtesy Dr Geza Terezhalmy)

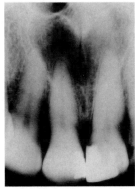

**Figure 32.4. Nasopalatine duct cyst:** classic midline, heart-shaped lesion with sclerotic margins. Central incisors tested vital. (Courtesy Dr Olaf Langland)

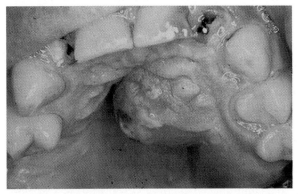

**Figure 32.5. Periapical abscess** arising from the nonvital maxillary lateral incisor.

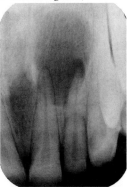

**Figure 32.6. Periapical abscess** producing a large radiolucent lesion and palatal swelling.

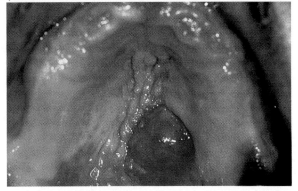

**Figure 32.7. Lymphoid hyperplasia** arising at the junction of hard and soft palate and irritated by denture shown in Figure 32.8. (Courtesy Dr Dale Miles)

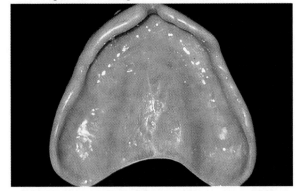

**Figure 32.8. Lymphoid hyperplasia** and inappropriate management with a denture that accommodates the nodule shown in Figure 32.7. (Courtesy Dr Dale Miles)

# Swellings of the Palate

**Necrotizing Sialometaplasia (Figs. 33.1 and 33.2)** Necrotizing sialometaplasia is a benign reactive lesion, chiefly of accessory palatal salivary glands, that has histologic features suggestive of malignancy. The inflammatory lesion begins after trauma as a rapidly growing nodular swelling on the lateral aspect of the hard palate, particularly in men older than age 40. Tissue infarction as a result of vasoconstriction and ischemia has been implicated in the pathogenesis. Rarely the soft palate or buccal mucosa is involved; bilateral cases have been reported.

Necrotizing sialometaplasia first appears as a small painless nodule that eventually enlarges and causes pain. Within a few weeks it ulcerates and the pain diminishes. The size of the soft tissue swelling varies, and growth to a diameter of 2 cm is possible. A deep central ulcer with a grayish pseudomembrane is characteristic. The ulcer is irregular and pebbly, the border is often rolled. Healing occurs spontaneously over 4 to 8 weeks or after a biopsy. The latter is recommended to rule out similar-appearing lesions such as salivary gland tumors and malignant lymphoma. Histologically it demonstrates squamous metaplasia of ductal epithelium, which may be misdiagnosed as mucoepidermoid carcinoma or adenocarcinoma.

**Benign Accessory Salivary Gland Neoplasm (Figs. 33.3 and 33.4)** The pleomorphic adenoma, or benign mixed tumor, is the most common benign neoplasm of accessory salivary glands. It occurs in major or minor salivary glands; the palate is the most common location when accessory salivary glands are affected. Occurrences are most frequent in women between the ages of 30 and 60 years. These neoplasms tend to occur lateral to the midline and distal to the anterior third of the hard palate.

The classic clinical presentation of the pleomorphic adenoma is a firm, painless, nonulcerated, irregularly dome-shaped swelling. Palpation may reveal isolated softer areas and a smooth or lobulated surface. Slow persistent enlargement over a period of years is typical, and lesions may achieve sizes greater than 1.5 cm in diameter. Histologically it shows epithelial cells in a nest-like arrangement, with pools of myxoid, chondroid, and mucoid material. A distinct fibrous connective tissue capsule containing tumor cells surrounds and usually limits the extension of the tumor. Thorough excisional biopsy is the recommended treatment because the condition frequently recurs after simple enucleation or incomplete excision. Tumorous involvement of the capsule may play a role in recurrence.

The basal cell (monomorphic) adenoma is a benign salivary gland tumor that can develop in the palate. It consists of a regular glandular pattern, usually one cell type, and lacks a mesenchymal component as seen in pleomorphic adenoma. Treatment is surgical excision.

**Malignant Accessory Salivary Gland Neoplasm (Figs. 33.5 and 33.6)** Adenoid cystic carcinoma (cylindroma) and mucoepidermoid carcinoma are the two most common intraoral malignant accessory salivary gland neoplasms. Persons between the ages of 20 and 50 years are most frequently affected by mucoepidermoid carcinoma; the adenoid cystic carcinoma usually occurs after age 50 years. The adenoid cystic carcinoma also occurs in respiratory, gastrointestinal, and reproductive tissues, whereas mucoepidermoid carcinoma may occur in the skin; respiratory tract; or centrally within bone, particularly the mandible.

Malignant accessory salivary gland neoplasms occur frequently in the posterior palate. These neoplasms are usually asymptomatic, firm, dome-shaped swellings that occur lateral to the midline. The overlying tissue appears normal in the early stages, but the mucosa later becomes erythematous, with several small telangiectactic surface vessels. These neoplasms grow more quickly and are more painful than benign salivary gland tumors. Induration and eventual spontaneous ulceration are common. A bluish appearance or a mucus exudate emanating from the ulcerated tumor surface are distinctive features of mucoepidermoid carcinoma.

Treatment is usually radical excision. The prognosis varies depending on the degree of histologic differentiation, the extent of the lesion, and the presence of metastasis. Adenoid cystic carcinoma rarely metastasizes but is an infiltrating malignant condition with a propensity for distant spread by perineural invasion; thus, lifetime follow-up is necessary. In contrast, the mucoepidermoid tumor infrequently metastasizes and is more easily cured by surgical means. Other, less common, malignant accessory salivary gland neoplasms include the adenocarcinoma, carcinoma ex pleomorphic adenoma, carcinosarcoma, and metastasizing mixed tumor.

**Primary Lymphoma of the Palate (Figs. 33.7 and 33.8)** Malignant lymphomas are solid neoplastic growths of lymphocytes or histiocytes that are classified into Hodgkin's or non-Hodgkin's lymphoma and subdivided between nodal and extranodal disease. Primary non-Hodgkin's lymphoma may develop at any site at which lymphoid tissue is present, including the cervical lymph nodes, mandible, and palate. Primary palatal lesions are sometimes called lymphoproliferative disease of the palate. Rarely, lymphoma may affect the gingiva.

Primary lymphomas of the palate occur most commonly in patients older than age 60 years but may be seen in younger patients, especially those with the acquired immunodeficiency syndrome. Primary lymphomas may be solitary or associated with widespread disease, although they usually precede disseminated disease. Clinical examination shows that the lesion arises slowly at the junction of the hard and soft palates. The palatal swelling is asymptomatic, soft, spongy, and nonulcerated and rarely affects the underlying palatal bone. The surface is often lumpy and pink to blue-purple. Early recognition and biopsy is important because the disease may be confined entirely to the palate in the early stages. Irradiation is used to treat palatal lymphomas, whereas chemotherapy is used for disseminated disease.

# Swellings of the Palate

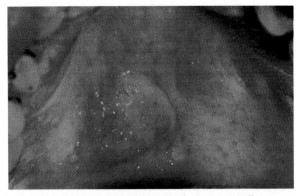

Figure 33.1. Necrotizing sialometaplasia: a rapidly growing and painful swelling of the lateral hard palate. (Courtesy Dr Dale Buller)

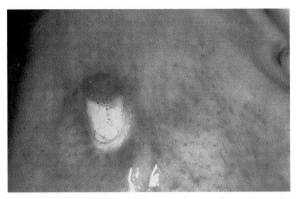

Figure 33.2. Necrotizing sialometaplasia: ulceration occurs within a few weeks. (Courtesy Dr J. L. Jensen)

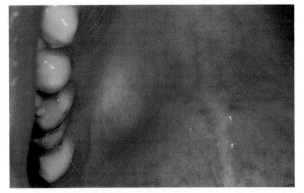

Figure 33.3. Pleomorphic adenoma: slow growing, strikingly firm nodule. (Courtesy Dr James Cottone)

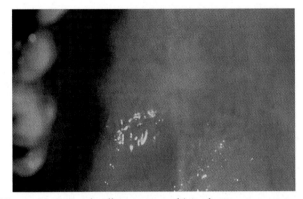

Figure 33.4. Basal cell (monomorphic) adenoma: asymptomatic tumor in a 25-year-old woman. (Courtesy Dr S. Brent Dove)

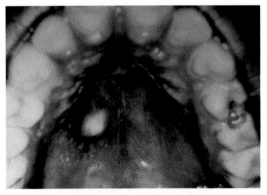

Figure 33.5. Mucoepidermoid carcinoma: a whitish mucous exudes from the tumor. (Courtesy Dr Jack Sherman)

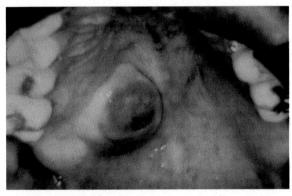

Figure 33.6. Adenoid cystic carcinoma: rapidly growing neoplasm with surface ulceration.

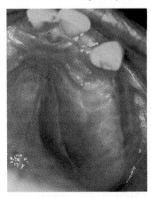

Figure 33.7. Primary lymphoma of the palate: unilateral mass interfering with a partial denture. (Courtesy Dr D. B. Smith)

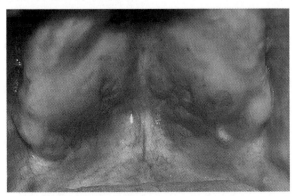

Figure 33.8. Primary lymphoma of the palate: bilateral purplish swelling with superficial telangectasia.

# Swellings of the Face

**Odontogenic Infection (Figs. 34.1–34.8)** Orofacial infections arise when microbes, most commonly bacteria, have sufficient substrate to replicate and overwhelm the local immune response. The infection may be promoted by poor health and systemic disease, poor oral hygiene, or traumatic surgery. Oral infections are called "odontogenic" when they are tooth-related. Most odontogenic infections arise as a consequence of pulpal necrosis, sulcular and apical periodontitis, and pericoronitis. Almost all odontogenic infections are polymicrobial, consisting of anaerobes (65%) and aerobes (35%). Obligate Gram-negative anaerobes (such as *Bacteroides*, *Fusobacterium* species), anaerobic Gram-positive organisms (such as *Peptostreptococcus* species), and facultative anaerobic Gram-positive streptococci (such as *Streptococcus milleri*) are the organisms most frequently identified in odontogenic infections. Other contributors are *Lactobacillus*, *Diphtheroids*, *Actinomyces*, and *Eikenella* species. Infections classically produce four features: calor (heat), dolor (pain), rubor (redness), and tumor (swelling).

An odontogenic infection generally begins as a slowly enlarging swelling that may be accompanied by dull pain and a bad taste. It may remain localized for a long time or progress to an abscess, parulis, cellulitis, or space infection. An **abscess** is an acute swelling that contains pus and necrotic debris. It appears as a well-localized swelling that is soft and occasionally pointed. It is visible in or outside the mouth and drains spontaneously or when incised. The **parulis** is similar to the abscess, but the bacterial infection drains through a sinus tract onto the mucosal surface as a yellow-red papule. In most cases the parulis represents chronic infection and is asymptomatic. **Cellulitis** is an early feature of a spreading odontogenic infection; it represents a diffuse inflammatory response that has not yet localized. Cellulitis produces a diffuse, red, warm, hard swelling (generally over the cheek or mandible) that is firm and tender to palpation. It may mature into an abscess and drain or may become aggressive and spread. The spread of an odontogenic infection beyond normal anatomic boundaries through fascial (spaces) planes is called a **space infection**.

**Buccal Space Infection (Figs. 34.1 and 34.2)** Buccal space infection is most often caused by an odontogenic infection that has spread externally to the cortical plate, laterally to the buccinator muscle, and anteriorly to the masseter muscle. It frequently arises from lateral migration of organisms that infect the periapex of a maxillary or mandibular molar. Entry into the space is usually gained at the posterior insertion of the buccinator muscle. Radiographs of the posterior quadrant usually reveal chronic periapical inflammation of a mandibular molar. Pain, swelling, and fever are the most prominent features.

**Masseteric (Submasseteric) Space Infection (Figs. 34.3 and 34.4)** A masseteric space infection is generally the result of an odontogenic infection that has spread posteriorly from an infected mandibular molar or buccal space to a region between the masseter muscle and the lateral aspect of the ramus. The swelling is firm and nonfluctuant and overlies the angle of the mandible. Masseteric muscle involvement produces marked trismus (difficulty in opening). Computed tomography and magnetic resonance imaging are useful in defining this condition.

**Infraorbital Space Infection (Figs. 34.5 and 34.6)** Infraorbital space infection is a microbial infection that has spread superiorly from an infected maxillary tooth (usually a tooth anterior to the first molar) to a region lateral to the nasal ala and below the eye. Grave concern is raised when the infection encroaches on the eyelid or affects vision, because the ophthalmic (angular) veins lack valves and spread of infection to the brain is possible. **Cavernous sinus thrombosis** is a severe infection resulting from spread of infection via the angular veins to the brain.

Treatment of odontogenic infection involves four steps: 1) removal of the source of the infection, 2) establishment of drainage, 3) provision of antibiotics when needed, and 4) provision of supportive care. The infection is often controlled by instituting root canal therapy or extraction of the offending tooth when the source of infection is localized (for example, parulis, apical periodontitis). These treatments provide a pathway for pus and exudate drainage and reduce or remove the microbial load. Alternatively, incision and drainage can be performed to drain an abscess. If the condition is diffuse, as in cellulitis or pericoronitis, incision and drainage are generally unsuccessful and not recommended. Root canal therapy or extraction are used to treat cellulitis caused by a nonvital tooth, whereas pericoronitis is generally first managed with irrigation and antibiotics. When the pain of pericoronitis remits, extraction is performed. Guidelines for prescribing antibiotics for odontogenic infection include presence of spreading infection (regional lymphadenopathy, fever, swelling beyond anatomic boundaries) in combination with inability to establish drainage. Penicillin VK is the drug of choice, generally prescribed as 500 mg orally four times daily for 7 days.

**Ludwig's Angina (Figs. 34.7 and 34.8)** Ludwig's angina is a severe and spreading infection that involves the submandibular spaces, submental spaces, and sublingual spaces bilaterally. These spaces are located between the tongue, hyoid bone, and lingual cortical plates of the mandible. It generally arises from an infected mandibular molar or a fractured (and infected) mandible. Spreading infection forces the tongue superiorly and posteriorly and forces submandibular tissues apically. This impinges on the airway and can result in airway obstruction. Aggressive use of antibiotics, culture, sensitivity, multiple incision, and drainage may be required to control the infection. In some patients, emergency procedures, such as a tracheostomy, may be needed to sustain life.

# Swellings of the Face

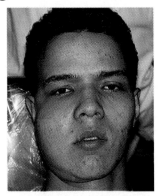

**Figure 34.1. Buccal space infection:** a rapidly spreading and painful infection of the buccal space from an infected first mandibular molar.

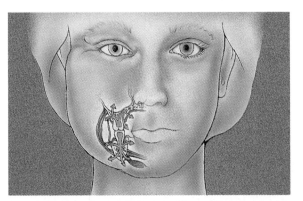

**Figure 34.2. Buccal space infection:** illustration of spread into the buccal space from an infected mandibular molar.

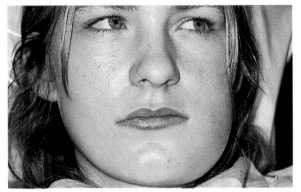

**Figure 34.3. Masseteric space infection:** slowly spreading infection below the masseter muscle adjacent to the ramus.

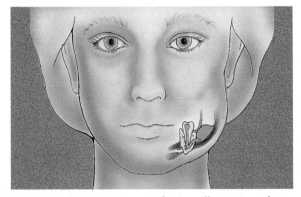

**Figure 34.4. Masseteric space infection:** illustration of spread into the space between the masseter muscle and mandibular ramus.

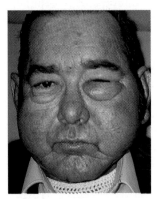

**Figure 34.5. Infraorbital space infection:** severe infection from the maxillary first premolar that has impinged on the patient's eye.

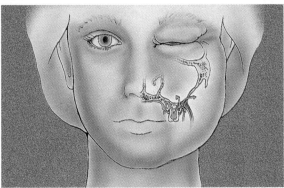

**Figure 34.6. Infraorbital space infection:** illustration of spread of infection into the soft tissue space over the maxillary sinus toward the eye.

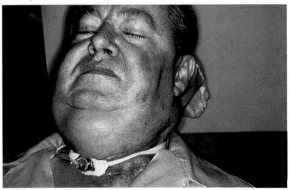

**Figure 34.7. Ludwig's angina:** massive swelling of the submandibular, submental, and sublingual spaces requiring tracheostomy. (Courtesy Dr Geza Terezhalmy)

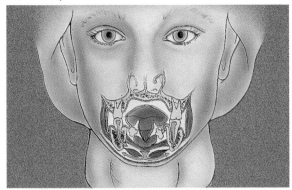

**Figure 34.8. Ludwig's angina:** illustration of spread of infection from an infected molar.

# Swellings of the Face

**Sialadenosis (Figs. 35.1)** Sialodenosis is the asymptomatic, noninflammatory enlargement of major salivary glands. The condition indicates an underlying systemic disorder, such as alcoholism, anorexia nervosa, bulimia, diabetes mellitus, drug reaction, malnutrition, or HIV infection. Most cases arise as slowly growing, painless swellings of the parotid gland. The condition usually develops bilaterally but sometimes occurs unilaterally. Salivary flow may be reduced, and autonomic innervation to the gland may be disrupted. Microscopy shows hypertrophied acinar cells and infiltration of fat. Treatment is directed toward controlling the systemic disease, with the goal of minimizing gland growth.

**Warthin's Tumor (Papillary Cystadenoma Lymphomatosum) (Fig. 35.2)** Warthin's tumor is a benign salivary gland tumor that usually occurs after age 60 and almost exclusively occurs in the parotid gland. The cause of the tumor is unknown, but smokers have more than 5 times the risk as nonsmokers. There is a slight predilection for men. Warthin's tumors arise mostly in the tail of the parotid gland as a slowly growing, firm, nodular mass. About 10% of tumors occur in parotid glands bilaterally; the submandibular gland and minor salivary glands are rarely affected. Microscopy shows that the tumor is composed of bilayered, oncocytic ductal epithelium and a lymphoid stroma, which form many papillae and invaginate into a cystic space. Biopsy and surgical excision are recommended. Recurrence and malignant transformation are rare.

**Sjögren's Syndrome (Inflammatory Exocrinopathy) (Fig. 35.3)** Sjögren's syndrome is a chronic disease characterized by progressive lymphocytic infiltration and eventual dysfunction of the exocrine glands. Current theory suggests that it is an autoimmune disease associated with certain histocompatibility antigens or Epstein-Barr virus infection. The disease affects 1 in 2000 persons, occurs in women in 80% of cases, and generally manifests between the ages of 35 and 50 years. In its primary form, **sicca syndrome**, the condition is limited to the salivary and lacrimal glands; producing dry eyes (xerophthalmia) and dry mouth (xerostomia). Oral and ocular disease accompanied by systemic disease (ie, rheumatoid arthritis, systemic lupus erythematosus, and infiltrative disease of gastrointestinal exocrine glands), is known as **secondary Sjögren's syndrome**. The syndrome usually develops slowly and involves progressive enlargement of the major salivary glands, particularly the parotid glands bilaterally. The glands are generally firm and nonpainful. Involvement of the pancreas or gall bladder can result in abdominal symptoms and difficulty digesting food. The diagnosis is supported when biopsy specimens of minor salivary glands show multiple inflammatory aggregates adjacent to salivary acini. The presence of antinuclear antibodies (anti-SS-A and anti-SS-B) and rheumatoid factor help to confirm the diagnosis of secondary Sjögren's syndrome. Management of dryness is attempted with use of artificial tears and saliva. Pilocarpine, fluoride, and chlorhexidine are also important in minimizing the consequences of xerostomia. Periodic evaluation is important because of the patients' increased risk for the development of lymphoma.

**Cushing's Disease and Syndrome (Fig. 35.4)** Cushing's disease is the persistent elevation of cortisol blood levels caused by hypersecretion of cortisol by the adrenal gland. It is usually induced by a pituitary adenoma. The cortisol elevation results in fluid retention, hypertension, and hyperglycemia. Clinical features include truncal obesity, a round (moon-shaped) face with plethora (red), facial and truncal acne, a buffalo hump at the back of the neck, and purple abdominal striae. These features are caused by collagen wasting, dermal weakening, capillary fragility and fluid accumulation. Treatment is directed toward eradicating tumors and correcting daily cortisol levels.

**Masseter Hypertrophy (Fig. 35.5)** Masseter hypertrophy occurs as a result of chronic muscle activity induced by tooth clenching, gum chewing, or bruxism. The muscles are firm and nontender. Enlargement is most prominent over the angle of the mandible.

**Neurofibromatosis (von Recklinghausen's Disease) (Fig. 35.6)** Neurofibromatosis is primarily an autosomal dominant disease associated with multiple tumors (neurofibromas) of the skin, mouth, bone, and gastrointestinal tract and with pigmentations of the skin (café au lait), iris (Lisch nodules), and axilla (axillary freckling or Crowe's sign). The tumors appear after puberty as papules, nodules, or pendulous growths. Those affecting the mandible may expand the mandibular canal and cortical plates, thereby producing facial swelling, or may rarely undergo malignant transformation.

**Cystic Hygroma (Cystic Lymphangioma) (Fig. 35.7)** Cystic hygroma is a hamartoma of lymphoid vessels (lymphangioma) that fail to communicate with the normal lymphatic system. As a result, lymph collects within the numerous dilated vessels. Cystic hygromas most often appear in the neck and axilla as a soft, compressible swelling. Airway obstruction may be a concern. Surgical excision is generally successful, but recurrence is common.

**Ewing's Sarcoma (Fig. 35.8)** Ewing's sarcoma is a malignant tumor derived from hematopoietic stem cells or primitive mesenchymal cells that usually arises in bone. Persons under age 30 are most often affected. Most sarcomas arise in the femur and pelvic bones; fewer than 5% arise in the jaws. They are sometimes found in soft tissue without bony involvement. In the jaws, the mandible is most often involved. Patients present with swelling and pain, paresthesia, loose teeth, fever, leukocytosis, and an elevated sedimentation rate. The mass is often soft when the tumor has penetrated the bony cortical plate. Radiographs show displaced teeth and a osteolytic radiolucent mass with ill-defined tumor margins. Metastasis to lung, liver, and lymph nodes occurs frequently. Survival rates of 50–75% have been achieved with the combined use of radiation, surgery, and chemotherapy.

# Swellings of the Face

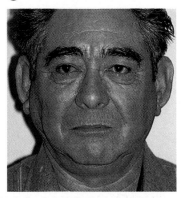

Figure 35.1. **Sialadenosis:** bilateral, asymptomatic enlargement of the parotid glands in a man with type II diabetes mellitus.

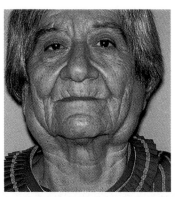

Figure 35.2. **Warthin's tumor:** bilateral tumorous enlargement within the tail of the parotid glands. Tumors slowly evolved over many years.

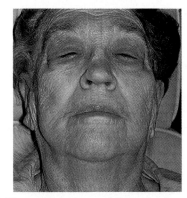

Figure 35.3. **Sjögren's syndrome:** bilateral enlargement of parotid glands and redness of the eyelids caused by frequent rubbing of dry eyes.

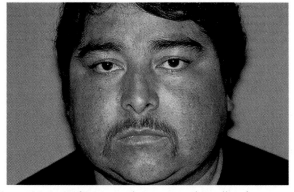

Figure 35.4. **Cushing's syndrome:** round swollen face caused by prolonged use of a corticosteroid drug. Acne is another feature of this syndrome.

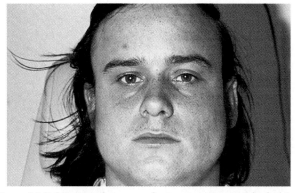

Figure 35.5. **Masseter hypertrophy** in a young man who habitually clenched his teeth.

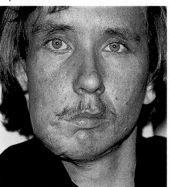

Figure 35.6. **Neurofibromatosis:** asymmetrical enlargement of the right mandible caused by a neurogenic tumor.

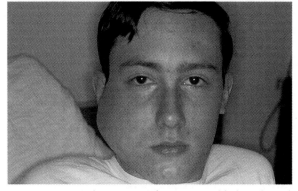

Figure 35.7. **Cystic hygroma:** soft, compressible lymphatic hamartoma that has been present since birth.

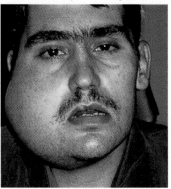

Figure 35.8. **Ewing's sarcoma:** an aggressive and rapidly growing malignant tumor that has extended through the mandibular cortical plate.

# Conditions Peculiar to the Face

**Angioedema (Fig. 36.1)** Angioedema is a hypersensitivity reaction characterized by the accumulation of fluid within the facial tissues. The resulting tissues are soft, swollen, and itchy. Angioedema can be triggered by mechanical trauma, stress, infection, or an allergen. Most cases are acquired and result from IgE-mediated mast-cell degranulation and release of histamine after exposure to antigenic stimuli (such as food) or physical contact. Histamine mediates capillary permeability and the leakage of plasma into the soft tissues. Less commonly, infections and autoimmune disease trigger capillary permeability via the formation of antigen-antibody complexes or elevation in the number of circulating eosinophils.

Angioedema produces facial swelling that develops within minutes or over a few hours. The swellings are usually uniform, diffuse, and symmetric. The lips are commonly affected, producing overly full, stretched, pliable swellings. Generally the skin tone remains normal in color or is slightly red. The tongue, floor of the mouth, eyelids, face, and extremities may also be affected. Acquired angioedema is usually recurrent and self-limiting and poses little threat to the patient. Symptoms are limited to burning or itching. Management involves prescription of antihistamines, identification and withdrawal of allergenic stimuli, and stress reduction.

In the rare hereditary form, angioedema is transmitted by an autosomal dominant pattern. It involves the activation of the complement pathway caused by an enzyme deficiency (type I) or a dysfunctional enzyme (type II). Treatment involves avoidance of violent physical activity and trauma and prophylaxis with androgenic drugs, such as danocrine (Danazol). Angiotension-converting enzyme drugs have also been implicated as causing angioedema resulting from increased bradykinin levels. Histamine is not released, and management involves substitution of other types of antihypertensive agents.

**Emphysema (Fig. 36.2)** Emphysema is defined as the abnormal presence of air in tissue. In dentistry, emphysema is most commonly caused by a dentist during a surgical procedure. The condition results when compressed air from a high-speed handpiece is forced under a mucoperiosteal flap, through an open pulp chamber, or intralveolarly. The air becomes entrapped in subcutaneous tissue or a fascial plane. Under these circumstances, the soft tissues become distended adjacent to the surgical site within minutes of the procedure. The swelling is soft or mildly firm and yields a distinctive crackling sound upon palpation. The entrapped air can migrate along fascial planes through the neck to the sternum, into the prevertebral fascia and mediastinum, toward the temporal and orbital regions, or into the vascular system. Emphysema is associated with risks for infection, air embolism, and death. Broad-spectrum antibiotics are recommended to prevent infection. Signs suggestive of embolic sequelae, such as sudden vision changes, dyspnea, altered heart rate, or loss of consciousness, warrant immediate transfer to an emergency care facility.

**Postoperative Bleeding (Figs. 36.3–36.6)** Bleeding is the result of trauma and surgery of the oral soft tissues. Facial swelling can result from orofacial bleeding when there is excess bleeding or blood that does not have an escape route through the epithelium. The end result is **purpura**, the accumulation of blood within the subcutaneous or submucosal tissues. Purpura is classified according to the size of the severed vessel and the size of the lesion produced. Rupture of capillaries produces punctate bleeds called **petechiae**. Subcutaneous bleeding that produces a nonraised lesion up to 1 cm in diameter is called an **ecchymosis** (bruise). A large (greater than 1 cm) area of subcutaneous bleeding that distends soft tissues is a **hematoma**.

In dentistry, hematomas are commonly caused by the inadvertent penetration of the needle into the posterior superior alveolar vein. Swelling occurs without pain within seconds or minutes of the trauma. The swelling grows uniformly and without color change in the posterior cheek region, over and in front of the mandibular ramus. The hematoma is slightly firm and compressible. It may cause tissue tenderness, nerve paresthesia, and muscle trismus. Pressure and ice should be applied to the hematoma during the first 24 hours. Thereafter, heat should be applied to dissipate the blood. Depending on its size, the lesion may take over 1 week to resolve and may discolor the skin. During the healing phase, the skin color fades from purple to brown, then tan and yellow. Antibiotics should be considered if the hematoma is caused by severance of a vessel with a contaminated instrument.

**Bell's Palsy (Figs. 36.7 and 36.8)** Bell's palsy is unilateral paralysis of the seventh cranial nerve. The condition results in the inability to move the muscles of facial expression on the affected side. Trauma to the facial nerve caused by surgery, tooth extraction, infection, or exposure to cold is the most frequent cause. Some cases have been linked to the inflammatory response caused by reactivation of herpesvirus in the geniculate ganglion. All persons are susceptible, but the condition is seen most often in middle-aged adults (slightly more often in women). The classic characteristics are abrupt onset of inability to raise the forehead skin, close the eye, and lift the corner of the mouth of the affected side. Eye watering (crocodile tears), mouth drooling, and loss of taste are common consequences. The palsy may be temporary or permanent. In 70% of patients with idiopathic Bell's palsy, normal function returns within 6 weeks. Cases lasting longer than 1 year usually persist indefinitely. Palliative care should be provided to protect the eye from corneal ulceration. Corticosteroids and surgical decompression of the facial nerve have lessened the severity and duration of symptoms in some patients.

# Conditions Peculiar to the Face

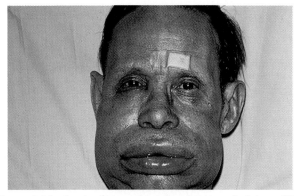

**Figure 36.1. Angioedema:** abrupt and severe facial swelling caused by contact with latex rubber.

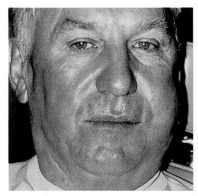

**Figure 36.2. Air emphysema:** compressible swelling that produced a crackling sound upon palpation; caused by air forced under a mucoperiosteal flap from high-speed handpiece use during surgery.

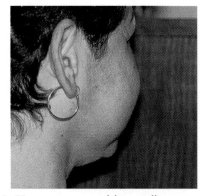

**Figure 36.3. Hematoma** caused by needle penetration of the posterior alveolar vein during administration of local anesthesia.

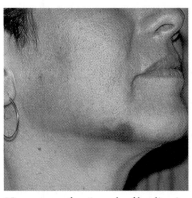

**Figure 36.4. Hematoma** after 1 week of healing in same patient shown in Figure 36.3.

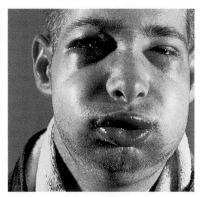

**Figure 36.5. Surgical trauma:** facial swelling 2 days after third molars were surgically extracted.

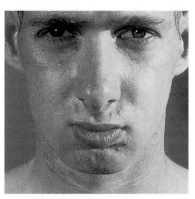

**Figure 36.6. Healing of postsurgical swelling** 2 weeks after surgery in same patient shown in Figure 36.5.

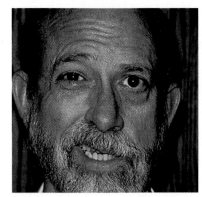

**Figure 36.7. Bell's palsy:** inability to raise skin and muscles of left side of face.

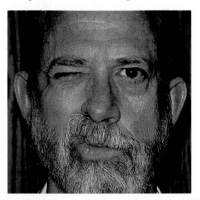

**Figure 36.8. Bell's palsy:** inability to close left eyelids in same patient shown in Figure 36.7.

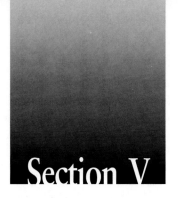

# Section V

# Intraoral Findings by Color Changes

# White Lesions

**Fordyce's Granules (Figs. 37.1 and 37.2)** Fordyce's granules are ectopic sebaceous glands found within the mouth that are considered a variation of normal oral mucosal anatomy. These granules consist of individual sebaceous glands that are 1–2 mm in diameter. Characteristically they appear on the buccal mucosa as white, creamy white, or yellow slightly raised papules. They usually occur in multiples, forming clusters, plaques, or patches. Enlarged clusters may feel rough to palpation and to the patient's tongue. They are sometimes an isolated finding. Less common locations include the lip, labial mucosa, retromolar pad, attached gingiva, tongue, and frenum.

Fordyce's granules arise from sebaceous glands embryologically entrapped during fusion of the maxillary and mandibular processes. They become more apparent after sexual maturity as the sebaceous system develops. Rarely, an intraoral hair may be seen in association with the condition.

Fordyce's granules occur in approximately 80% of adults, and no predilection in race or sex has been reported. Histologic examination shows rounded nests of clear cells, 10–30 per nest; darkly staining, small, centrally located nuclei are found encapsulated in the lamina propria and submucosa. The clinical appearance is adequate for diagnosis of Fordyce's granules; biopsy is not usually required.

**Linea Alba Buccalis (Figs. 37.3 and 37.4)** The linea alba buccalis is a common intraoral finding that appears as a raised white wavy line of variable length and prominence located at the level of the occlusion on the buccal mucosa. Generally, this asymptomatic cornified entity is 1–2 mm wide and extends from the second molar to the canine region of the buccal mucosa. The lesion is usually found bilaterally and cannot be rubbed off. The thickened epithelial changes consist of hyperkeratotic tissue that is a response to frictional activity of the teeth. The condition is often associated with crenated tongue and may be a sign of bruxism, clenching, or negative oral pressure. The clinical appearance is diagnostic and requires no treatment.

**Leukoedema (Figs. 37.5 and 37.6)** Leukoedema is a common mucosal variant associated with dark-pigmented persons but may be seen infrequently in lighter-pigmented persons. The incidence of leukoedema tends to increase with age, and 50% of African-American children and 92% of African-American adults are affected. Leukoedema usually appears bilaterally on the buccal mucosa as an opalescent, milky-white, or gray thin surface film. The labial mucosa, soft palate, and floor of the mouth are less common locations of occurrence.

Leukoedema is often faint and may be difficult to see. Prominence of the lesion is related to the degree of underlying melanin pigmentation, level of oral hygiene, and amount of smoking. Close examination of leukoedema reveals fine white lines, wrinkles, or overlapping folds of tissue. The borders of the lesion are irregular and diffuse; they fade into adjacent tissue, which makes it difficult to determine where the lesion begins and ends. The condition is diagnosed by stretching the mucosa, which causes the white appearance to significantly diminish or disappear in some cases. Wiping the lesion fails to remove it. The cause of leukoedema is unknown, although it is more severe in smokers and diminishes with smoking cessation. Histologic examination of biopsy specimens shows increased epithelial thickness with prominent intracellular edema of the spinous layer. No serious complications are associated with this lesion, and no treatment is required.

**Morsicatio Buccarum (Mucosal Chewing) (Figs. 37.7 and 37.8)** Morsicatio buccarum (cheek biting or chewing) is a common nervous habit that produces a progression of mucosal changes. Slightly raised white plaques and folds initially appear in a diffuse pattern that cover areas of trauma. Increased injury produces a hyperplastic response that increases the size of the plaque. A linear or striated pattern is sometimes observed, with thick and thin areas seen side by side. Persistent injury leads to interadjacent traumatic erythema and ulceration.

Mucosal chewing is usually seen on the buccal mucosa and less frequently on the labial mucosa. The lesions may be unilateral or bilateral and can occur at any age. No sex or race predilection has been reported. Diagnosis requires visual or verbal confirmation of the nervous habit. Although morsicatio buccarum has no malignant potential, patients should be advised of the mucosal alterations. Because of the similar clinical appearance, speckled leukoplakia and candidiasis should be ruled out. Microscopy shows a normal maturing epithelial surface with a corrugated parakeratotic surface and minor subepithelial inflammation.

# White Lesions

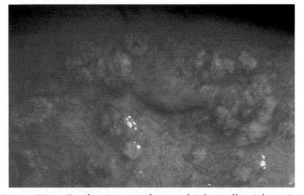

Figure 37.1. **Fordyce's granules:** multiple, yellowish, raised papules on buccal mucosa. (Courtesy Dr Linda Otis)

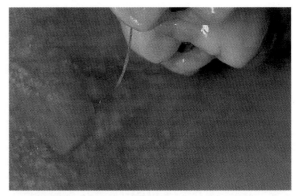

Figure 37.2. **Fordyce's granules:** creamy white with a rare intraoral hair. (Courtesy Dr Bill Baker)

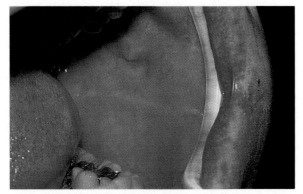

Figure 37.3. **Linea alba buccalis:** faint, white wavy line on buccal mucosa below parotid papilla.

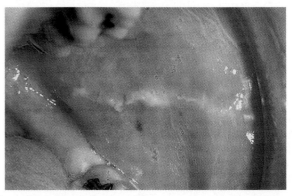

Figure 37.4. **Linea alba buccalis:** prominent, raised white wavy line with mild unrelated leukoedema. (Courtesy Dr Dale Miles)

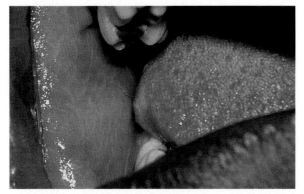

Figure 37.5. **Leukoedema:** grayish white film of the buccal mucosa that disappears on stretching.

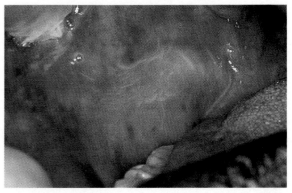

Figure 37.6. **Leukoedema:** milky-white film of the buccal mucosa in a patient who smokes.

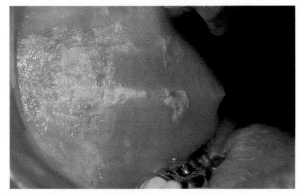

Figure 37.7. **Morsicatio buccarum:** raised white plaques caused by cheek biting.

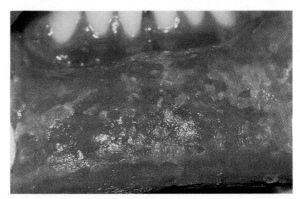

Figure 37.8. **Morsicatio buccarum** of the labial mucosa. (Courtesy Dr Kenneth Abramovitch)

# White Lesions

**White Sponge Nevus (Familial White Folded Dysplasia) (Figs. 38.1 and 38.2)** White sponge nevus is a relatively uncommon genodermatosis that usually appears at birth or in early childhood but persists throughout life. It is characterized by mucosal lesions that are asymptomatic, white, folded, and spongy. The lesions often exhibit a symmetric wavy pattern. The most common location is the buccal mucosa bilaterally, followed by the labial mucosa, alveolar ridge, and floor of the mouth. This condition may involve the entire oral mucosa or may be distributed unilaterally as discrete white patches. The gingival margin and dorsal tongue are almost never affected, although the soft palate and ventral tongue are commonly involved. The size of the lesions varies from patient to patient and from time to time.

White sponge nevus exhibits no race or sex predilection; however, because of this condition's autosomal dominant pattern of transmission, several family members may manifest the disorder. Extraoral mucosal sites may involve the nasal cavity, esophagus, larynx, vagina, and rectum. Concurrent skin lesions exclude the diagnosis. Causation has been attributed to a basic defect in epithelial maturation and exfoliation. Microscopy shows prominent parakeratosis, thickening and clearing of the spinous layer, and perinuclear tangles of keratin tonofilaments. No treatment is required, and the lesions are harmless.

**Traumatic White Lesions (Acute Trauma, Chemical Burns, and Peripheral Scar) (Figs. 38.3–38.6)** Traumatic white lesions can be caused by many physical and chemical irritants, such as frictional trauma, heat, prolonged use of aspirin, and excessive use of mouthwash or other caustic liquids. In particular, frictional trauma is often noted on the attached gingiva. It is caused by excessive tooth brushing, movement of oral prostheses, and chewing on the edentulous ridge. With time the mucosa becomes thickened and develops a roughened white surface. Pain is characteristically absent, and histologic examination reveals hyperorthokeratosis.

Severe trauma can produce a white lesion if the superficial layers of mucosal epithelium are lost. Underneath the white slough is a raw, red, or bleeding surface. Acute traumatic lesions usually appear as punctate white patches with diffuse and irregular borders. Moveable mucosa is more susceptible to trauma than is attached mucosa. Pain frequently lasts several days.

Trauma involving the subjacent dermal layers may induce a fibrous healing response or scar. Scars are often asymptomatic, linear, whitish-pink, and sharply delineated. A thorough history may reveal previous injury,

recurrent ulcerative disease, seizure disorder, self-mutilating behavior, or previous surgery.

**Leukoplakia (Figs. 38.7 and 38.8)** Leukoplakia is a clinical term for a white plaque or patch on the oral mucosa that cannot be scraped off and cannot be classified as any other clinically diagnosable disease. Persons of any age may be affected, but most cases occur in men between the ages of 45 and 65 years. Recent incidence figures indicate that the male to female ratio is decreasing; women are being affected almost as frequently as men.

Leukoplakias are protective reactions against chronic irritants. Tobacco, alcohol, syphilis, vitamin deficiency, hormonal imbalance, galvanism, chronic friction, and candidiasis have been implicated in the cause of these lesions. Leukoplakias vary considerably in size, location, and clinical appearance. The preferential sites for leukoplakia are the lateral and ventral tongue, floor of the mouth, alveolar mucosa, lip, soft palate–retromolar trigone, and mandibular attached gingiva. The lesional surface may appear smooth and homogeneous, thin and friable, fissured, corrugated, verrucoid, nodular, or speckled. The lesions can vary in color, from faintly translucent white to gray or brown-white.

A classification system offered by the World Health Organization recommends two divisions for oral leukoplakias: homogeneous and nonhomogeneous. Nonhomogeneous leukoplakias have been further subdivided into erythroleukoplakia, nodular, speckled, and verrucoid.

Most leukoplakias (80%) are benign, and the rest are dysplastic or cancerous. The clinical challenge lies in determining which leukoplakias are premalignant or malignant, especially because 4–6% of all leukoplakias progress to squamous cell carcinoma within 5 years. High-risk sites of malignancy include the floor of the mouth, lateral and ventral tongue, uvulo-palatal complex, and lips.

Leukoplakias with localized red areas also confer a high risk for carcinoma. For example, nonhomogeneous leukoplakias, particularly oral speckled leukoplakias, represent epithelial dysplasia in about half of the cases and have the highest rate of malignant transformation among intraoral leukoplakias. *Candida albicans*, a fungal organism often associated with oral speckled leukoplakias, may have a role in the dysplastic changes seen.

The initial step in the treatment of leukoplakia is to eliminate any irritating and causative factors and then observe for healing. The lesion may or may not disappear. When an unexplained oral leukoplakia is persistent, biopsy is mandatory. Several biopsy sites may be necessary for diffuse lesions. Nonhomogeneous or reddish areas of the lesion should always be selected for biopsy because they are associated with a higher risk for dysplasia and malignant transformation.

# White Lesions

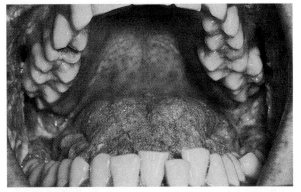

**Figure 38.1. White sponge nevus** affecting the buccal mucosa, soft palate, and retromolar pad.

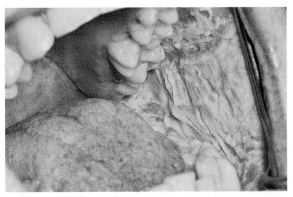

**Figure 38.2. White sponge nevus:** thickened, white, folded plaques seen on buccal mucosa of patient in Figure 38.1.

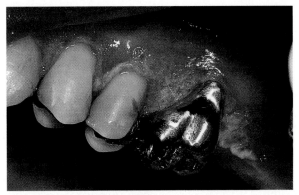

**Figure 38.3. Traumatic white lesion (frictional keratosis)** caused by vigorous tooth brushing.

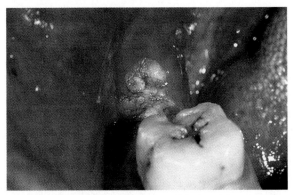

**Figure 38.4. Traumatic white lesion (frictional keratosis)** from a supraerupted maxillary molar.

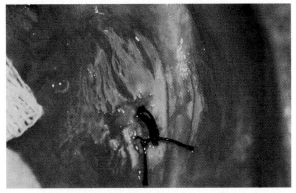

**Figure 38.5. Traumatic white lesion:** chemical burn from aspirin placement at a biopsy site.

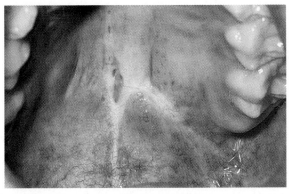

**Figure 38.6. Traumatic white lesion.** This scar on soft palate resulted from a traumatic laceration at age 2 years.

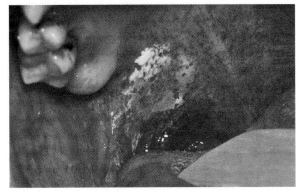

**Figure 38.7. Leukoplakia** of the soft palate. Biopsy revealed hyperorthokeratosis.

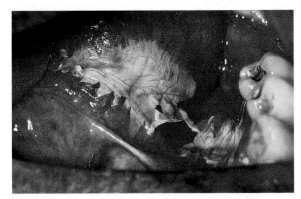

**Figure 38.8. Leukoplakia** of the floor of the mouth and ventral tongue; biopsy revealed mild epithelial dysplasia.

# Tobacco-Associated White Lesions

**Cigarette Keratosis (Figs. 39.1 and 39.2)** Cigarette keratosis is a specific reaction evident in persons who smoke nonfiltered or marijuana cigarettes to a very short length. The lesions, which approximate each other upon lip closure, involve the upper and lower lips at the location of cigarette placement. These keratotic patches are about 7 mm in diameter and invariably are located lateral to the midline. Raised white papules are evident throughout the patch, producing a roughened texture and firmness to palpation. Cigarette keratoses may extend onto the labial mucosa, but the vermilion border is rarely involved. Elderly men are most commonly affected. Smoking cessation usually brings about resolution. The development of ulcer and crust formation should raise the suspicion of neoplastic transformation.

**Nicotine Stomatitis (Pipe Smoker's Palate) (Figs. 39.3 and 39.4)** Nicotine stomatitis is a response of oral ectodermal structures to prolonged pipe and cigar smoking. It is usually found in middle-aged and elderly men, posterior to the palatal rugae, on the soft palate, and sometimes extending onto the buccal mucosa. Rarely, the dorsum of the tongue is affected; these tobacco-associated changes of the tongue have been termed glossitis stomatitis nicotina.

Nicotine stomatitis shows progressive changes with time. The irritation initially causes the palate to become diffusely erythematous. The palate eventually becomes grayish-white secondary to hyperkeratosis. Multiple discrete keratotic papules with depressed red centers develop that correspond to dilated and inflamed excretory duct openings of the minor salivary glands. The papules enlarge as the irritation persists but fail to coalesce, producing a characteristic cobblestone (parboiled) appearance of the palate. Isolated but prominent red-centered papules are common. Whether the lesion arises as a consequence of heat or of tobacco is a matter of debate. Pipe smoking and reverse cigarette smoking, a habit of some women, produces similar findings. Smoking cessation usually results in regression. Biopsy is rarely needed to confirm the diagnosis.

**Snuff Dipper's Patch (Tobacco Chewer's Lesion, Snuff Keratosis) (Figs. 39.5 and 39.6)** A wrinkled yellow-white area on the gingival mucosal flexure and mandibular buccal or labial mucosa suggests intraoral use of unburned tobacco. The hard palate, floor of the mouth, and ventral tongue may also be affected if tobacco is placed in the maxillary vestibule or beneath the tongue. Smokeless tobacco has various forms (snuff, dip, plug, or quid) and leaves its characteristic mark at the preferential site of tobacco placement. Posterior sites are commonly used for dip, plug, or quid, whereas anterior sites are preferred for snuff. Persons whose intraoral sites vary have multiple, less prominent lesions. Male teenagers are most frequently affected, largely because of intensive marketing, peer and sports associations.

Early snuff dipper's patches are pale pink, and the surface appears corrugated and wrinkled. The color may progress to white, yellow-white, and yellow-brown as hyperkeratosis and exogenous staining occur.

Long-term use of smokeless tobacco is associated with periodontal alterations, caries, epidermal dysplastic changes, and verrucous carcinoma. To achieve resolution, cessation of use is recommended. If normal appearance does not return 14 days after cessation, biopsy is necessary.

**Verrucous Carcinoma (of Ackerman) (Snuff Dipper's Cancer) (Figs. 39.7 and 39.8)** Verrucous carcinoma most frequently arises in association with long-term use of smokeless tobacco. However, it is a less common form of oral cancer than squamous cell carcinoma. It is a variant malignant squamous cell tumor that is considered low-grade and nonmetastasizing. The carcinoma appears as a warty, exophytic, reddish-white mass that is firm to palpation. Some would describe it as cauliflower-like or papulonodular. The buccal mucosa and mandibular gingiva are the most common locations. Men older than age 60 years who have used smokeless tobacco for many years are most often affected. The disease is rare in persons younger than age 40 years and in persons who do not use tobacco. Human papillomavirus infection is associated with this type of cancer in 30% of cases.

Verrucous carcinoma has a distinctive surface appearance. A characteristic feature is a white keratotic surface with pink-red pebbly papules throughout. Lateral growth leads to an increase in mass, and the tumor can achieve a diameter of several centimeters. Large lesions can be locally destructive by invading and eroding the underlying alveolar bone. Similar-appearing lesions include verrucous epithelial hyperplasia, pyostomatitis vegetans, and proliferative verrucous leukoplakia.

Recommended treatment for verrucous carcinoma is wide surgical excision. Radiation therapy is contraindicated because of the risk for anaplastic transformation to squamous cell carcinoma. The long-term prognosis of affected patients improves after use of smokeless tobacco is discontinued.

# Tobacco-Associated White Lesions

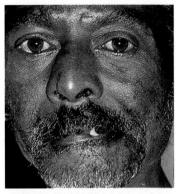

**Figure 39.1. Cigarette keratosis** in a 65-year-old man who smoked unfiltered cigarettes.

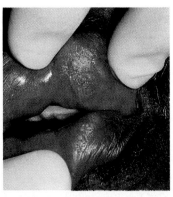

**Figure 39.2. Cigarette keratosis** on labial mucosa of same patient shown in Figure 39.1.

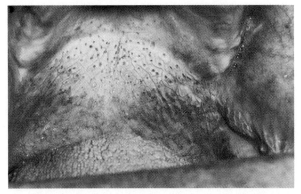

**Figure 39.3. Nicotine stomatitis** prominent on hard and soft palate, extending onto the buccal mucosa.

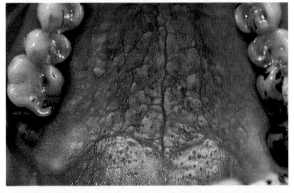

**Figure 39.4. Nicotine stomatitis:** cobblestone appearance and red accessory salivary duct openings in a reverse smoker.

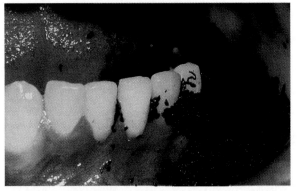

**Figure 39.5. Snuff dipper's patch:** typical placement of chewing tobacco.

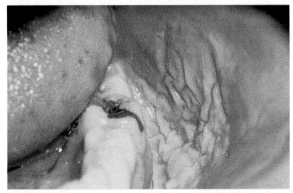

**Figure 39.6. Snuff dipper's patch:** typical white wrinkled appearance.

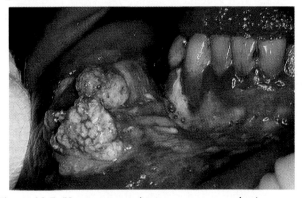

**Figure 39.7. Verrucous carcinoma:** warty, exophytic mass of the labial mucosa after many years of tobacco chewing. (Courtesy Dr Spencer Redding)

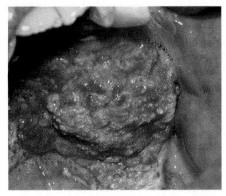

**Figure 39.8. Verrucous carcinoma:** alveolar ridge and palatal involvement in a patient who routinely placed snuff in the maxillary vestibule. (Courtesy Dr James Cottone)

# Red Lesions

## Purpura (Petechiae, Ecchymoses, Hematoma) (Figs. 40.1–40.4)

Purpura is characterized by the pooling of extravasated blood in soft tissue. The stimulating factor can be iatrogenic, factitial, or accidental trauma to vascular tissues contained within the dermis or submucosa. In circumstances in which trauma is not involved, quantitative or qualitative deficits in the platelets, clotting factors, or capillary fragility should be suspected. Purpura initially appears bright red but tends to discolor with time, becoming purplish-blue and later brown-yellow. Because these lesions consist of extravasated blood, they do not blanch on pressure.

The three types of purpura—petechiae, ecchymoses, and hematoma—are classified according to size and cause. Petechiae are pinpoint, nonraised circular red spots. The soft palate is the most common intraoral location for multifocal petechiae. Palatal petechiae may represent an early sign of infectious mononucleosis, scarlet fever, leukemia, bleeding diatheses, or blood dyscrasia. They may also indicate rupture of palatal capillaries caused by coughing, sneezing, vomiting, or fellatio. "Suction petechiae" under a maxillary denture are not true purpura. They evolve as a result of candidal infection and the resulting inflammation of the orifices of accessory salivary glands, not because of denture-created negative pressure as previously believed.

An area of extravasated blood usually greater than 1 cm in diameter is called an ecchymosis (common bruise). Careful physical evaluation may reveal the cause to be mechanical trauma; hemostatic disorders; Cushing's disease; neoplastic disease; primary idiopathic or secondary thrombocytopenic purpura; or use of such anticoagulant drugs as aspirin, bishydroxycoumarin, warfarin, or heparin.

Hematomas are large pools of extravasated blood resulting from traumatic vascular severance. They occur most commonly in the oral cavity as a result of a blow to the face, tooth eruption, or rupture of the posterior superior alveolar vein during administration of local anesthesia. They are usually dark red-brown or blue and tender to palpation. Purpurae fade with time and require no specific treatment. Determining the underlying cause is the prime consideration.

## Varicosity (Varix) (Fig. 40.5)

A varix is a red-purple fluctuant swelling frequently seen in elderly persons. The swelling represents a venous dilatation caused by reduced elasticity of the vascular wall as a result of aging or by an internal blockage of the vein. The ventro-lateral surface of the anterior two thirds of the tongue is a common location. The lip and labial commissure are other common sites. Labial varices appear dark red to blue-purple. They are usually single, round, dome-shaped, and fluctuant. Palpation of the lesion disperses the blood from the vessel and flattens the surface appearance; thus, the lesions are diascopy-positive.

Varices are benign and asymptomatic and require no treatment. If they are of cosmetic concern to the patient, varices can be surgically removed without significant bleeding. Varices are sometimes slightly firm because of fibrotic changes. Thrombosis is a rare complication that produces a firm nodule within the varix. When several veins on the ventral tongue are prominent, the condition is called phlebectasia linguae, or "caviar tongue."

## Thrombus (Fig. 40.6)

The series of events that includes trauma, activation of the clotting sequence, and formation of a blood clot typically results in the cessation of bleeding. Several days later clot breakdown occurs and normal blood flow resumes. In certain cases, if the clot does not dissolve, blood flow stagnates and a thrombus is formed.

Thrombi appear as raised red-brown or blue round nodules, typically in the labial mucosa. They are firm to palpation and may be slightly tender. No sexual predilection is evident, but thrombi are most commonly seen in patients older than age 30. Thrombi concentrically enlarge to occlude the entire lumen of the vessel or mature and calcify to form a phlebolith. Phleboliths are rare oral findings that develop in the cheek, lips, or tongue. Radiography shows phleboliths to be doughnut-like, circular radiopaque foci with a radiolucent center.

## Hemangioma (Figs. 40.7 and 40.8)

Hemangiomas are benign, enlarged, vascular hamartomas that may be seen in any soft-tissue intraoral location. They occur early in life and somewhat more commonly in females than in males. The dorsum of the tongue, gingiva, and buccal mucosa are common locations. On histologic examination they may be capillary or cavernous.

Hemangiomas, when situated deep within the connective tissue, do not alter the color of the mucosal surface. Superficial hemangiomas, in contrast, are red, blue, or purple; flat or slightly elevated; smooth-surfaced; and somewhat firm. Hemangiomas are positive to diascopy and may vary in size from a few millimeters to several centimeters. The borders are usually diffuse, and lobular surfaces are infrequent. Single hemangiomas are most common, whereas multiple lesions are seen in Maffucci's syndrome. Facial and oral hemangiomas form a component of Sturge-Weber's syndrome.

Large soft tissue hemangiomas present management problems. Surgical excision, sclerosing agents, cryotherapy, and radiation therapy have been used to eliminate these lesions. A hemangioendothelioma is the malignant counterpart to the hemangioma, whereas Kaposi's sarcoma is another malignant vascular tumor seen in about 25% of patients with the acquired immune deficiency syndrome (AIDS).

# Red Lesions

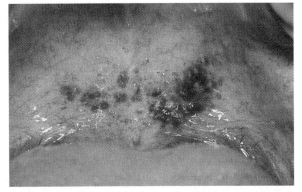

Figure 40.1. **Petechiae:** discrete red spots of the soft palate caused by trauma (in this case, viral illness and repeated coughing).

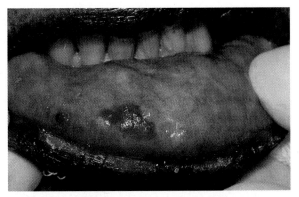

Figure 40.2. **Ecchymosis** developing after lip trauma in a patient receiving heparin.

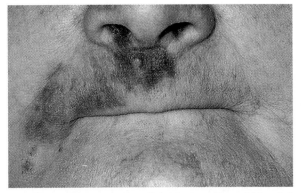

Figure 40.3. **Hematoma:** purplish-blue pooling of blood that occurred after patient fell on her face.

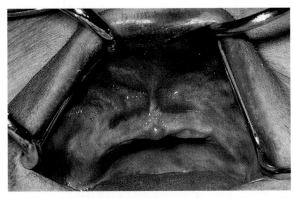

Figure 40.4. **Hematoma:** same patient shown in Figure 40.3; denture flange caused oral trauma.

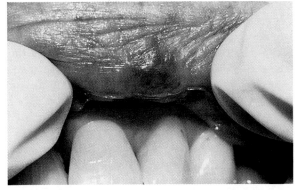

Figure 40.5. **Varix:** purplish papule that blanched upon diascopy. (Courtesy Dr Linda Otis)

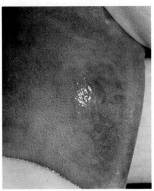

Figure 40.6. **Thrombus** of the labial mucosa that organized within a varix. (Courtesy Dr Ed Heslop)

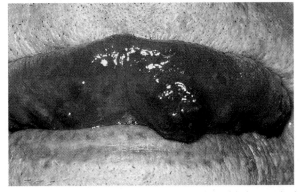

Figure 40.7. **Hemangioma:** dome-shaped, reddish-purple lesion of the ventral tongue. (Courtesy Dr Tom Razmus)

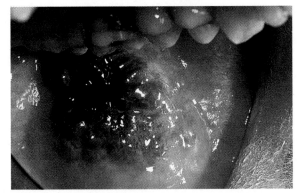

Figure 40.8. **Hemangioma:** multinodular, solitary, bluish-purple lesion of the buccal mucosa.

# Red Lesions

## Hereditary Hemorrhagic Telangiectasia (Osler-Weber-Rendu Syndrome) (Figs. 41.1–41.4)

Hereditary hemorrhagic telangiectasia is a genetic disease inherited as an autosomal dominant trait. The disease is characterized by multiple telangiectasias, which are purplish red macules or slightly red papules representing permanently enlarged end capillaries of the skin, mucosa, and other tissues. The lesions are usually 1–3 mm, lack central pulsation, and blanch upon diascopy. After puberty the size and number of lesions tend to increase with age. Males and females are affected equally. Bleeding is a prominent feature of this disease, and epistaxis is often a presenting feature.

History, clinical appearance, and histologic features are important in making the diagnosis of hereditary hemorrhagic telangiectasia. The lesions of this disease are located immediately subjacent to the mucosa and are easily traumatized, resulting in rupture, hemorrhage, and ulcer formation. Skin lesions are less subject to rupture because of the overlying cornified epithelium. The most common locations on the skin are the palms, fingers, nail beds, face, and neck. Mucosal lesions can be found on the lips, tongue, nasal septum, and conjunctivae. The gingiva and the hard palate are less commonly involved. Some complications include epistaxis from drying or irritation of involved nasal mucosa or from nasotracheal intubation; gastrointestinal bleeding, melena, and iron deficiency caused by rupture of telangiectasias of gastrointestinal mucosa and prolonged bleeding; and hematuria caused by rupture of telangiectasia within the urinary tract. Other complications include cirrhosis of the liver, pulmonary arteriovenous fistulae, and brain abscesses. Precautions are recommended with the use of inhalation analgesia, general anesthesia, oral surgical procedures, and hepatotoxic and antihemostatic drugs. Rupture of a telangiectasia may cause hemorrhage that is best controlled by pressure packs. Because brain abscesses form in a small percentage of patients, antibiotic prophylaxis before invasive dental treatment may be beneficial to these patients.

## Sturge-Weber Angiomatosis (Sturge-Weber or Encephalotrigeminal Syndrome) (Figs. 41.5–41.8)

Sturge-Weber angiomatosis is a rare nonhereditary, congenital disorder that manifests venous angiomas of the leptomeninges of the brain, ipsilateral macular hemangiomas of the face, neuromuscular deficits, and oculo-oral lesions. The macular hemangioma of the facial skin, also called "port-wine stain" or "nevus flammeus," is the most striking feature of the syndrome. The facial hemangioma is well demarcated, flat or slightly raised, and red to purple. It blanches under pressure. It is present at birth, is distributed along a branch of the trigeminal nerve, and typically extends to the patient's midline without crossing to the other side. However, the contralateral side may be involved. The ophthalmic division of the trigeminal nerve is most frequently affected. No tenderness or inflammation is associated with the hemangioma, and it does not enlarge with age. In many patients with solitary congenital port wine angiomas of the face, lesions regress spontaneously at puberty. Approximately 30% of persons with facial port wine stains have Sturge-Weber angiomatosis. Involvement of the ophthalmic branch of the trigeminal nerve appears to be most predictive of full involvement of the syndrome.

The altered venous blood flow caused by an angioma of the leptomeninges can result in cerebral cortical degeneration, seizures, mental retardation, and hemiplegia. On lateral skull radiographs, gyriform calcifications characteristically appear as double-contoured "tramlines." Approximately 30% of patients have ocular abnormalities including angiomas, colobomas, or glaucoma.

Vascular hyperplasia involving the buccal mucosa and lips is the most frequent oral finding. The palate, gingiva, and floor of the mouth may also be affected. The bright red oral patches are located on areas supplied by the branches of the trigeminal nerve. Like facial lesions, these patches stop abruptly at the midline. Involvement of the gingiva may produce edematous tissue and cause difficulty with hemostasis when surgical procedures involving these tissues are performed. Abnormal tooth eruption, macrocheilia, macrodontia, and macroglossia are sequelae of large vascular overgrowths. Gingival hyperplasia may result from phenytoin therapy, which is given because these patients are subject to seizures. Careful assessment of the enlarged gingiva on the ipsilateral side, including biopsy, may be required to establish vascular involvement or the drug-induced gingival hyperplasia. In areas of vascular hyperplasia, oral surgery should be performed in accordance with strict hemostatic measures.

# Red Lesions

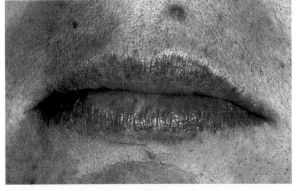

**Figure 41.1. Hereditary hemorrhagic telangiectasia:** multiple, tiny red spots representing dilated capillaries.

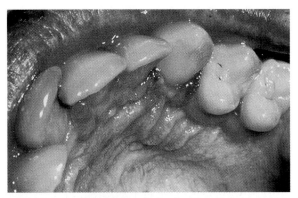

**Figure 41.2. Hereditary hemorrhagic telangiectasia:** gingival telangiectasias in same patient shown in Figure 41.1.

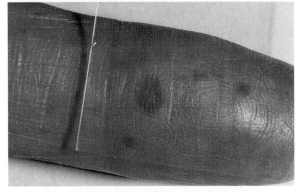

**Figure 41.3. Hereditary hemorrhagic telangiectasia:** skin telangiectasias under a glass slide. (Courtesy Dr Margot van Dis)

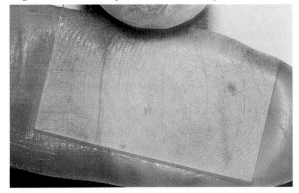

**Figure 41.4. Hereditary hemorrhagic telangiectasia:** blanching of lesions on diascopy. (Courtesy Dr Margot van Dis)

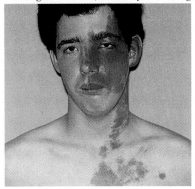

**Figure 41.5. Sturge-Weber angiomatosis:** port wine stain affecting ophthalmic and maxillary division of trigeminal nerve. (Courtesy Dr Larry Skoczylas)

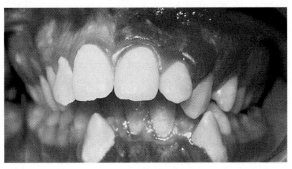

**Figure 41.6. Sturge-Weber angiomatosis:** unilateral gingival involvement in same patient shown in Figure 41.5. (Courtesy Dr Larry Skoczylas)

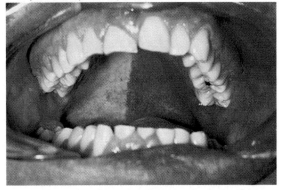

**Figure 41.7. Sturge-Weber angiomatosis:** palatal lesion stops at midline; generalized phenytoin-induced gingival hyperplasia.

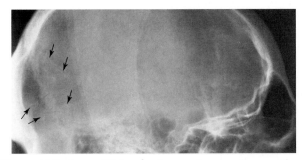

**Figure 41.8. Sturge-Weber angiomatosis:** tram-line gyriform calcifications seen on lateral skull radiograph in same patient shown in Figure 41.7.

# Red and Red-White Lesions

**Erythroplakia (Figs. 42.1–42.4)** Erythroplakia is defined as a persistent red patch that cannot be characterized clinically as any other condition. This term, like "leukoplakia," has no histologic connotation; however, most erythroplakias are histologically diagnosed as epithelial dysplasia or worse and thus have a much higher propensity for progression to carcinoma than leukoplakia. Erythroplakias appear most prevalent in the mandibular mucobuccal fold, oropharynx, and floor of the mouth. The redness of the lesion is a result of atrophic mucosa overlying a highly vascular submucosa. The border of the lesion is usually well demarcated. There is no sexual predilection, and patients older than age 60 are most commonly affected.

Three clinical variants of erythroplakia have been recognized: 1) the homogenous form, which is completely red; 2) erythroleukoplakia, which has red patches interspersed with occasional leukoplakic areas; and 3) speckled erythroplakia, which contains white specks or granules scattered throughout the lesion. Biopsy is mandatory for all types of erythroplakia because 91% of erythroplakias represent severe dysplasia, carcinoma in situ, or invasive squamous cell carcinoma. Close inspection of the entire oral cavity is also required because 10–20% of these patients have several erythroplakic areas, a phenomenon known as field cancerization.

**Erythroleukoplakia and Speckled Erythroplakia (Fig. 42.5)** Erythroleukoplakia and speckled erythroplakia, or "speckled leukoplakia," as some authors prefer, are precancerous red and white lesions. Erythroleukoplakia is a red patch with isolated leukoplakic areas, whereas speckled erythroplakia is a red patch that contains white speckles or granules throughout the entire lesion. A variant red-white lesion that has a nodular appearance is called proliferative verrucous leukoplakia.

Erythroleukoplakia and speckled erythroplakia have a male predilection, and most lesions are detected in patients older than age 50 years. They may occur at any intraoral site but frequently affect the lateral border of the tongue, buccal mucosa, and soft palate. These lesions are often associated with heavy smoking, alcoholism, and poor oral hygiene.

Fungal infections are common in speckled erythroplakias. *Candida albicans*, the predominant organism, has been isolated in most cases; thus, the management of these lesions should include analysis for candida. The cause-and-effect relationship between candidiasis and speckled leukoplakia is unknown, but erythroplakia with leukoplakic regions confers a greater risk for atypical cytologic changes. Because of the increased risk for carcinoma, biopsy of all red-white lesions is mandatory.

**Squamous Cell Carcinoma (Figs. 42.5–42.8)** Squamous cell carcinoma is a malignant neoplasm of mucosal origin. It is the most common type of oral cancer, accounting for more than 90% of all malignant neoplasms of the oral cavity. Oral cancer may occur at any age, but it is primarily a disease of the elderly; more than 95% of oral cancers occur in persons older than age 40 years. In the past, the prevalence was much higher in males, but the male to female ratio has dramatically decreased in recent years to approximately 2:1 because of the increased number of women who smoke.

The exact cause of oral squamous cell carcinoma is unknown but probably involves loss of genes that regulate cell proliferation and apoptosis. Cytologic atypism and mutagenesis are most frequently associated with excessive use of tobacco and alcohol, infection by human papillomavirus, and immune dysregulation. Other contributory factors are those associated with aging and exposure to a variety of biologic, chemical, and physical agents, such as infection with *Treponema pallidum*, herpes simplex virus, or *C. albicans*; nutritional deficiency states; oral neglect; chronic trauma; and radiation.

In the U.S., the most common site of intraoral squamous cell carcinoma is the lateral border and ventral surface of the tongue, followed by the oropharynx, floor of the mouth, gingiva, buccal mucosa, lip, and palate. The buccal mucosa is a common site in persons of developing countries who have chronically used quid tobacco. The occurrence of squamous cell carcinoma of the lip has decreased dramatically in the past decade because of the increased use of protective sunscreening agents. The dorsal surface of the tongue is almost never affected.

The appearance of squamous cell carcinoma is variable; more than 90% of the cases are erythroplakic, and about 60% are leukoplakic. A combination of colors and surface patterns, such as a red and white lesion that is exophytic, infiltrative, or ulcerated, indicates instability of the oral epithelium and is highly suggestive of carcinoma. Early lesions are often asymptomatic and slow-growing. As the lesion develops, the borders become diffuse and ragged, and induration and fixation ensue. If the mucosal surface becomes ulcerated, the most frequent oral symptom is that of a persistent sore or irritation. Not uncommonly, patients may report numbness or a burning sensation, swelling, or difficulty in speaking or swallowing. Lesions can extend to several centimeters in diameter if treatment is delayed; this delay permits large lesions to invade and destroy vital osseous structures.

Squamous cell carcinoma spreads by local extension or by way of the lymphatic vessels. Staging of the tumor according to the TNM system—size (T), regional lymph nodes (N), and distant metastases (M)—allows assessment of the extent of disease. Surgery and radiation therapy have been the principal forms of treatment for oral cancer. The prognosis for oral cancer depends, in large measure, on the site involved, the clinical stage at the time of diagnosis, the width of the tumor at its greatest diameter, the patient's access to adequate health care, and the patient's ability to cope and mount an immunologic response. Because early treatment is paramount, biopsy should be done if neoplasia is suspected.

# Red and Red-White Lesions

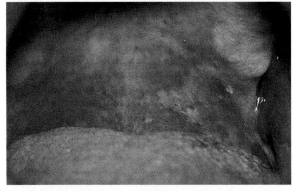

Figure 42.1. **Erythroplakia** not discernible until the tongue is depressed (as shown in Figure 42.2).

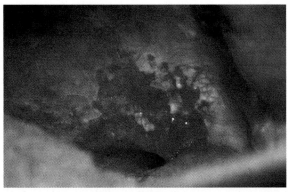

Figure 42.2. **Erythroplakia** with leukoplakic border; biopsy revealed epithelial dysplasia.

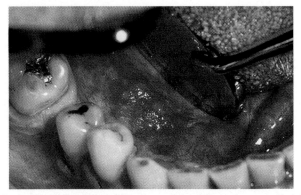

Figure 42.3. **Erythroplakia** along the sublingual caruncle; biopsy revealed carcinoma in situ. (Courtesy Dr Robert Craig)

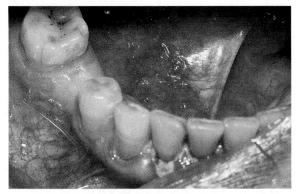

Figure 42.4. **Erythroplakia** of the floor of the mouth; biopsy revealed squamous cell carcinoma

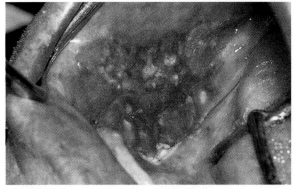

Figure 42.5. **Erythroleukoplakia:** biopsy revealed squamous cell carcinoma.

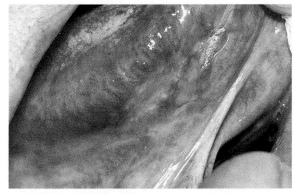

Figure 42.6. **Squamous cell carcinoma** of the tongue adjacent to area shown in Figure 42.5; example of **field cancerization.**

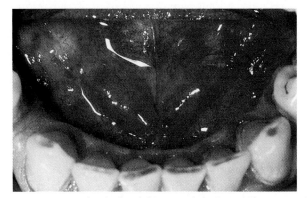

Figure 42.7. **Erythroleukoplakia:** a subtle lesion that proved to be squamous cell carcinoma. (Courtesy Dr Robert Craig)

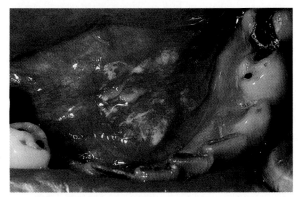

Figure 42.8. **Speckled erythroplakia:** biopsy revealed squamous cell carcinoma. (Courtesy Dr Robert Craig)

# Red and Red-White Lesions

**Lichen Planus (Figs. 43.1–43.6)** Lichen planus is a common skin disease that can have mucosal manifestations. The cause and pathogenesis are unknown, although evidence suggests that lichen planus is an immunologic disorder in which T lymphocytes destroy the basal cell layer of the affected epithelium. Both CD4 and CD8 T-cell subsets have been identified in the submucosal lymphocyte population. Nervous, high-strung persons and persons infected with hepatitis C virus are predisposed to lichen planus. Most patients are women older than age 40. The disease exhibits a protracted course with periods of remission and exacerbation.

The skin lesions of lichen planus initially consist of small, flat-topped, red papules with a depressed central area. The lesions may enlarge and become polygonal in shape or coalesce into larger plaques. The papules progressively acquire a violaceous hue and surface lichenification, which consists of fine white striae. The lesions usually itch and may change color to yellow or brown before resolution. Bilateral distribution on the flexor surfaces of the extremities is common, occasionally involving the fingernails. Patients with characteristic purple, polygonal, pruritic papules on the skin often have concurrent intraoral lesions. The vulva or glans penis are sometimes involved.

Oral lesions of lichen planus may have one of four appearances: atrophic, erosive, striated (reticular), or plaquelike. More than one form may affect a single patient. The most frequently affected site is the buccal mucosa. The tongue, lips, palate, gingiva, and floor of the mouth may also be affected. Bilateral and relatively symmetrical lesions are common. Patients with reticular oral lichen planus characteristically have several delicate white lines or tiny papules arranged in a lacy, web-like network known as Wickham's striae. The glistening white areas are often asymptomatic but may be of cosmetic concern. They may involve large areas.

Atrophic lichen planus results from atrophy of the epithelium and predominantly appears as a red, nonulcerated mucosal patch. Wickham's striae are often present at the border of the lesion. When the attached gingiva is affected, the term "desquamative gingivitis" has been used.

Erosive lichen planus occurs if the surface epithelium is completely lost and erosion results. The buccal mucosa and tongue are commonly affected sites. A vesicle or bulla may initially appear; this eventually breaks down and produces an erosion. Mature lesions have irregular red borders, a yellowish necrotic central pseudomembrane, and an annular white patch, often at the periphery. The condition is intermittently painful and may develop rapidly. All of these features are helpful in differentiating oral lichen planus from other lesions with a similar clinical appearance, such as leukoplakia, erythroplakia, candidiasis, lupus erythematosus, pemphigoid, and erythema multiforme.

The least common type of lichen planus is the asymptomatic plaque form. This lesion is a solid white plaque or patch that has a smooth to slightly irregular surface and an asymmetric configuration. Lesions are commonly found on buccal or glossal mucosa. Patients may be unaware of these lesions.

In many cases, clinical appearance alone can confirm the diagnosis of oral lichen planus, and biopsy is not necessary. Asymptomatic intraoral lesions can be left alone. Biopsy of the atrophic or erosive form should be performed at the border of the lesion, away from areas of ulceration.

The oral lesions of lichen planus tend to be more persistent than those of the skin. A vacation, change in routine, or discharge of psychologically burdensome problems can bring about abrupt and dramatic resolution of the lesions. Chronic, symptomatic, erosive lichen planus lesions are best managed with topical or systemic steroids and immunosuppressant agents. A few patients with oral lichen planus are diabetic and should be tested for glucose intolerance. Carcinomatous transformation has been reported (in fewer than 100 cases) to have an association with erosive lichen planus and tobacco use. The true cause-and-effect relationship, however, has yet to be established for squamous cell carcinoma and lichen planus.

**Electrogalvanic White Lesion (Lichenoid Mucositis, Oral Lichenoid Reaction) (Figs. 43.7 and 43.8)** Electrogalvanic white lesions closely resemble the hypertrophic form of lichen planus. This disorder is more apparent after age 30 years and frequently occurs on the buccal mucosa, immediately adjacent to a metallic material (usually a restoration). Mild cases are asymptomatic, whereas erosive cases can cause a burning type of pain. The histologic features of this lesion mimic those of lichen planus. Electric microcurrents induced by dissimilar restorations is one explanation for this phenomenon. A more recent theory suggests that the disorder results from a delayed hypersensitivity reaction to antigens in various metals, particularly mercury. Interestingly, lichenoid drug reactions, which are similar in appearance to electrogalvanic white lesions, can be caused by the systemic administration or application of the same metals (mercury and gold) found in dental restorations. When systemically used drugs produce these lesions they are called oral lichenoid reactions or lichenoid drug eruptions (see Figs. 44.6–44.8). Treatment consists of replacing the restoration with a different restorative material, preferably gold, porcelain, glass ionomer, or composite materials. The prognosis is excellent, and healing occurs within weeks of removing the offending agent.

# Red and Red-White Lesions

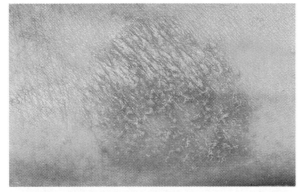

**Figure 43.1. Lichen planus:** violaceous skin plaque with lichenification on flexor surface of wrist.

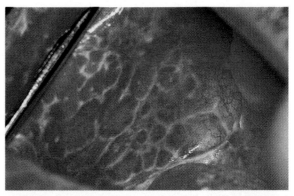

**Figure 43.2. Reticular lichen planus:** characteristic Wickham's striae and tiny white papules. (Courtesy Dr Birgit Glass)

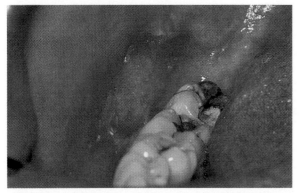

**Figure 43.3. Erosive lichen planus:** painful denuded erosion with central yellowish pseudomembrane.

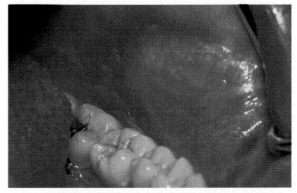

**Figure 43.4. Erosive lichen planus:** bilateral occurrence of erosion in same patient shown in Figure 43.3.

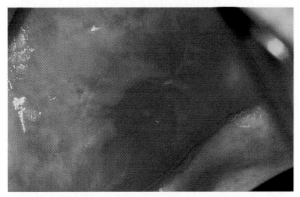

**Figure 43.5. Atrophic lichen planus:** a red patch on buccal mucosa after biopsy. (Courtesy Dr Tom Razmus)

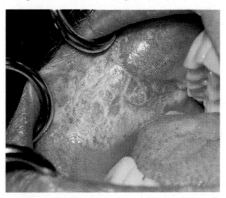

**Figure 43.6. Plaque form of lichen planus** with a few Wickham's striae.

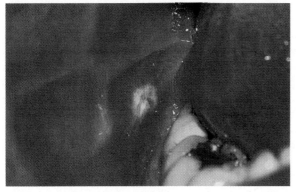

**Figure 43.7. Lichenoid mucositis (electrogalvanic white lesion)** that has a configuration coincident with the adjacent class V alloy restoration.

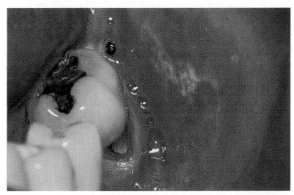

**Figure 43.8. Lichenoid mucositis (electrogalvanic white lesion)** on the opposite side of the same patient shown in Figure 43.7.

# Red and Red-White Lesions

**Lupus Erythematosus (Figs. 44.1–44.4)** Lupus erythematosus exists in three forms: chronic discoid lupus erythematosus, also known as chronic cutaneous lupus erythematosus, which only involves the skin; systemic lupus erythematosus, in which multiple organ systems are involved; and subacute cutaneous lupus erythematosus, a cutaneous variant with mild systemic symptoms. The cause of all three types is unknown.

Chronic discoid lupus erythematosus, the benign form of the disease, is a purely mucocutaneous disorder. It may appear at any age but predominates in women older than age 40 years. The condition is classically characterized by the appearance of a red butterfly rash symmetrically distributed across the bridge of the nose. Other prominent photosensitive areas of the face, including the cheeks, malar areas, forehead, scalp, and ears, may be involved.

The lesions of lupus erythematosus are chronic, with periods of exacerbation and remission. Mature lesions exhibit three zones: an atrophic center lined by a hyperkeratotic middle zone, which is surrounded by an erythematous periphery. Many patients have a hypopigmented lesion that results from melanocyte damage at the epidermal-dermal junction. Telangiectasias, blackheads, and a fine scale are common dermal findings. The lesions are usually limited to the upper portion of the body, particularly the head and neck.

Twenty–40% of patients with lupus erythematosus have oral lesions. These lesions may develop before or after skin lesions develop. Lip lesions are red with a white to silvery, scaly margin. A sun-exposed lower lip at the vermilion border is a common site, whereas the upper lip is usually involved as a result of direct extension of dermal lesions. Intraoral lesions are frequently diffuse and erythematous, with ulcerative and white components.

Chronic discoid lupus erythematosus sometimes appears as isolated white plaques. The buccal mucosa is the most frequent intraoral site, followed by the tongue, palate, and gingiva. The oral lesions are characterized by a central, red atrophic area sometimes covered by a fine stippling of white dots; at the periphery, alternating red and keratotic white lines extend for a short length up to about 1 cm in a radial pattern. These lesions may mimic lichen planus, but concurrent ear involvement helps to exclude the diagnosis of lichen planus. Ulcerative lesions are painful and require treatment. Avoidance of emotional stress, cold, sunlight, and hot spicy foods is necessary. The use of sunscreens, topical steroids, systemic steroids, and antimalarial agents have proven effective. Patients using antimalarial agents require close ophthalmologic follow-up.

Systemic lupus erythematosus, an autoimmune collagen disease, is characterized by the production of antinuclear and anti-DNA antibodies that participate in immunologically mediated tissue injury. Patients often report fatigue, fever, and joint pain. Generalized nontender lymphadenopathy is often present. Hepatomegaly, splenomegaly, peripheral neuropathy, and hematologic abnormalities may also be seen. Strict avoidance of sun exposure is necessary because sunburn can trigger acute reactions. Involvement of the kidneys and heart is a common occurrence that may prove fatal. Skin and oral lesions may accompany the condition, but there is little chance of conversion from discoid to systemic lupus. Patients with systemic lupus erythematosus often concurrently have other autoimmune collagen-vascular diseases, such as Sjögren's syndrome and rheumatoid arthritis. Allergic mucositis, candidiasis, leukoplakia, erythroleukoplakia, and lichen planus must be considered in the differential diagnosis of oral lupus erythematosus lesions. Biopsy and histologic examination with immunofluorescence confirm the diagnosis. Precautions are advised in the dental treatment of patients with lupus erythematosus, who may be taking high doses of systemic steroids, because of their predisposition to delayed wound healing, their risk for infection, and the possibility of stress-induced adrenal crisis characterized by cardiovascular collapse. These patients are also at risk for cardiomyopathy, which requires antibiotic prophylaxis.

**Lichenoid and Lupus-like Drug Eruption (Figs. 44.5–44.8)** Stomatitis medicamentosa is a general term for an oral hypersensitivity reaction to drugs. Two subcategories of oral hypersensitivity, called lichenoid drug eruption and lupus-like drug eruption, produce reticular or erosive lesions similar in appearance to lichen planus and lupus erythematosus. Although the appearance may vary, white linear plaques with red margins are common. The lesions may erupt upon immediate use or after prolonged use of a drug. Persistent inflammatory changes may result in large erythematous areas, eventual mucosal ulceration, and pain. Drug-induced lupus erythematosus is often associated with arthritis, fever, and renal disease. Hydralazine and procainamide are the most common instigators of lupus-like drug eruptions. Other drugs known to cause lupus-like eruptions include gold, griseofulvin, isoniazid, methyldopa, penicillin, phenytoin, procainamide, streptomycin, and trimethadione. Drugs known to induce lichenoid eruptions include the following: chloroquine, dapsone, furosemide, gold, mercury, methyldopa, palladium, penicillamine, phenothiazines, quinidine, thiazides, certain antibiotics, and heavy metals. Consultation with a physician and withdrawal of the offending medication leads to regression of the lesion. A substitute drug is usually selected to manage the patient's systemic problem.

# Red and Red-White Lesions

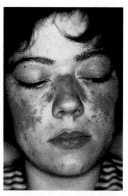

Figure 44.1. **Chronic discoid lupus erythematosus:** butterfly rash.

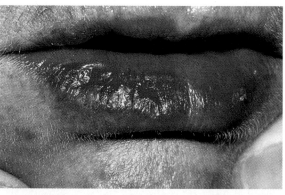

Figure 44.2. **Chronic discoid lupus erythematosus:** red scaly lip lesion. (Courtesy Dr James Cottone)

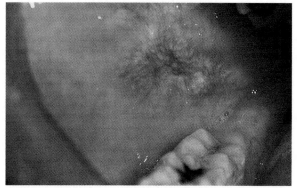

Figure 44.3. **Chronic discoid lupus erythematosus:** alternating red and white lines in a peripheral radiating pattern.

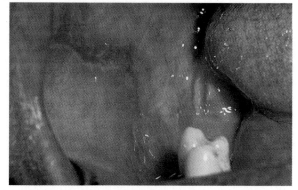

Figure 44.4. **Chronic discoid lupus erythematosus:** central red atrophic area with radiating striae. (Courtesy Dr James Cottone)

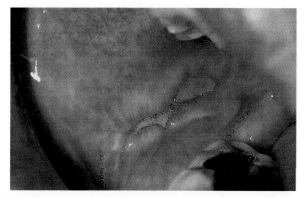

Figure 44.5. **Lupus-like drug eruption** that occurred after the administration of amitriptyline.

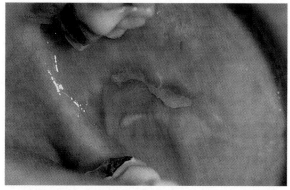

Figure 44.6. **Lupus-like drug eruption:** opposite buccal mucosa in same patient shown in Figure 44.5.

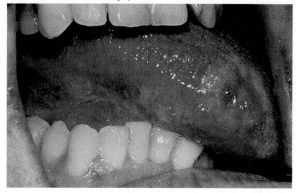

Figure 44.7. **Lichenoid drug eruption:** white plaques and striae developing after furosemide therapy.

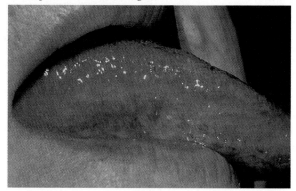

Figure 44.8. **Lichenoid drug eruption:** withdrawal of furosemide resulted in complete resolution in same patient shown in Figure 44.7.

# Red and Red-White Lesions

**Acute Pseudomembranous Candidiasis (Thrush) (Figs. 45.1 and 45.2)** Acute pseudomembranous candidiasis, an opportunistic infection, is caused by an overgrowth of the superficial fungus *Candida albicans*. It appears as diffuse, curdy, or velvety white mucosal plaques that can be wiped off, leaving a red, raw, or bleeding surface. The organism is a common inhabitant of the oral cavity, gastrointestinal tract, and vagina. Infants whose mothers have vaginal thrush at the time of birth and adults who have experienced an upset in the normal oral microflora because of antibiotics, steroids, or systemic alterations such as diabetes, hypoparathyroidism, immunodeficiency, or chemotherapy are frequently affected. There is no racial or gender predilection.

Acute pseudomembranous candidiasis is usually found on the buccal mucosa, tongue, and soft palate. On clinical examination the white plaques appear in clusters that have an erythematous border. In patients with asthma who use a steroid inhaler, the pattern appears as a circular or oval reddish-white patch at the site of aerosol contact on the palate. Diagnosis can be made by clinical examination, fungal culture, or direct microscopic examination of tissue scrapings. A cytologic smear treated with potassium hydroxide, Gram's, or periodic acid-Schiff stain will reveal budding organisms with branching pseudohyphae. Topical application of antifungal medication for 2 weeks usually produces resolution.

**Chronic Hyperplastic Candidiasis (Candidal Leukoplakia) (Figs. 45.3 and 45.4)** Chronic hyperplastic candidiasis is caused by candidal organisms that penetrate the mucosal surface and stimulate a hyperplastic response. Chronic irritation, poor oral hygiene, and xerostomia are predisposing factors; thus, smokers and persons who wear dentures are commonly affected. Chiefly involved are the dorsum of the tongue, palate, buccal mucosa and labial commissures. The lesion invariably has a distinctive raised border and a white, pebbly surface with an occasional red area; thus, the condition may resemble leukoplakia or erythroleukoplakia. The scattered erythematous components are a result of destruction of the mucosal cell layer.

The white patch of chronic hyperplastic candidiasis cannot be peeled off; thus, the diagnosis must be made by biopsy. On microscopy, the organisms may be identified by routine hematoxylin and eosin stain or, more appropriately, by the periodic acid-Schiff stain. With adequate topical application of an antifungal agent, the condition usually resolves. In some instances surgical stripping may be required. All patients with chronic keratotic candidiasis should be followed closely because this form may be related to speckled erythroplakia, a lesion that is often premalignant or worse.

**Acute Atrophic Candidiasis (Antibiotic Sore Mouth) (Fig. 45.5)** The use of broad-spectrum antibiotics, particularly tetracyclines, or topical steroids can result in the oral condition acute atrophic candidiasis. This fungal infection is the result of an imbalance in the oral ecosystem between *Lactobacillus acidophilus* and *Candida albicans*. Antibiotics taken by the patient reduce the *Lactobacillus* population and permit candidal organisms to flourish. The infection produces desquamated areas of surface mucosa that appear as diffuse, nonelevated red patches. Burning pain is the most frequent symptom. The distribution of the patches of acute atrophic candidiasis sometimes indicates the cause. Lesions affecting the buccal mucosa, lips, and oropharynx often suggest the systemic administration of antibiotics, whereas redness of the tongue and palate are more common after the use of antibiotic troches. When the tongue is affected, a surface devoid of filiform papillae is common. Candidiasis rarely affects the attached gingiva; if this is the clinical finding, severe immune suppression is a distinct possibility. The diagnosis of a candidal infection should be confirmed by demonstration of budding organisms or hyphal forms on a stained cytologic smear. Treatment is with antifungal agents.

**Angular Cheilitis (Fig. 45.6)** Angular cheilitis is a chronic painful condition involving the labial commissures caused by *Candida albicans*. On clinical examination, angular cheilitis appears red, fissured and centrally ulcerated. Erythema crusting, and brownish granulomatous nodules may be apparent along the peripheral margins. Discomfort caused by opening the mouth may limit normal oral function. Predisposing factors include nutritional deficiency, loss of vertical dimension, and high sucrose intake. Treatment involves antifungal agents and correction of the predisposing factors.

**Chronic Atrophic Candidiasis (Denture Stomatitis) (Figs. 45.7 and 45.8)** Chronic atrophic candidiasis is the most common form of chronic candidiasis. It is present in 15–65% of complete and partial denture wearers, particularly elderly women who wear their dentures at night; rarely, dentate patients may also be affected. The mandible, however, is rarely involved. Misnomers for this disease are "denture sore mouth" and "denture base allergy."

Chronic atrophic candidiasis is caused by candidal organisms located under the denture base. There are three stages of mucosal alterations. The earliest lesions are red pinpoint areas of hyperemia limited to the orifices of the palatal minor salivary glands. Progression produces a diffuse erythema of the hard palate that is sometimes accompanied by epithelial desquamation. **Papillary hyperplasia** is the third stage. It may be generalized or restricted to relief areas. With time, the papules may enlarge to form red nodules on the palate. Effective therapy requires antifungal treatment of the mucosa and denture base. Traumatic influences, such as the rocking action of the denture, should be eliminated to expedite healing.

# Red and Red-White Lesions

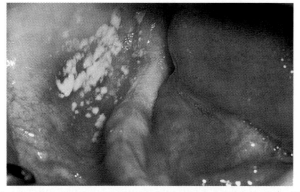

Figure 45.1. **Acute pseudomembranous candidiasis** in a 47-year-old edentulous woman with uncontrolled diabetes.

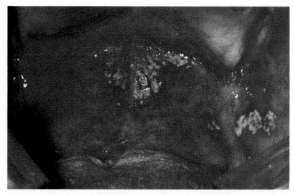

Figure 45.2. **Acute pseudomembranous candidiasis** in a patient who uses a steroid inhaler. (Courtesy Dr Geza Terezhalmy)

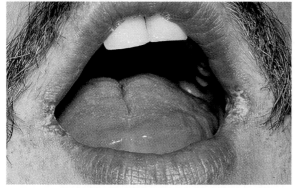

Figure 45.3. **Chronic hyperplastic candidiasis** at the labial commissure that extends onto the buccal mucosa.

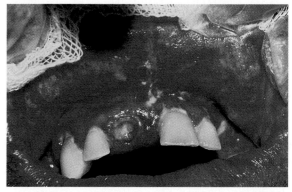

Figure 45.4. **Chronic hyperplastic candidiasis** in a debilitated patient.

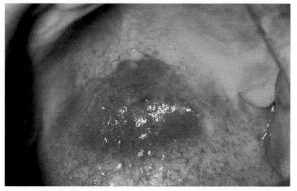

Figure 45.5. **Acute atrophic candidiasis** that is limited to non-denture-bearing area and is caused by use of inhaled steroids.

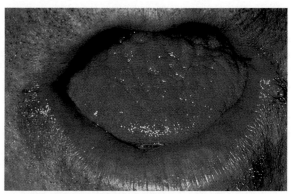

Figure 45.6. **Angular cheilitis:** with involvement of the tongue after antibiotic therapy. (Courtesy Dr James Cottone)

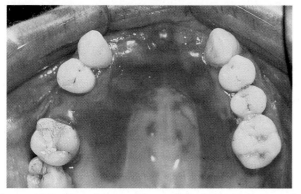

Figure 45.7. **Chronic atrophic candidiasis** limited to partial denture-bearing area. (Courtesy Dr Nancy Mantich)

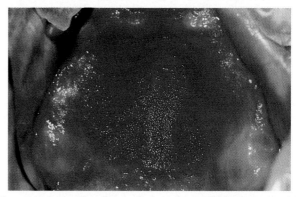

Figure 45.8. **Papillary hyperplasia:** a form of denture stomatitis characterized by multiple red inflamed papules. (Courtesy Dr Ken Abramovitch)

# Pigmented Lesions

**Melanoplakia (Fig. 46.1)** Melanoplakia is a generalized and constant dark pigmentation of the oral mucosa, commonly seen in dark-skinned persons (melanoderms). The condition is physiologic, not pathologic, and results from increased amounts of melanin, an endogenous pigment, that are deposited in the basal layer of the mucosa and lamina propria. The most common site for observing melanoplakia is the attached gingiva. It often appears as a diffuse, ribbon-like, dark band with a well-demarcated and curvilinear border that separates it from the alveolar mucosa. The region is characteristically symmetric and asymptomatic. The degree of pigmentation varies from light brown to dark brown and infrequently may appear blue-black. Other sites of occurrence are the buccal mucosa, hard palate, lips, and tongue. At these sites the deposition of pigment is often multifocal and diffuse. Melanoplakia should be differentiated from similar-appearing conditions that produce oral pigmentations, such as Addison's disease, Albright's syndrome, Peutz-Jeghers syndrome, heavy metal pigmentation, and use of antimalarial drugs.

**Tattoo (Figs. 46.2–46.5)** Tattoos are caused by intentional or accidental implantation of exogenous pigments into the mucosa. The most common intraoral type is the amalgam tattoo, which has been referred to as focal argyrosis. The amalgam tattoo appears as a blue-black, nonelevated discoloration that is usually irregular in shape and variable in size. It results from the entrapment of amalgam in a soft tissue wound such as an extraction socket or a gingival abrasion from a rotating bur. Deterioration of the silver compounds of the amalgam impart the characteristic blue-black color. Focal discolorations may occasionally appear green to dark gray because of the deposition of high copper alloys.

Amalgam tattoos are usually seen in the gingiva in posterior areas adjacent to a large amalgam restoration or gold casting. These lesions are not limited to the gingiva and may also be seen on the edentulous ridge, vestibular mucosa, palate, buccal mucosa, and floor of the mouth. The clinical diagnosis of an amalgam tattoo can be confirmed by finding radiographic evidence of the foreign metal in the paradental tissue. The radiographic appearance may vary from no demonstrable particles to pinpoint or globular radiopacities several millimeters in diameter. If radiographs fail to demonstrate suspected metallic particles, a biopsy is required to rule out more serious pigmented lesions.

Other types of tattoos seen in the oral cavity are the graphite pencil wound and India ink tattoos. The graphite pencil wound appears after trauma as a focal, slate-gray macule frequently located on the palate. The nature of the lesion can be easily ascertained by questioning the patient. Ordinary India ink tattoos are occasional findings on the labial mucosa of the lower lip. In general, tattoos are harmless and of no clinical significance; however, they may be indistinguishable from more potentially ominous lesions.

**Ephelis (Freckle) (Fig. 46.6)** An ephelis is a light to dark-brown macule that appears on the lip or skin after active deposition of melanin triggered by exposure to sunlight. Unlike some pigmentations, this lesion remains essentially unchanged in size with time, darkens in response to sunlight, and has a predilection for light-skinned or red-headed persons. A single freckle is clinically distinguished from an oral melanotic macule by the history of a traumatic or inflammatory episode that precedes the development of the latter condition. On microscopic examination, an ephelis shows an increase in melanin pigment without an increase in the number of melanocytes. Multiple freckles on the lip should be distinguished from the identical lip ephelides seen in conjunction with palmar pigmentations and intestinal polyposis of Peutz-Jeghers syndrome. Ephelides may be of cosmetic concern and require surgical removal; otherwise, observation is normally recommended.

**Smoker's Melanosis (Tobacco-Associated Pigmentation) (Figs. 46.7 and 46.8)** Smoking tobacco imparts smoker's melanosis, a characteristic change in color to exposed mucosal surfaces. The condition is not a normal physiologic process but instead results primarily from the deposition of melanin in the basal cell layer of the mucosa. The relationship of smoker's melanosis and inflammatory changes that result from heat, smoke inhalation, and the absorption of exogenous pigments has not been determined.

Smoker's melanosis affects older persons who are heavy smokers. It appears as a diffuse brown patch up to several centimeters in size. The mandibular anterior gingiva and buccal mucosa are the most frequently affected sites; other susceptible sites include the labial mucosa, palate, tongue, floor of the mouth, and lips. The degree of pigmentation ranges from light to dark brown and appears to be directly related to the amount of tobacco consumed. Dark-brown foci are usually distributed asymmetrically throughout an ill-defined, light-brown patch. Brown-stained teeth and halitosis usually accompany the condition. Smoker's melanosis itself is not premalignant; however, the clinician should closely inspect the adjacent tissues for other tobacco-induced lesions.

# Pigmented Lesions

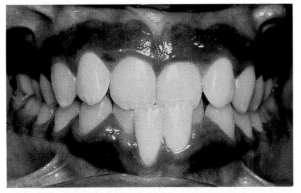

**Figure 46.1. Melanoplakia** distributed along the attached gingiva.

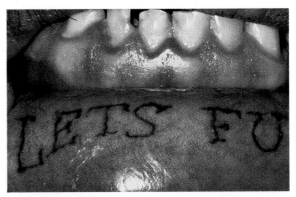

**Figure 46.2. Tattoo** made with India ink. (Courtesy Dr David Freed)

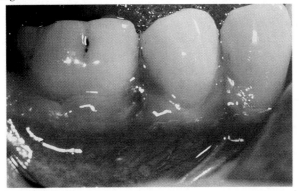

**Figure 46.3. Amalgam tattoo:** blue-gray macule. (Courtesy Dr Linda Otis)

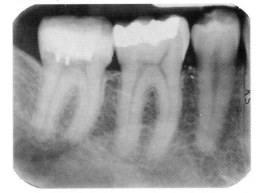

**Figure 46.4. Amalgam tattoo:** radiograph of same patient shown in Figure 46.3 reveals radiopaque amalgam particles between the first molar and second bicuspid that confirm the diagnosis.

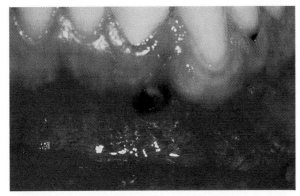

**Figure 46.5. Focal argyrosis** from failed silver-point endodontic therapy.

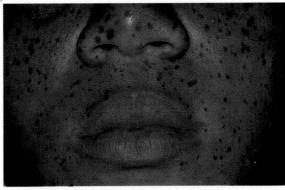

**Figure 46.6. Ephelides:** multiple freckles of the face and lips.

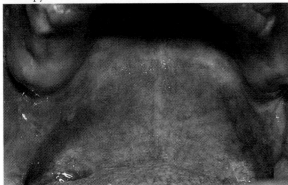

**Figure 46.7. Smoker's melanosis:** lateral regions of the soft palate.

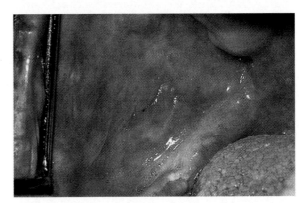

**Figure 46.8. Smoker's melanosis** of the buccal mucosa in same patient shown in Figure 46.7.

# Pigmented Lesions

**Oral Melanotic Macule (Focal Melanosis) (Figs. 47.1 and 47.2)** Within the lip and mouth, an increased amount of melanin deposited as a single, flat, well-circumscribed discoloration usually less than 1 cm in diameter is termed an oral melanotic macule. These endogenous pigmentations are common in light-skinned persons between the ages of 25 and 45 years and probably represent posttraumatic or inflammatory pigmentation, a condition analogous to postinflammatory hypermelanosis on the skin. The most common site is the lower lip close to the midline. Other sites include the gingiva, buccal mucosa, and palate. The color is uniform and may be blue, gray, brown, or black. Biopsy is recommended unless the lesion has been present for many years without visible change and periodic observation is provided.

**Nevus (Figs. 47.3–47.6)** The nevus is commonly seen on the skin and may, in rare instances, occur in the mouth. Although the histogenesis of the nevus is controversial, authorities suggest that it has a melanocyte or Schwann cell derivation. There are many types of nevi, which are broadly classified as either congenital or acquired. Congenital nevi are present at birth and are also known as birthmarks or "garment trunk" nevi. They are usually larger than acquired nevi and have a higher incidence of malignant transformation.

Acquired nevi, or moles, occur later in life and usually appear as dark, slightly raised papules or dome-shaped nodules. They vary in pigment and can be brown, gray, blue, or black. Occasionally nevi are amelanotic and appear pink. In the mouth, nevi are a rare finding. They are usually small, pigmented, well-circumscribed, dome-shaped papules or flat macules that occur more frequently on the palate and buccal mucosa of females. Their size tends to remain constant after puberty. These asymptomatic lesions do not blanch on pressure.

Benign nevi have been classified into four subtypes according to the histologic appearance and location of the nevus cells, which are arranged in nests, or theques. The following nevi are listed in order of decreasing frequency: intramucosal nevus, blue nevus, compound nevus, and junctional nevus.

The **intramucosal nevus,** the most common nevus found in the mouth and the body, has ovoid nevus cells located in the connective tissue only. This entity is analogous to the intradermal nevus, which appears as a dark raised papule on the skin, often seen with a hair growing from it. It is rare, however, to find a hair associated with the intramucosal nevus of the mouth. The intramucosal nevus is usually brown, and raised and ranges from 0.4 to 0.8 cm in diameter.

The second most common intraoral nevus is the **blue nevus.** The name originates from the typical blue or blue-black color imparted by the spindle-shaped nevus cells located deep in the connective tissue. These cells are derivatives of neural crest cells that fail to migrate from the region. A small, well-circumscribed blue macule is the typical appearance, although the nevus often fades with age. The palate is the most common location. Malignant transformation of intraoral blue nevi has never been reported.

The **compound nevus,** as the name implies, is composed of nevus cells located in the epithelium and the lamina propria. The compound nevus rarely undergoes malignant transformation. The **junctional nevus** is a subtype of acquired nevus in which nevus cells are located at the junctional layer of the epithelium and the lamina propria. These lesions are the rarest type of oral nevus and usually appear flat and brown and have a diameter less than 1 cm. The palate and buccal mucosa are common locations.

On rare occasions the **melanotic freckle of Hutchinson** (lentigo maligna) is found in the mouth. The melanotic freckle is usually seen on the face of persons older than age 50 years. This lesion is flat, irregularly shaped, and dirty gray-brown. It may spread superficially in a horizontal direction and undergo malignant transformation.

Nevi may be difficult to distinguish from their malignant counterparts; thus, all intraoral pigmented lesions should be surgically removed and submitted for histopathologic examination, especially if they are exposed to chronic irritation.

**Melanoma (Figs. 47.7 and 47.8)** Melanomas are malignant neoplasms of melanocytes that may occur in the oral cavity. They occur approximately twice as frequently in males as in females and mostly in persons older than age 50 years. Approximately 30% of melanomas have been reported to arise from previously existing pigmented lesions, particularly ones with a history of trauma. Like the nevus, melanomas may be flat or raised, nonpigmented or pigmented. When pigmented, their color is usually deep and may be brown, gray, blue, or jet black. The most frequent sites for occurrence are the maxillary alveolar ridge, palatal tissues, anterior gingivae and labial mucosa.

Melanoma begins as a small superficial or slightly raised patch that grows slowly and laterally over several months. Early recognizable signs are: A, asymmetrical lesion; B, border irregularity; C, color variegation within the lesion; and D, diameter enlarging. Eventually a prominent, nonmovable, dark lesion develops. The clinician should be alert to features that include multiple colors (the combination of red together with blue-black and white is particularly ominous); change in size; satellite lesions arising at the periphery of the lesion; and signs of inflammation, such as a peripheral zone of erythema. Late signs include bleeding and ulceration, firmness to palpation, and rock hard regional lymph nodes. Intraoral melanomas are extremely dangerous and more serious than their cutaneous counterpart because of early and wide metastasis, which results in very poor prognosis. Early diagnosis when tumors are less than 1.5 mm in size and complete resection are critical to long-term survival.

# Pigmented Lesions

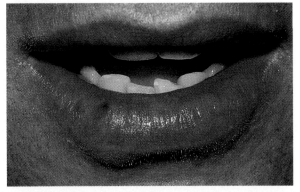

**Figure 47.1. Oral melanotic macule** at its most common site in the lower lip.

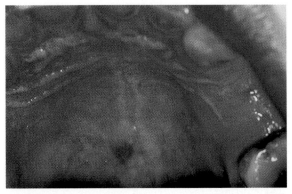

**Figure 47.2. Oral melanotic macule:** a brown lesion of the hard palate.

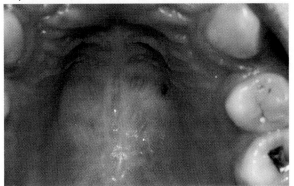

**Figure 47.3. Blue nevus** of the hard palate. (Courtesy Dr Nancy Mantich)

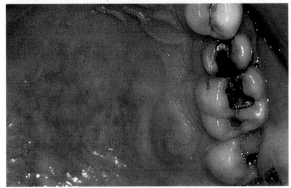

**Figure 47.4. Blue nevus:** a brown-purple lesion on the lateral palatal vault. (Courtesy Dr Tom McDavid)

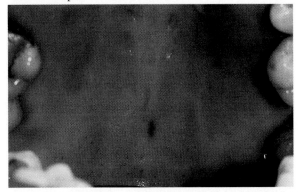

**Figure 47.5. Compound nevus:** a brown macule on the anterior palate. (Courtesy Dr Dale Miles)

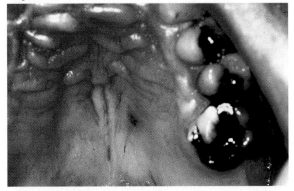

**Figure 47.6. Amelanotic intramucosal nevus:** raised pink nodule adjacent to first maxillary molar. (Courtesy Dr Curt Lundeen)

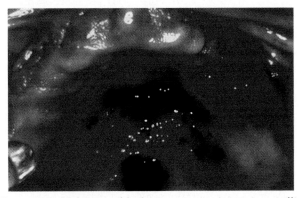

**Figure 47.7. Melanoma:** black pigmentation, pinpoint satellite lesions, and peripheral erythema characteristic of this malignant disease. (Courtesy Dr Geza Terezhalmy)

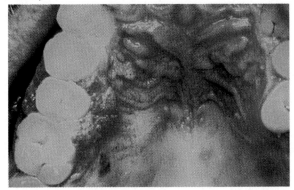

**Figure 47.8. Amelanotic melanoma:** vegetative, pink nodular tumor of palate and alveolar ridge adjacent to second premolar. (Courtesy Dr A.M. Abrams and Dr John Tall)

# Pigmented Lesions

**Peutz-Jeghers Syndrome (Hereditary Intestinal Polyposis) (Figs. 48.1 and 48.2)** Peutz-Jeghers syndrome is an autosomal dominant condition associated with multiple melanotic mucocutaneous macules and gastrointestinal polyposis. These multiple benign intestinal polyps are hamartomatous tissue growths that usually occur in the ileum but may also be found in the stomach and colon. Symptoms such as intermittent colicky pain and reports of obstruction may be concurrent. The perioral pigmentations must be distinguished from multiple ephelides and lentigenes of the LEOPARD syndrome.

The multiple, asymptomatic, melanotic discolorations are usually small, flat, brown ovals that do not darken with exposure to the sun as freckles do. These macules are most often found on the skin around the eyes, nose, mouth, lips, perineum, oral mucosa, gingiva, and palmar and plantar surfaces of the hands and feet. The most common intraoral locations for these pigmentations are the lips and buccal mucosa. In contrast to their cutaneous counterparts, the intraoral spots tend to persist into adulthood, whereas the dermal macules may fade with age. No treatment is necessary for the macules, which on microscopic examination are shown to contain hyperpigmentation of the basal cell layer and lamina propria. Although the macules are benign, they are of considerable clinical significance because a small percentage of affected patients are prone to develop gastrointestinal adenocarcinoma and are at an increased risk for tumors of the reproductive system. The diagnosis of Peutz-Jeghers syndrome therefore necessitates prompt medical evaluation.

**Addison's Disease (Adrenal Cortical Insufficiency, Hypoadrenocorticism) (Figs. 48.3 and 48.4)** Addison's disease most commonly results from autoimmune-induced destruction of the adrenal gland. Other causes include infectious diseases, adrenalectomy, gram-negative sepsis, pituitary insufficiency, and tumor invasion. Progression of the disease results in anemia, anorexia, diarrhea, hypotension, lethargy, nausea, and weight loss.

A complication associated with this disorder is failure of the feedback loop from the adrenal gland to the pituitary gland. This causes an increase in adrenocorticotrophic hormone, which induces melanocyte-stimulating hormone and the deposition of melanin in the skin, especially in sun-exposed areas. Classically the skin acquires a bronze tan that persists after sun exposure. Darkening may be initially noted on the knuckles, elbows, palmar creases, and intraoral mucosa.

In the mouth, the disease is characterized by hypermelanosis that is similar in appearance to melanoplakia. The pattern is not unique and may consist of multiple focal brown to blue-black spots or generalized, diffuse streaks of dark-brown pigmentation. The pigmented areas are usually macular, nonraised, brown, and varied in shape.

The buccal mucosa and gingiva are most commonly affected, but the pigmentation may also extend onto the tongue and lips. Biopsy is not diagnostic, and serum cortisol tests are recommended. Replacement therapy with corticosteroids produces a gradual diminution of the hyperpigmentation; thus, the degree of oral pigmentation is a sensitive indicator of therapeutic effectiveness. Transient changes in pigmentation in a treated patient may indicate inadequate therapy.

**Heavy Metal Pigmentation (Figs. 48.5–48.8)** Excessive ingestion of heavy metals (bismuth, lead, mercury, silver) and certain drugs (antimalarial agents, antipsychotic agents, birth control pills) can produce mucocutaneous pigmentations. Bismuth is commonly found in diarrhea medications, which if used over a long term result in diffuse deposition of the metal in the gingiva. The discoloration is confined to the marginal gingiva, particularly in areas where inflammation is present. The "bismuth line" usually appears blue to black in a linear distribution along the gingival sulcus. A metallic taste and burning mucosa are common symptoms.

Lead poisoning, or plumbism, is usually a result of occupational exposure to excessive doses of lead used in paints, batteries, or plumbing. The most prominent intraoral change and early diagnostic sign is a gray-black "lead line" that occurs from the deposition of lead sulfide in the marginal gingiva. Spotty gray macules on the buccal mucosa, a coated tongue, tremor of the extended tongue, and hypersalivation are other intraoral findings. The condition is reversible if exposure to lead is eliminated.

Mercury poisoning, or acrodynia, can be acquired by absorption, inhalation, or ingestion. Although uncommon today, acrodynia was the result of treatment for syphilis earlier in the century. Inadequate mercury hygiene measures, such as handling mercury, breathing mercury vapors, and spilling mercury, place dental personnel at risk for acrodynia. Like bismuth and lead intoxication, mercury poisoning produces a dark mercury gingival line. In addition, the disease is often accompanied by many signs and symptoms, including abdominal pain, anorexia, headaches, psychological symptoms, vertigo, oral ulcerations, hemorrhage, a metallic taste, sialorrhea, burning mouth, and periodontal destruction.

Silver pigmentation, or argyria, is a rare occurrence that most often results from prolonged exposure to silver-containing ocular or nasal medications. Asymptomatic pigmentations accumulate in the sun-exposed areas of the skin, along with the hair, fingernails, and oral mucosa. A blue-gray pigmentation is characteristic; once evident, the pigmentation is irreversible. Nasal inhalation of solutions containing silver salts have a propensity to deposit in the palatal mucosa, imparting a color similar to that seen on the skin. Treatment is immediate withdrawal of the medication.

# Pigmented Lesions

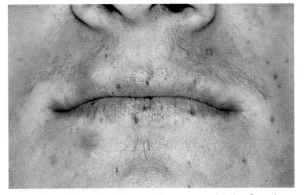

Figure 48.1. Peutz-Jeghers syndrome: multiple flat, brown freckle-like pigmentations of the lips and perioral skin.

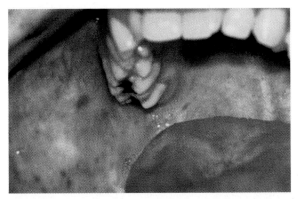

Figure 48.2. Peutz-Jeghers syndrome: brown macules on the buccal mucosa and tongue in same patient shown in Figure 48.1.

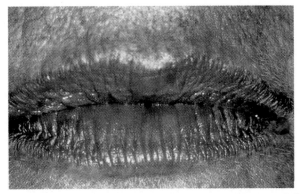

Figure 48.3. Addison's disease: brown pigmentations of the lips.

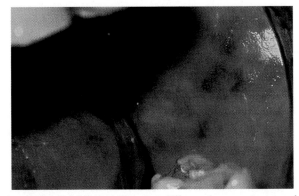

Figure 48.4. Addison's disease: diffuse pigmentation on the buccal mucosa and tongue in same patient shown in Figure 48.3.

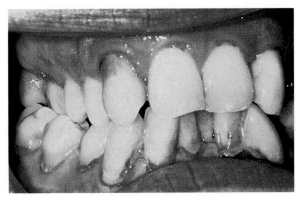

Figure 48.5. Heavy metal pigmentation: lead line distributed along mandibular anterior marginal gingiva.

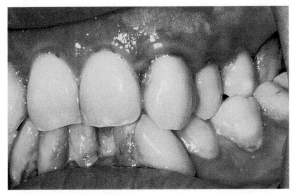

Figure 48.6. Heavy metal pigmentation: lead line in same patient shown in Figure 48.5.

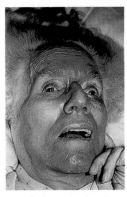

Figure 48.7. Heavy metal pigmentation (argyria): extreme manifestation with long-term use of silver-containing nasal drops. (Courtesy Dr Charles Morris)

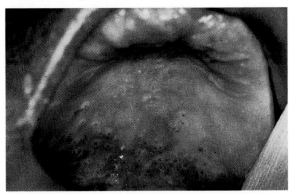

Figure 48.8. Heavy metal pigmentation (argyria): bluish-gray pigmentation of palate in a pipe smoker who used nose drops. (Courtesy Dr Charles Morris)

Section VI

# Intraoral Findings by Surface Change

# Nodules

**Retrocuspid Papilla (Figs. 49.1 and 49.2)** Not all persons have a retrocuspid papilla. It consists of a firm, round, fibroepithelial papule, usually 1–4 mm in diameter, located on the attached gingiva lingual to the mandibular cuspids just below or several millimeters below the marginal gingiva. The surface mucosa is usually pink, soft, and smooth. Rarely, the structures may be pedunculated and the stalk can be lifted off the gingiva by a periodontal probe. This finding is a variation of normal and is frequently found bilaterally. Some authorities state that the retrocuspid papilla is a developmental anomaly that represents a variant form of fibroma. The retrocuspid papilla seems to be present in most children but regresses with maturity; thus, the incidence and size decrease with increasing age. The retrocuspid papilla has no gender predilection, and no treatment is necessary unless interference with a removable prosthesis is anticipated.

**Oral Lymphoepithelial Cyst (Figs. 49.3 and 49.4)** The oral lymphoepithelial cyst is an encapsulated, fluid-filled dermal or submucosal mass that arises from epithelium entrapped in lymphoid tissue that has undergone cystic transformation. It is usually asymptomatic but may enlarge and spontaneously fistulate. Most appear in children and young adults. No sex predilection has been demonstrated.

When the lymphoepithelial cyst is derived from degenerative tissue of the second branchial arch, it is referred to as a cervical lymphoepithelial cyst and appears on the lateral aspect of the neck just anterior and deep to the superior third of the sternocleidomastoid muscle near the angle of the mandible. The cyst may occur in the proximity of the parotid gland. The extraoral lymphoepithelial cyst is a well-circumscribed, soft, fluctuant mass that is rubbery to the touch.

Common sites for the oral lymphoepithelial cyst are the floor of the mouth, lingual frenum, ventral tongue, posterior lateral border of the tongue, and, rarely, the soft palate. These small swellings, rarely exceeding 1 cm in diameter, are characteristically well circumscribed, soft, doughy, yellow when superficial, and pink when deeper. Palpation yields a slightly moveable nodule. When located in the anterior floor, the lesion may resemble a mucus-retention cyst. Infrequently, multiple lymphoepithelial cysts can be found.

Histologic examination shows that lymphoepithelial cysts are usually lined with stratified squamous epithelium; occasionally, pseudostratified, columnar, or cuboidal epithelium is found. A fibrous connective tissue wall surrounds the lesion, which contains dark-staining lymphoid aggregates with prominent germinal centers. The luminal fluid is yellow and viscous because of a cheesy keratinaceous content. Excisional biopsy should be performed to provide histologic confirmation. Lymphoepithelial cysts rarely recur.

**Torus, Exostosis, and Osteoma (Figs. 49.5–49.8)** Tori, exostoses, and peripheral osteomas are readily recognizable bony hard nodules that appear histologically identical. The term used depends on location, appearance, and systemic associations.

Bony protuberances of the jaws, localized to the palatal midline or mandibular lingual attached gingiva, are called tori. They are the most common intraoral lesions that are exophytic by nature. Females are most frequently affected. Tori have smooth rounded contours, normal-appearing or slightly pale mucosa, and a sessile base. Tori are often found to have a lobulated surface. Internally they are composed of cortical bone with occasional areas of spongy bone.

Bony outgrowths in alternate locations are termed exostoses. The facial aspect of the maxillary and mandibular alveolar ridge are common sites. Infrequently, the palatal alveolar ridge adjacent to maxillary molars is affected. Most exostoses are multiple hard nodules that demonstrate crease-like folds between distinct nodules. The surface mucosa is firm, taut, and white to pale pink.

Tori and exostoses tend to increase slowly in size with increasing age but remain asymptomatic unless traumatized. After a traumatic incident, patients may be concerned about neoplasia and state that the bony mass is enlarging or that it was not present before the injury. Removal is generally unnecessary unless prompted by cosmetic, prosthodontic, psychological, or traumatic considerations.

Osteomas are considered to be neoplastic growths that are distinct from the developmental lesions, tori and exostoses, because osteomas have more growth potential, tend to be larger, and may be confined to soft tissue. Patients with osteomas should be examined radiographically for multiple impacted supernumerary teeth, which may indicate the presence of Gardner's syndrome. This autosomal dominant condition is characterized by osteomas, dermal cysts, multiple impacted and supernumerary teeth, and intestinal polyposis with a high propensity for malignant transformation. Most patients with Gardner's syndrome demonstrate malignant polyposis by age 40 years; thus, all patients with this condition require close medical management.

# Nodules

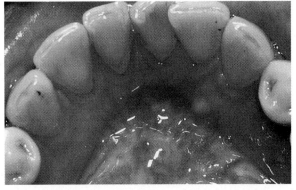

Figure 49.1. **Retrocuspid papilla** appearing as a pink papule.

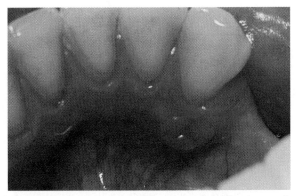

Figure 49.2. **Retrocuspid papilla;** unusual clefting in a unilateral papilla.

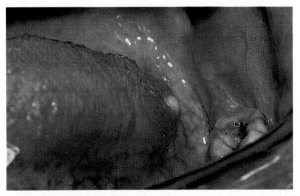

Figure 49.3. **Oral lymphoepithelial cyst** on the margin of the tongue; the cyst is yellow because of keratin cystic contents.

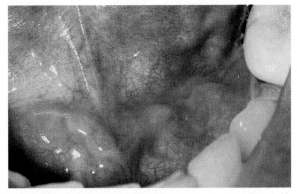

Figure 49.4. **Oral lymphoepithelial cyst:** telangiectatic surface vessels cover the pink nodule in the floor of mouth.

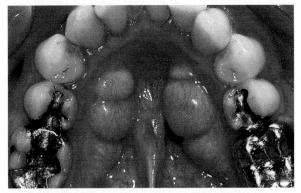

Figure 49.5. **Mandibular tori:** lobulated, bony hard, and bilaterally symmetric.

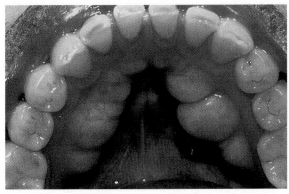

Figure 49.6. **Mandibular tori:** multinodular and usual pale pink color.

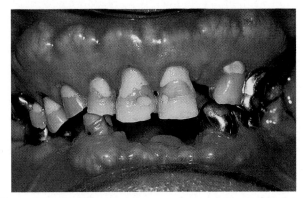

Figure 49.7. **Exostoses** apparent at the mucogingival junction of the maxilla and mandible.

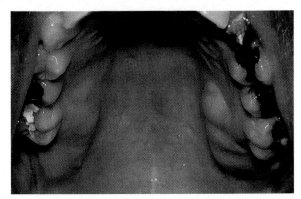

Figure 49.8. **Exostoses:** bilaterally on the palate adjacent to molar-premolar region. (Courtesy Dr Tom McDavid)

# Nodules

**Irritation Fibroma (Fig. 50.1)** The irritation fibroma is one of the most common benign lesions of the oral cavity. It results from reactive hyperplasia caused by a chronic irritant; thus, this lesion is not a true neoplasm as the term "fibroma" seems to imply. True neoplastic fibromas are a rare intraoral finding. The irritation fibroma typically appears as a well-defined, pale pink, slow-growing papule that enlarges to form a nodule. This smooth and symmetrically round lesion is firm and painless to palpation. Infrequently, a leukoplakic, roughened, or ulcerated surface is present because of repeated trauma. The base is usually sessile. This growth can arise on any soft tissue location in the mouth, including the buccal mucosa, labial mucosa, gingiva, or tongue. Histologic examination shows an interlacing mass of dense collagenous tissue subjacent to thinned epithelium. Fibromas are treated by removing the source of the irritation together with conservative surgical excision. Fibromas occur mostly in adults. They recur infrequently if treated properly. Multiple intraoral fibromas may be associated with tuberous sclerosis, a disorder characterized by seizures, mental deficiency, and sebaceous adenomas that are in fact fibromas.

**Peripheral Odontogenic Fibroma** The peripheral odontogenic fibroma is clinically similar to the irritation fibroma but is characterized by its unique location and tissue of origin (arising from cells of the periodontal ligament). Accordingly, it is generally found in the region of the interdental papilla. An example is shown in Fig. 21.7.

**Giant Cell Fibroma (Fig. 50.2)** The giant cell fibroma is a pink papule or nodule that has a sessile base and smooth or slightly pebbly surface. It represents a variant of the irritation fibroma and is distinguished mostly by its histologic appearance. The giant cell fibroma has many large, polynucleated stellate-shaped fibroblasts scattered among a loosely arranged vascular connective tissue; the irritation fibroma does not. Most giant cell fibromas occur before age 35; the mandibular gingiva, tongue, and palate are common sites. Excision is recommended, and recurrence is rare.

**Lipoma (Figs. 50.3 and 50.4)** The lipoma is a common dermal tumor but a rare intraoral finding. This slow growing benign neoplasm is composed of mature fat cells surrounded by a thin, fibrous connective tissue wall. Adults older than age 30 are commonly affected, and no gender predilection exists. In the mouth, the lipoma appears as a well-circumscribed, smooth-surfaced, dome-shaped, or diffusely elevated nodule that is yellow to pale pink. Lipomas are sometimes polypoid, pedunculated, or lobulated. They occur on the buccal mucosa, tongue, floor of the mouth, alveolar fold, and lip. The palate is a rare site of involvement. Palpation reveals a soft, movable, and compressible submucosal mass that has a slightly doughy consistency. Therapy consists of surgical removal, which includes the base of the lesion. Lipomas rarely recur.

**Lipofibroma (Fig. 50.5)** The lipofibroma is a rare benign intraoral neoplasm of mixed connective tissue origin. Microscopy shows a well-demarcated submucosal mass that consists of mature lipid-containing cells with a significant fibrous connective tissue component. Clinical examination shows a blend of a fibroma and lipoma. It is generally found on labial and buccal mucosa. On palpation the lesion is nonindurated, movable, painless, and soft or firm depending on the lipoid-to-collagen content. These lesions grow slowly but can grow to several centimeters in diameter.

**Traumatic Neuroma (Amputation Neuroma) (Fig. 50.6)** The traumatic neuroma results from a hyperplastic response to nerve damage after severance of a large nerve fiber. In the mouth, the traumatic neuroma is frequently encountered in the mandibular mucobuccal fold in the region adjacent to the mental foramen. Other locations include the area facial to the mandibular incisors, the area lingual to the retromolar pad, and the ventral tongue. The size of the lesion depends on both the degree of insult and the degree of hyperplastic response.

Traumatic neuromas are usually small nodules, measuring less than 0.5 cm in diameter. Visualization may be difficult if the lesion is located deep below normal oral mucosa. Neuromas are painful when palpated. Pressure applied to the neuroma elicits a response often described as an "electric shock." Multiple neuromas discovered on the lips, tongue, or palate may indicate the possibility of multiple endocrine neoplasia type IIb. Treatment of the traumatic neuroma is surgical excision or intralesional injection with corticosteroids. Excision may further damage the nerve and lead to recurrence.

**Neurofibroma (Figs. 50.7 and 50.8)** Neoplastic proliferation of all of the elements of a peripheral nerve, including the sheath of Schwann, results in neurofibroma, a benign tumor. Neurofibromas most commonly appear as firm pink nodules. On clinical examination neurofibromas may be solitary or diffuse or exceed 1000 in number. Solitary nodules are rare. More commonly, multiple large neurofibromas are encountered, which are associated with neurofibromatosis (von Recklinghausen's disease). See Swellings of the Face (Figs. 35.6 and 35.7).

Intraoral neurofibromas may be located on the dental arches, buccal mucosa, tongue, and lips. Most soft tissue neurofibromas are asymptomatic, but those arising within deeper tissues or bone may produce pain and paresthesia. Diffuse neurofibromas are striking for their firmness and irregular nodular surface that often results in physical deformity. In some cases, neurofibromas undergo sarcomatous change, which necessitates close follow-up. Solitary neurofibromas not associated with von Recklinghausen's disease have no tendency for malignant transformation.

# Nodules

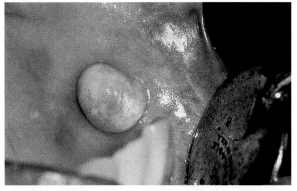

Figure 50.1. **Irritation fibroma:** a large pink nodule on the buccal mucosa.

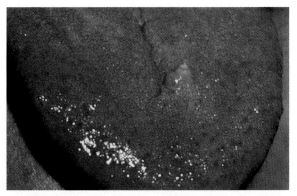

Figure 50.2. **Giant cell fibroma** on the dorsum of the tongue.

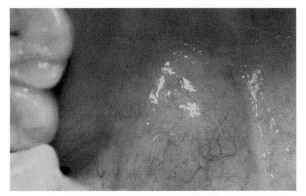

Figure 50.3. **Lipoma** arising at the junction of the hard and soft palates. (Courtesy Dr Dale Miles)

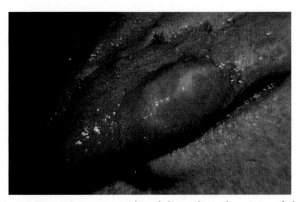

Figure 50.4. **Lipoma:** ovoid nodule on lateral margin of the tongue.

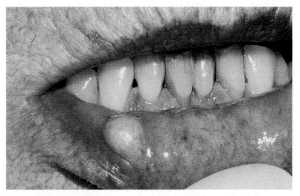

Figure 50.5. **Lipofibroma:** pale pink nodule on labial mucosa. (Courtesy Dr Birgit Glass)

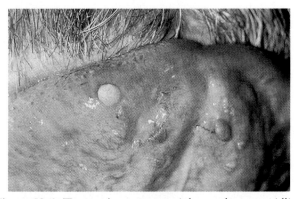

Figure 50.6. **Traumatic neuroma:** pink papule near midline and a whitish papilloma. (Courtesy Dr Jerry Cioffi)

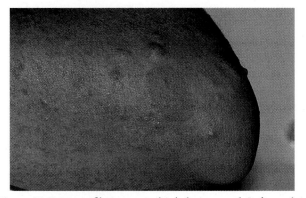

Figure 50.7. **Neurofibromas:** multiple lesions and Café-au-lait spots in von Recklinghausen's disease.

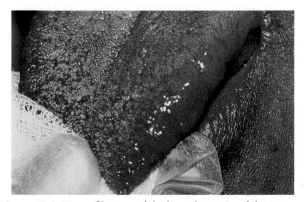

Figure 50.8. **Neurofibroma** of the lateral margin of the tongue.

# Papulonodules

**Oral Squamous Papilloma (Papilloma) (Figs. 51.1 and 51.2)** Papillomas are the most common benign epithelial neoplasm of the oral cavity, especially on the tongue and palate. They appear as small, pink-white, exophytic masses that are usually less than 1 cm in diameter. The surface of the papule may be smooth, pink, and pebbly or have numerous small finger-like projections. The base is pedunculated and well circumscribed. Intraoral lesions are typically soft, whereas keratin-producing lesions are rough or scaly. Lesions are generally solitary, but multiple lesions are occasionally seen. Human papillomavirus (HPV) types 6 and 11 have been detected in more than 50% of papillomas examined and are generally accepted as the cause of this disease.

The mean age of occurrence of papilloma is 35 years; both sexes are affected equally. The most common location is the uvulopalatal complex, followed by the tongue and frenum, lips, buccal mucosa, and gingiva. Other HPV-induced lesions, such as the condyloma acuminatum, focal epithelial hyperplasia (Heck's disease), and verruca vulgaris, share similar clinical features but are microscopically distinct. Histologic features of papilloma are finger-like projections and a fibrovascular core. Treatment is complete excision, including the base. Recurrence is rare. No cases of malignant transformation have been reported; thus, any rapidly advancing papillomatous lesion should be suspected to be a more aggressive lesion.

**Verruca Vulgaris (Fig. 51.3)** Verruca vulgaris is a common skin growth that seldom occurs intraorally. The etiologic agents are HPV types 2, 4, 6 and 11. Virally induced cellular changes result in the characteristic clinical findings. The lesional surface is typically rough and raised, with white finger-like projections. The whiteness of intraoral verrucae varies depending on the amount of surface keratinization. Pink areas are not unusual at the lesional base. Verrucae are commonly located on the skin, vermilion border, labial and buccal mucosa, tongue, and attached gingiva. The base of the lesion is broad, but the size is usually less than 1 cm. On clinical examination a verruca may appear identical to a papilloma, although the clefts are more shallow and the mass more sessile. Viral inclusion bodies are frequently seen on histologic examination. Patients with skin verrucae are more likely to have oral lesions as a result of autoinoculation. A lesion may sometimes regress spontaneously. If not, treatment is complete excision or ablation with a carbon dioxide laser using high-speed evacuation.

**Focal Epithelial Hyperplasia (Heck's Disease) (Fig 51.4)** Focal epithelial hyperplasia is a virus-induced disease associated with multiple papulonodular growths of the oral mucosa, particularly the tongue and labial and buccal mucosa. It was first described in Native Americans and Eskimos but now has been reported in many populations. The etiologic agents have been identified as HPV types 13 and 32. The virus is transmitted during kissing. Virus replication in epithelial cells produces soft papular growths in children and teenagers. Lesions are initially small, discrete, flat papules that are pink or whitish-pink. Later lesions enlarge, become papillary or cobblestoned, and can coalesce. Some lesions undergo spontaneous regression; surgical excision can be performed for those that do not regress.

**Condyloma Acuminatum (Venereal Wart) (Figs. 51.5 and 51.6)** The condyloma acuminatum is a transmissible papillomatous growth that may look identical to the papilloma or fibroma except for several distinguishing features. The oral condyloma occurs much less frequently than the papilloma. It is seen more commonly in sexually active persons and is much more likely to be multiple. The warm, moist, intertriginous areas of the anogenital skin and mucosa are frequent sites of growth.

Condyloma acuminata are usually small and pink to dirty gray. The surface may be flat but is more often pebbly and resembles a cauliflower. The base is sessile and the borders are raised and rounded. Contagious spread may occur between the host and sexual partners. When multiple lesions are present, proliferation of adjacent condylomas can form extensive clusters that may appear as a single mass. Any oral mucosal surface may be affected, but the labial mucosa is the most common site. Other sites include the tongue, lingual frenum, gingiva, and soft palate. Histologic examination shows parakeratosis, cryptic invagination of cornified cells, and koilocytosis. In more than 85% of condyloma acuminata, HPV types 6 and 11 DNA is present in the epithelium. Treatment is wide excision because these lesions have a high rate of recurrence. Occasional oncogenic transformation of long-standing anogenital growths has been reported, but this is not the case with oral lesions.

**Lymphangioma (Figs. 51.7 and 51.8)** Lymphangiomas are benign hamartomas of lymphatic channels that develop early in life with no sex predilection. They may occur on the skin or mucous membrane. In the oral cavity, a frequent site, the dorsal and lateral surface of the anterior portion of the tongue, lips, and labial mucosa are commonly affected.

Small superficial lymphangiomas have irregular papillary projections that resemble a papilloma. They are soft and compressible and vary from normal pink to whitish, slightly translucent, or blue. Deep-seated lesions cause diffuse enlargement and stretching of the surface mucosa. Macroglossia, macrocheilia, and cystic hygroma are clinical deformities that result from the diffuse swelling. Aspiration or diascopy is mandatory before surgical excision of a lymphangioma to prevent complications associated with the similar-appearing hemangioma. Patients with a large, diffuse lesion often require hospitalization to monitor postoperative edema and possible airway obstruction. Lymphangiomas do not undergo malignant change. Some lymphangiomas, especially congenital types, regress spontaneously during childhood.

# Papulonodules

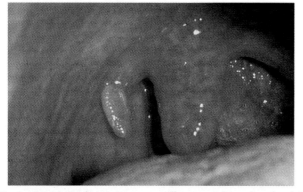

Figure 51.1. Oral squamous papilloma: pedunculated, pink papule with corrugated surface on soft palate. (Courtesy Dr Curt Lundeen)

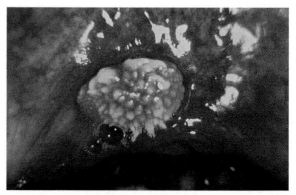

Figure 51.2. Oral squamous papilloma with cauliflower-like projections. (Courtesy Dr Tom McDavid)

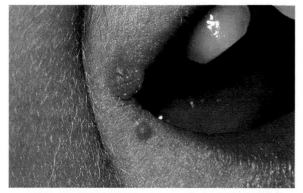

Figure 51.3. Verrucae vulgaris: several warts at commissure of the lips from autoinoculation of warts on the fingers.

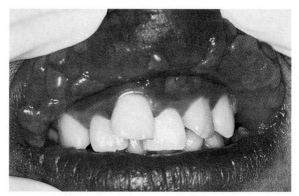

Figure 51.4. Focal epithelial hyperplasia: multiple, soft, flat papules on labial mucosa.

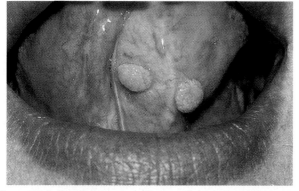

Figure 51.5. Condyloma acuminata: soft pink-gray appearance on ventral tongue; patient also had a genital lesion.

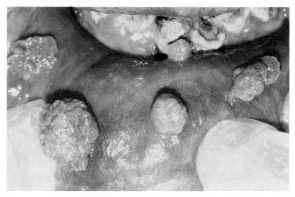

Figure 51.6. Condyloma acuminata: multiple cauliflower-like pinkish warty lesions.

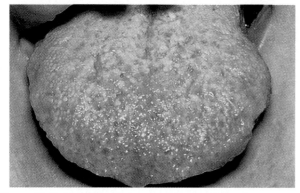

Figure 51.7. Lymphangioma causing macroglossia.

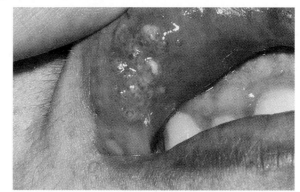

Figure 51.8. Lymphangioma: papulonodular lesion of lip in same patient shown in Figure 51.7.

113

# Vesiculobullous Lesions

**Primary Herpetic Gingivostomatitis (Figs. 52.1–52.3)** Herpes simplex virus (HSV) types 1 and 2 belong to the family Herpesviridae, which includes eight viruses (cytomegalovirus, varicella-zoster virus, Epstein-Barr and human herpes virus VI, VII, and VIII). Approximately 80–90% of the adult human population have been infected with HSV. Transmission occurs by direct mucocutaneous contact of infected secretions, resulting in more than half of a million cases of primary herpetic gingivostomatitis annually in the United States. In most cases, HSV-1 is the causative organism; however, HSV-2, which has a propensity to infect the skin below the waist, can cause herpetic gingivostomatitis by oral-genital or oral-oral contact.

The manifestations of the primary infection may be trivial or fulminating. Trivial infections may produce subclinical signs of infection that often go unrecognized or may produce flu-like symptoms. When symptomatic, the infection is called primary herpetic gingivostomatitis. The infection usually affects children younger than age 10; the second most affected group is young adults aged 15 to 25. The acute inflammatory response of the primary HSV infection usually follows a 3- to 10-day incubation period. The infected patient reports fever, malaise, and irritability. Focal areas of the marginal gingiva initially become fiery red and edematous. The swollen interdental papillae bleed after minute trauma because of capillary fragility and increased permeability. Widespread inflammation of the marginal and attached gingiva develops, and small clusters of vesicles rapidly erupt throughout the mouth. The vesicles burst, forming yellowish ulcers that are individually circumscribed by a red halo. Coalescence of adjacent lesions forms large ulcers of the buccal mucosa, labial mucosa, gingiva, palate, tongue and lips. Shallow erosions of the perioral skin and hemorrhagic crusts of the lips are characteristic. Headache, lymphadenopathy, and pharyngitis are usually present; some reports indicate preferential pharyngeal involvement in young adults.

A significant problem in patients with primary herpetic gingivostomatitis is the pain caused by the mouth ulcers. Mastication and deglutition may be impaired, resulting in dehydration and subsequent elevation of temperature. Viral culturing, serum antibody levels, and results of cytologic testing are confirmatory. Treatment is supportive and should include acyclovir in severe cases. Patients with a high temperature (exceeding 101°F) should also receive nonaspirin antipyretic drugs.

Primary herpetic gingivostomatitis is a contagious disease that usually regresses spontaneously within 12–20 days without scarring. Complications associated with the primary infection include autoinoculation of other epidermal sites, producing keratoconjunctivitis and herpetic whitlow; extensive epidermal infection in the atopic patient, which is called Kaposi's varicelliform eruption; and meningitis, encephalitis, and disseminated infections in immunosuppressed patients. Immunity to HSV is relative, and patients previously infected with the virus may be reinfected with a different strain of HSV.

**Recurrent Herpes Simplex (Figs. 52.4–52.7)** After the initial infection, HSV infects sensory nerve fibers, migrates to a regional neuronal ganglia, and becomes stably associated with the nucleus of the infected cell in a latent and undetectable manner. Reactivation of virus, replication of progeny particles, and clinical recurrence occurs in approximately 40% of persons who harbor the latent virus. Recurrences are often precipitated by a triggering event such as sunlight, heat, stress, trauma, or immunosuppression. Normal immune mechanisms are required to eliminate reactivated HSV, and asymptomatic shedding of virus into saliva in the absence of oral lesions occurs in 10% of any given HSV-infected population.

Recurrent herpes simplex tends to produce clusters of vesicles that ulcerate. The vesicles repeatedly develop at the same site, following the distribution of the infected nerve. Recurrences on the vermilion border of the lip (recurrent herpes labialis) are clinically more apparent than intraoral recurrences (recurrent herpetic stomatitis). The lesions of recurrent herpes labialis are characterized by the appearance of small clusters of vesicles that erupt, coalesce, ulcerate, form a scab, and heal without scarring. Spread to perioral skin is common, especially with use of greasy lip ointments that permit horizontal weeping of vesicular fluid. Contact of vesicular fluid at other epidermal sites can result in spread of the infection. In relatively healthy persons, recurrent herpetic stomatitis produces small ulcers with red halos that are limited to periosteal-bound, keratinized mucosa consisting of the attached gingiva and hard palate. Recurrences on the buccal mucosa and tongue are infrequent unless the patient is immunosuppressed.

Most patients with recurrent herpes simplex report pain. Prodromal neurogenic symptoms such as tingling, throbbing, and burning often precede the eruption of lesions by 24 hours. Sunscreens are effective in the prevention of recurrences. Management also includes lysine, vitamin C, and antiviral drugs (acyclovir, famciclovir, and penciclovir).

**Herpangina (Fig. 52.8)** Herpangina is a self-limiting infection involving the oral cavity that is caused by group A and sometimes group B Coxsackie viruses. This infection is seen mainly in children during the warmer months of summer and is highly contagious. Young adults are occasionally affected. Herpangina produces light-gray papillary vesicles that rupture to form multiple, discrete, shallow ulcers. The ulcers have an erythematous border and are limited to the anterior pillars of the fauces, soft palate, uvula, and the tonsils. Diffuse pharyngeal erythema, dysphagia, and sore throat are common features, as are fever, malaise, headache, lymphadenitis, abdominal pain, and vomiting. Convulsions rarely occur. Treatment is palliative, and spontaneous healing occurs within 1–2 weeks.

# Vesiculobullous Lesions

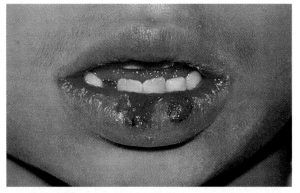

**Figure 52.1. Primary herpetic gingivostomatitis:** hemorrhagic crusts on the lips in a 7-year-old boy.

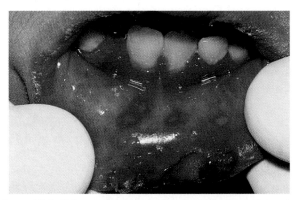

**Figure 52.2. Primary herpetic gingivostomatitis:** vesicles that break down and produce ulcers with red halos (same patient as shown in Figure 52.1).

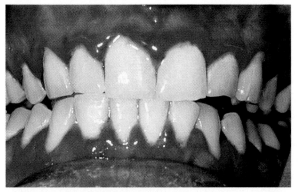

**Figure 52.3. Primary herpetic gingivostomatitis:** producing painful gingivitis in a 27-year-old man.

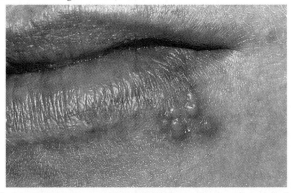

**Figure 52.4. Recurrent herpes labialis:** a cluster of virus-laden vesicles. (Courtesy Dr James Cottone)

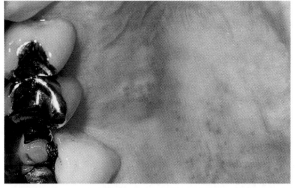

**Figure 52.5. Recurrent herpes simplex:** a cluster of pale vesicles on the palate.

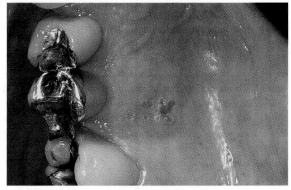

**Figure 52.6. Recurrent herpes simplex:** same patient shown in Figure 52.5 2 days later with broken down vesicles and absence of halos caused by minimal inflammation.

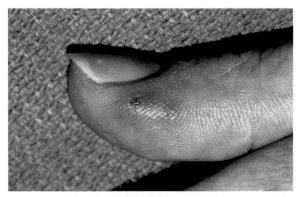

**Figure 52.7. Herpetic whitlow:** caused by autoinoculation from a lip lesion. (Courtesy Dr Linda Otis)

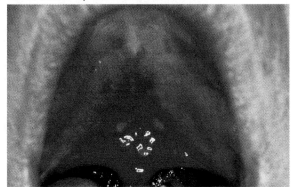

**Figure 52.8. Herpangina:** diffuse erythema of soft palate with multiple small ulcers. (Courtesy Dr Charles Morris)

# Vesiculobullous Lesions

## Varicella (Chickenpox) (Figs. 53.1 and 53.2)

Varicella and herpes zoster are caused by the same herpetic virus, varicella-zoster. Varicella is the highly contagious primary infection, whereas herpes zoster is the recurrent neurodermal infection. Typically, young children become infected with the virus during the late winter and spring months. After exposure to the virus and a 2- to 3-week incubation period, mild prodromal features appear.

Fever, malaise, and a distinctive red and very itchy rash on the trunk are the first recognizable signs of this disease. The pruritic rash quickly spreads to the neck, face and extremities and is followed shortly by the eruption of papules that form vesicles and pustules. Upon bursting, the pus-laden vesicles resemble a "dew drop on a rose petal" appearance. The first and largest skin lesion is called the "herald spot." It is often located on the face and, if scratched, may heal with scarring.

Intraoral lesions of varicella are few and often go unnoticed. They appear as vesicular lesions that break down and form ulcers with an erythematous halo. The soft palate is the predominant site, followed by the buccal mucosa and mucobuccal fold. Anorexia, chills, fever, nasopharyngitis, and musculoskeletal aches may accompany the course of the disease. Complications are infrequent, and vesicles eventually crust over and resolve spontaneously within 7–10 days. Infection during pregnancy poses a significant risk to the fetus. A live-attenuated vaccine (Varivax) is now available that prevents the development of chickenpox.

## Herpes Zoster (Shingles) (Figs. 53.3 and 53.4)

Herpes zoster is the recurrent infection of chickenpox. Unknown factors associated with aging, cancer, and immunosuppression result in reactivation of dormant varicella virus from sensory ganglia and migration of virus along the affected sensory nerves. Viral recrudescence usually affects adults older than age 50 years but may be seen in young adults or children. Before eruption, prodromal signs of itching, tingling, burning, pain, or paresthesia occur. Lesions are characterized by acutely painful vesicular eruptions of the skin and mucosa that are unilaterally distributed along nerve pathways and stop abruptly at the midline. Two areas are affected the most: 1) the trunk between vertebrae T3 and L2 and 3) the face along the ophthalmic division of the trigeminal nerve.

Cutaneous lesions of shingles begin as pruritic, erythematous macules that are followed by vesicular and pustular eruptions. Crust formation occurs within 7–10 days and persists for several weeks. Pain is intense but usually dissipates when the crusts fall off.

The intraoral lesions are vesicular and ulcerative with an intense red, inflammatory border. Ulcers may bleed; within several days, a large yellowish surface slough may form. The lips, tongue, and buccal mucosa may have unilateral ulcerative lesions if the mandibular branch of the trigeminal nerve is affected. Involvement of the second division of the trigeminal nerve typically produces unilateral palatal ulcerations that extend up to but not beyond the palatal raphe. Considerable malaise, fever, and distress accompany herpes zoster. Patients often present with intense pain 1–2 days before the viral vesicles erupt.

Herpes zoster usually heals without scar formation in about 3 weeks, but many patients may experience persistent pain after the lesions have faded. This condition, called **postherpetic neuralgia,** may continue for 6 months to 1 year before regressing. Immunosuppressed patients are particularly susceptible to shingles and have a high morbidity rate. In the past the rare occurrence of bilateral shingles was called the death sign because these victims inevitably died. Varicella-zoster virus infection is occasionally associated with the **Ramsay Hunt syndrome** (herpes zoster, unilateral facial paralysis, and ear eruptions) and **Reye's syndrome** (high fever, cerebral edema, liver degeneration, high mortality, and salicylate use in children). The antiviral agent, famciclovir (Famvir), is highly effective in blocking replication of varicella-zoster virus.

## Hand-Foot-and-Mouth Disease (Figs. 53.5–53.8)

Hand-foot-and-mouth disease is a mildly contagious disease caused by many Coxsackie A and B viruses. It usually affects children but may be seen in young adults. It typically occurs in spring and summer. As the name implies, it produces small ulcerative lesions in the mouth together with an erythematous and vascular rash on the dorsal and ventral surface of the hands, fingers, and soles of the feet. Multiple pinpoint vesicles that ulcerate and crust are characteristic. Patients may have several to more than 100 pinpoint lesions with distinctive erythematous halos.

Oral lesions of hand-foot-and-mouth disease are scattered mainly on the tongue, hard palate, and buccal and labial mucosa. In time they coalesce to form large eroded areas. The oropharynx is usually unaffected. The total number of intraoral lesions is usually less than 20. Pain is a common symptom, along with elevated temperature, malaise, and lymphadenopathy. The diagnosis can be made by viral culture and serum antibody studies; however, the classic distribution of lesions on the palms of hands, soles of feet, and oral mucosa is diagnostic in most instances. Healing occurs regardless of treatment in approximately 10 days.

# Vesiculobullous Lesions

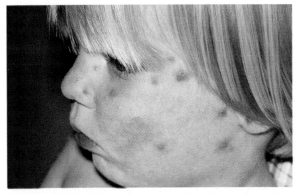

**Figure 53.1. Varicella (chickenpox):** early itchy, maculopapular facial rash; herald spot with scab evident lateral to eye at hairline.

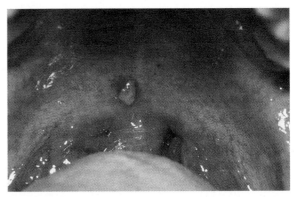

**Figure 53.2. Varicella (chickenpox):** intraoral vesicle in a common location.

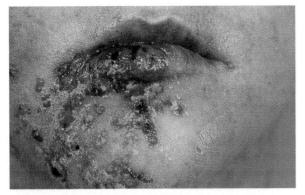

**Figure 53.3. Herpes zoster (shingles):** unilateral eruption along the mandibular branch of the trigeminal nerve.

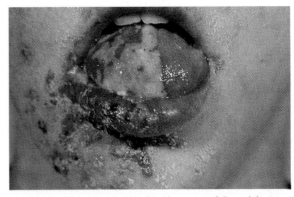

**Figure 53.4. Herpes zoster (shingles):** painful oral lesions in same patient shown in Figure 53.3.

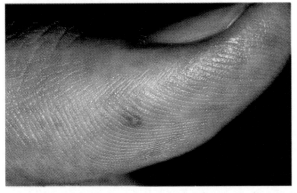

**Figure 53.5. Hand-foot-and-mouth disease:** typical pinpoint skin lesion in a young adult. (Courtesy Dr Birgit and Dr Tom Glass)

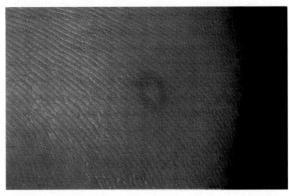

**Figure 53.6. Hand-foot-and-mouth disease:** erythematous border surrounding foot ulcer. (Courtesy Dr Birgit and Dr Tom Glass)

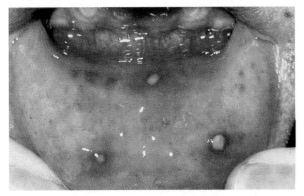

**Figure 53.7. Hand-foot-and-mouth disease** of the labial mucosa. (Courtesy Dr Birgit and Dr Tom Glass)

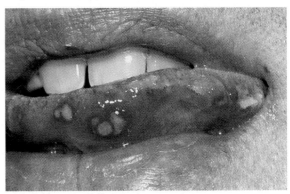

**Figure 53.8. Hand-foot-and-mouth disease:** painful clusters of vesicles that have ulcerated (same patient shown in Figures 53.5–53.8. (Courtesy Dr Birgit and Dr Tom Glass)

# Vesiculobullous Lesions

**Allergic Reactions (Figs. 54.1–54.8)** Allergy is a condition of hypersensitivity to certain substances acquired by repeated exposure to an allergen. Hypersensitivity reactions usually produce inappropriate tissue damage as a result of antigen-antibody reactions. Manifestations of allergy may be generalized or localized and may occur at any age. A genetic predisposition to allergy and persistent sensitivity are common features.

Hypersensitivity reactions have been classified into several types according to the following factors: the speed with which the symptoms occur (immediate or delayed); clinical appearance; and cellular and tissue response (type I: IgE-mediated immediate hypersensitivity; type II: antibody-dependent cytotoxic hypersensitivity; type III: complex-mediated hypersensitivity; type IV: cell-mediated, or delayed, hypersensitivity; and type V: stimulatory hypersensitivity). Reactions of clinical significance to the dentist include immediate hypersensitivity type I reactions (anaphylactic shock, urticaria, angioneurotic edema, allergic stomatitis) and delayed hypersensitivity type IV reactions (contact allergy).

**Localized Anaphylaxis (Figs. 54.1 and 54.2)** Localized anaphylaxis is an immediate allergic response mediated by IgE and histamine that occurs within minutes of exposure to an antigen. The localized condition produces vasodilation and increased permeability of superficial blood vessels, tissue swelling, and pruritis. Forms of localized anaphylaxis include individual wheals, urticaria or hives that arise after the ingestion of such foods as shellfish, citrus fruits, peanuts, chocolate, or systematically administered drugs.

**Generalized Anaphylaxis** Generalized anaphylaxis is an immediate and potentially life-threatening (type I) hypersensitivity reaction. It results from an antigen-antibody (IgE) interaction that produces mast cell degranulation and the release of vasoactive amines and mediators such as histamine. In fulminant cases, a generalized increase in vascular permeability and smooth-muscle contraction causes urticaria, dyspnea, hypotension, laryngeal edema, and vascular collapse. Mild localized immediate hypersensitivity reactions are treated with antihistamines, whereas epinephrine 1:1000 (0.3 mL–0.5 mL, subcutaneously) is required to effectively manage severe generalized anaphylactic reactions. Treatment should always include the elimination of the allergen.

**Allergic Stomatitis (Fig. 54.3)** Allergic stomatitis, also called allergic mucositis, is an oral type I hypersensitivity reaction to a systematically administered drug or food. The oral manifestations of drug-related eruptions are varied and may be clinically similar to erythema multiforme, lichen planus, or lupus erythematosus. In the mouth, a dry, glistening, red area is usually apparent. Focal white areas may be adjacent. The formation of multiple vesicles that break down and produce fibrin-covered ulcers eventually results. An erythematous, inflammatory border and a painful, burning sensation are common. The response may be limited to the buccal mucosa, gingiva, labial mucosa, lips, or tongue or may involve the entire oral cavity. Concurrent dermal lesions are possible. Treatment requires withdrawal of the allergen and administration of antihistamines.

**Angioedema (see Fig 36.1)** Angioedema is a hypersensitivity reaction characterized by the accumulation of serum within tissues, usually brought about by histamine-mediated vasodilation. Hereditary and acquired forms exist; the former is more serious because of possible visceral involvement. Swelling is the most prominent feature of angioedema. It appears rapidly and lasts for 24 to 36 hours. Sensations of warmth, tenseness, and itchiness are concurrent. The perioral and periorbital tissues are commonly affected. See page 66 for full discussion.

**Delayed Hypersensitivity (Figs. 54.4 and 54.5)** Delayed hypersensitivity or type IV hypersensitivity is a response of the immune system to a locally or systemically introduced allergen that usually develops slowly and reaches its maximum 24–48 hours after antigenic exposure. Topically applied allergens such as latex gloves or chemical disinfectants may produce a delayed hypersensitivity response evident as itchy, erythematous skin lesions (contact dermatitis) that eventually become inflamed and ulcerated at the site of contact. Delayed hypersensitivity is best treated with corticosteroids.

**Contact Stomatitis (Figs. 54.6 and 54.7)** Contact stomatitis is a form of delayed hypersensitivity that may occur at any intraoral mucosal site. It characteristically produces erythema at the site of contact with the topical allergen. Reactions to lipstick or sunscreen preparations may cause the lips to appear red, swollen, fissured, or dry; a sensation of burning may be present. Antiseptics, antibiotic lozenges, topical anesthetics, eugenol preparations, and mouthwashes may produce similar burning lesions. These appear on the alveolar mucosa, dorsum of the tongue, or palate as erythematous ulcers that are covered by a gray-white pseudomembrane. Cast alloy restorations and partial denture frameworks that contain heavy metals such as cobalt, mercury, nickel, or silver can also induce delayed hypersensitivity reactions of the mucosa adjacent to the restored area. The area is usually red and ulcerated and often burns. Allergy to the free monomer in dentures, once thought to be a common occurrence, is now known to be rare.

**Plasma Cell Gingivitis (Fig. 54.8)** Plasma cell gingivitis affects the gingiva, producing diffusely edematous and fiery red gingiva because of the flavoring ingredients (such as cinnamon) in some toothpastes and chewing gums. The lips and commissures are frequently involved, resulting in cheilitis. Microscopy shows that the tissue is infiltrated with plasma cells, a type of differentiated B cell that produces antibodies.

# Vesiculobullous Lesions

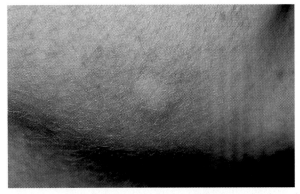

Figure 54.1. Immediate (type 1) hypersensitivity: wheal on the cheek developing immediately after the ingestion of Chinese food. (Courtesy Dr Michele Saunders)

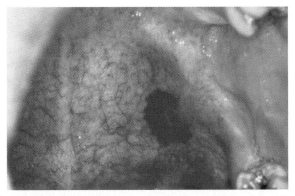

Figure 54.2. Immediate (type 1) hypersensitivity: bee-sting-induced palatal erythema. (Courtesy Dr Carson Mader)

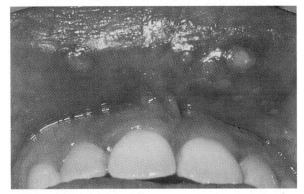

Figure 54.3. Immediate (type 1) hypersensitivity: allergic stomatitis, reaction to penicillin.

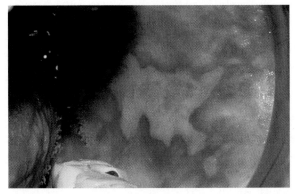

Figure 54.4. Delayed (type IV) hypersensitivity: lichenoid drug eruption with ulcerations that resolved after discontinuation of thiazide therapy.

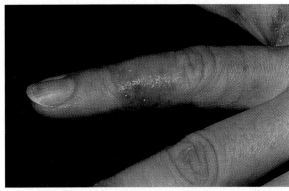

Figure 54.5. Delayed (type IV) hypersensitivity: contact dermatitis in a dental health care worker.

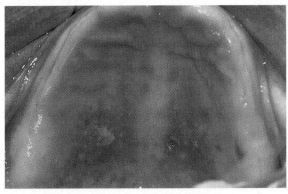

Figure 54.6. Delayed (type IV) hypersensitivity: contact stomatitis, an erythematous reaction to benzocaine.

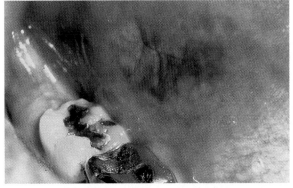

Figure 54.7. Delayed (type IV) hypersensitivity: contact stomatitis, a pigmented reaction to nickel in the adjacent cast alloy.

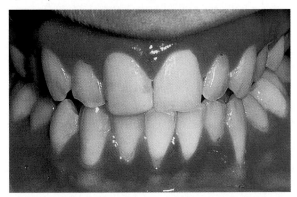

Figure 54.8. Plasma cell gingivitis: a form of delayed (type IV) hypersensitivity with red inflamed attached gingiva. (Courtesy Dr Steve Bricker)

# Vesiculobullous Lesions

**Erythema Multiforme** Erythema multiforme is a vesiculobullous disease of varied involvement of the skin and mucous membranes. It commonly affects young adults, particularly males, but may affect children and the elderly. Low-grade fever, malaise, and headache typically precede the emergence of lesions by 3–7 days. The cause is unknown. However, accumulating evidence suggests that circulating immune complexes that provoke complement-mediated cytopathic effects, combined with lymphocyte- and neutrophil-stimulated vascular injury, play a pathogenic role. Precipitating factors include infections with bacterial, fungal, and viral organisms such as herpes simplex and *Mycoplasma pneumoniae*; emotional stress; and allergy, especially to drugs containing sulfa or barbiturates. In about 50% of cases herpes simplex virus DNA has been identified in diseased tissue.

Erythema multiforme can be classified into four types according to its spectrum of clinical presentations. An association between ingested drugs and increasing severity of erythema multiforme has been recognized.

## Oral Erythema Multiforme (Figs. 55.1 and 55.2)

Oral erythema multiforme is the minimal manifestation of erythema multiforme. It is usually limited to the gingiva, but eruptions may also affect the tongue, lips or palate. A history of infection or drug therapy is common. Constitutional symptoms such as anorexia, malaise, and low-grade fever may or may not be present. As the name multiforme suggests, the lesions have a varied appearance. Affected gingiva appears fiery red, similar to the appearance of desquamative gingivitis, whereas mucosal surfaces of the tongue and lips often show several discrete irregular and bilateral ulcers. The borders of lesions are erythematous but seldom hemorrhagic, as is seen in pemphigoid, pemphigus and other forms of erythema multiforme.

## Erythema Multiforme (Fig. 55.3)

The hallmarks of classic erythema multiforme are the red-white, concentric, ring-like macules termed "target," "bulls-eye," or "iris" lesions that rapidly appear on the extensor surfaces of the arms, legs, knees, and palms of the hands. The trunk of the body is classically exempt from lesions, except in the most severe cases. The skin lesions are initially small, red, circular macules that vary in size from 0.5 to 2.0 cm in diameter. The macules then enlarge and develop a pale white or central clear area. Shortly thereafter the lesions form vesicles and bullae. The vesicles may go unnoticed until they rupture and become confluent forming large, raw, and shallow ulcers with erythematous borders. A necrotic slough and a fibrinous pseudomembrane typically cover the ulcers. Urticarial plaques that do not break down may also be present.

In the mouth, red macular areas, multiple ulcerations, and erosions with a gray-white fibrinous surface may be seen. These are generally limited to the buccal mucosa, labial mucosa, or tongue or involve all of those areas. The gingiva and palate are sometimes involved. Dark red-brown, hemorrhagic crusts are characteristically present on the lips, which helps establish the diagnosis. Lesions are usually short-lived and last about 2 weeks. Erythema multiforme rarely persists for more than 1 month. Recurrent and chronic forms exist but are rare.

Pain is the most common symptom. Oral hygiene may be neglected, resulting in secondary bacterial infection. Treatment consists of topical palliative rinses and, in some instances, low-dose systemic steroids. Complications resulting from erythema multiforme are uncommon unless the disease progresses to its major form, Stevens-Johnson syndrome.

## Stevens-Johnson Syndrome (Erythema Multiforme Major) (Figs. 55.4–55.6)

A severe form of erythema multiforme is termed erythema multiforme major or Stevens-Johnson syndrome, named for the two investigators who first described the clinical appearance of the disease in the early 1920s. It frequently affects children and young adults, predominantly males. The oral signs of Stevens-Johnson syndrome are similar to those of erythema multiforme; however the former is characterized by more widespread involvement of cutaneous and stomatologic structures, and more constitutional signs such as fever, malaise, headache, cough, chest pain, diarrhea, vomiting, and arthralgia.

The classic clinical triad of Stevens-Johnson syndrome consists of eye lesions (conjunctivitis), genital lesions (balanitis, vulvovaginitis), and stomatitis. Other features include the characteristic target skin lesions on the face, chest, and abdomen that later develop into painful "weeping" vesiculobullous lesions. Like erythema multiforme, the gingiva is less commonly affected by desquamating bullae than is the nonkeratinized mucosa. Extensive ulcerative and hemorrhagic lesions of the lips and denuded areas of oral mucosa are intensely painful and usually prevent affected patients from eating and swallowing. Inadequate nutritional intake, dehydration, and debilitation are common sequelae that necessitate hospitalization. Healing takes about 6 weeks.

## Toxic Epidermal Necrolysis (Figs. 55.7 and 55.8)

Toxic epidermal necrolysis is the most severe form of erythema multiforme. Its occurrence is rare, and most cases are associated with drug therapy. Unlike other forms of erythema multiforme, older persons are most commonly affected, especially women. The condition primarily affects the skin, eyes, and oral mucosa; the skin manifestations are especially severe. Large areas of the skin form coalescing bullae that eventually slough, leaving huge areas of denuded skin. Management is similar to that of a burn patient. Significant morbidity will occur if supportive therapy is not provided. Treatment consists of intravenous fluid, nutritional therapy, corticosteroids, anesthetic and antiseptic rinses, and prevention of secondary infection with antibiotics. All of the affected areas take longer to heal, and permanent eye damage is a frequent outcome. Both Stevens-Johnson syndrome and toxic epidermal necrolysis have been fatal.

# Vesiculobullous Lesions

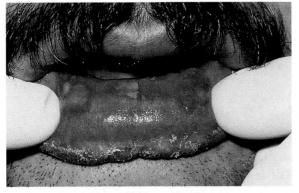

Figure 55.1. Erythema multiforme: irregular ulcers of the lips. (Courtesy Dr John McDowell)

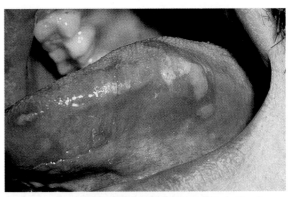

Figure 55.2. Erythema multiforme: ulcers of lateral and ventral tongue. (Courtesy Dr John McDowell)

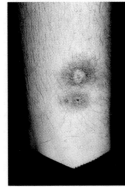

Figure 55.3. Erythema multiforme: classic "target" or "iris" skin lesion. (Courtesy Dr Tom McDavid)

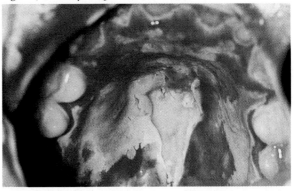

Figure 55.4. Stevens-Johnson syndrome: extensive, multicolored ulcerations of palate. (Courtesy Dr Tom McDavid)

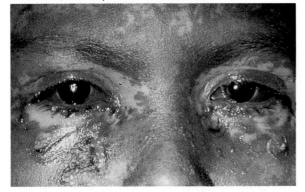

Figure 55.5. Stevens-Johnson syndrome: severe conjunctivitis and weeping skin lesions. (Courtesy Dr Tom McDavid)

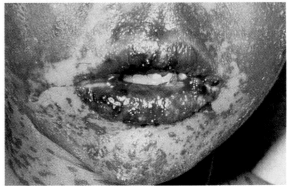

Figure 55.6. Stevens-Johnson syndrome: hemorrhagic and crusted lips of same child shown in Figure 55.5. (Courtesy Dr Tom McDavid)

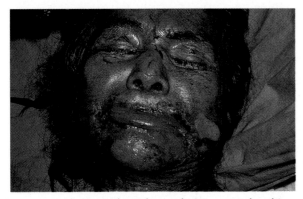

Figure 55.7. Toxic epidermal necrolysis: severe sloughing of facial skin. (Courtesy Dr Eric Kraus and Dr Herman Corrales)

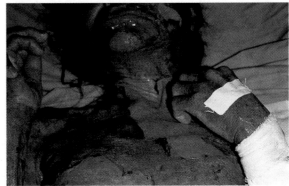

Figure 55.8. Toxic epidermal necrolysis: general sloughing of skin that resulted in dehydration (same patient shown in Figure 55.7) (Courtesy Dr Eric Kraus and Dr. Herman Corrales).

# Vesiculobullous Lesions

**Pemphigus Vulgaris (Figs. 56.1–56.4)** Pemphigus is a potentially fatal, vesiculobullous disease that has been categorized into four types: **vulgaris** and **vegetans,** which have intraoral manifestations, and **foliaceous** and **erythematosus,** which generally do not. Pemphigus vulgaris, the most common type of intraoral pemphigus, usually develops between the ages of 30 and 50 years; it may be seen in younger or older patients but rarely develops in patients older than 60 years. It is seen with equal frequency in men and women and is usually encountered in light-pigmented patients of Jewish or Mediterranean origin. Acute and chronic forms exist; the slow chronic form is the most common.

Pemphigus vulgaris involves autoimmune destruction of the pericellular adherence (cadherin) proteins that compose the desmosome. Cadherins are the intercellular glue-like substance that hold epithelial cells together. Their destruction causes cell-to-cell separation, particularly a separation of the basal cell layer from the stratum spinosum. This pathologic process produces multiple bullae that tend to rupture and leave erosions of the skin and oral mucous membranes. Lesions develop rapidly and in their early form consist of weeping bullae or clear gelatinous plaques. The bullae are extremely fragile and rapidly disintegrate, bleed, and crust. They tend to recur in the same area and later spread to adjacent regions. Light lateral pressure applied to a bulla causes it to enlarge by extension (Nikolsky's sign). A characteristic mucosal finding is the appearance of a whitish superficial covering, which is the roof of a collapsed bulla that can be easily stripped away. Desquamation of tissue is sometimes limited to the gingiva.

Pemphigus may appear as an epithelial slough with white tissue folds or as an aphthous or traumatic ulcer. It may also involve the lips, buccal mucosa, tongue, gingiva, palate, and oropharynx and resemble erythema multiforme. Individual lesions often have circular or serpiginous borders, whereas extensive erosions of the buccal mucosa are red and raw and have diffuse irregular borders. Frequent eruptions may be superimposed over healing lesions so that periods of remission are absent. The tongue is less commonly involved than other sites. Thick hemorrhagic lip crusts and fetor oris are characteristic of extensive disease. Severe pain is common.

The diagnosis of pemphigus is confirmed by positive Nikolsky's sign, biopsy, and immunofluorescent staining. Early recognition of oral lesions, which usually precede skin involvement by several months, is important because early diagnosis greatly enhances the initiation of treatment and the prognosis. Before the advent of corticosteroid and immunosuppressive therapy, dehydration and septicemia were fatal complications of this disease.

**Bullous Pemphigoid and Cicatricial (Benign Mucous Membrane) Pemphigoid (Figs. 56.5–56.8)** Pemphigoid is a chronic, self-limiting autoimmune disease of mucocutaneous structures that involves the oral cavity in about 90% of cases. It is more common in the oral cavity than is pemphigus but is associated with much less morbidity and mortality. Pemphigoid is caused by separation of the epithelium from the basement membrane. Two types of pemphigoid exist: bullous and cicatricial pemphigoid. They produce identical oral lesions and are distinguished by clinical and immunohistologic features.

Bullous pemphigoid, the less common of the two, affects both the skin and the oral cavity and has no sex or racial predilection. Skin folds of the axilla, inguinal, and abdominal regions are commonly affected. The disease occurs when autoantibodies (IgG or IgM) bind and destroy a 220-kilodalton basement protein within the hemidesmosome of the epithelium attachment apparatus. Detached epithelium separates from the connective tissue at the level of the lamina lucida and exposes the connective tissue.

Cicatricial pemphigoid is also called benign mucous membrane pemphigoid. It is limited to the mucous membranes and favors the ocular and oral mucosal membranes. It occurs twice as frequently in women than men and usually develops after age 50 years. Younger persons are sometimes affected. There is no racial predilection, and the antigen for cicatricial pemphigoid has not yet been identified.

Pemphigoid skin lesions usually precede oral lesions, tend to be desquamative and localized, and heal spontaneously. The lips are rarely affected. Intraoral bullae are usually small tense blebs that are yellow or hemorrhagic. They form slowly and tend to favor the palate, gingiva, and buccal mucosa. Because bullae of pemphigoid result from a subepithelial separation, they are thicker-walled, less fragile, and longer-lasting than those of pemphigus. Some patients may have bullae that persist for several days before rupture. Large, shallow ulcers can result from coalescence of several adjacent lesions. The ulcers are surrounded by an erythematous ring. They exhibit a symmetrical and curvilinear pattern and occasionally bleed.

When the condition is limited to the gingiva, which occurs frequently, the clinical term desquamative gingivitis has been used to describe the bright red, burning, and denuded gingiva. Desquamative gingivitis is a descriptive term and may represent several clinically similar conditions, such as erosive lichen planus, oral erythema multiforme, pemphigoid and pemphigus, for which a diagnosis has not yet been obtained.

Cicatricial pemphigoid may affect the anal, vaginal, and pharyngeal mucosa, but the most severe complication is ocular involvement producing conjunctivitis, occasional bullae, clouding of the cornea, and fibrous scarring. Blindness is a serious sequela of protracted eye disease. Although the condition is rarely fatal, close follow-up is suggested for progressive cases because rare reports of carcinoma of the rectum and uterus have been associated with pemphigoid. Moderate doses of corticosteriods, alone or in conjunction with immunosuppressive agents such as azathioprine, have provided effective management.

# Vesiculobullous Lesions

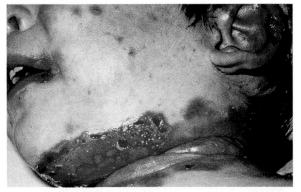

Figure 56.1. Pemphigus vulgaris: young child with extensive skin and oral erosions.

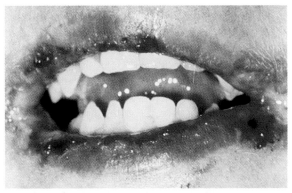

Figure 56.2. Pemphigus vulgaris: hemorrhagic lip crusts of same child shown in Figure 56.1.

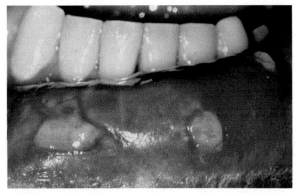

Figure 56.3. Pemphigus vulgaris: rare, intact bullae on labial mucosa. (Courtesy Dr Tom McDavid and Dr Martin Tyler)

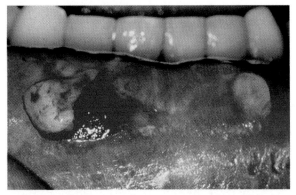

Figure 56.4. Pemphigus vulgaris: ruptured bullae in same patient shown in Figure 56.3. (Courtesy Dr Tom McDavid and Dr Martin Tyler)

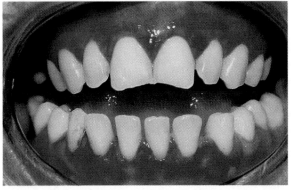

Figure 56.5. Cicatricial pemphigoid: manifesting solely as desquamative gingivitis.

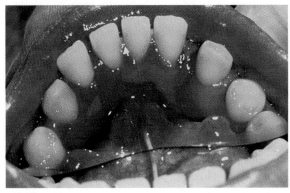

Figure 56.6. Cicatricial pemphigoid: whitish slough in desquamative gingivitis (same patient shown in Figure 56.5).

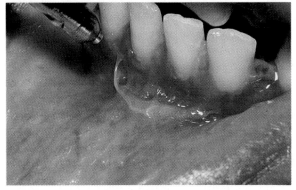

Figure 56.7. Cicatricial pemphigoid: positive Nikolsky's sign in same patient shown in Figures 56.5 and 56.6.

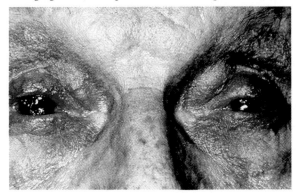

Figure 56.8. Cicatricial pemphigoid: corneal and conjunctival scarring.

# Ulcerative Lesions

**Traumatic Ulcer (Figs. 57.1–57.3)** Recurrent oral ulceration is a common condition caused by several factors, primarily trauma. Ulcers may occur at any age and in either sex. Likely locations for traumatic ulcers are the labial mucosa, buccal mucosa, palate, and peripheral borders of the tongue.

Traumatic ulcers may result from chemicals, heat, electricity, or mechanical force and are often classified according to the exact nature of the insult. Pressure from an ill-fitting denture base or flange or from a partial denture framework is a source of a decubitous or pressure ulcer. Trophic, or ischemic ulcers, occur particularly on the palate at the site of a previous injection. Dental injections have also been implicated in the traumatic ulcerations seen on the lower lip by children who chew their lip after dental appointments. In addition to factitial injury, young children and infants are prone to traumatic ulcers of the soft palate from thumb sucking, called Bednar's aphthae.

Ulcers may be precipitated by contact with a fractured tooth or restoration, a partial denture clasp, or inadvertent biting of the mucosa. The palate is often burned by food or drinks that are too hot. Other traumatic ulcers are caused by factitial injury from inappropriate use of fingernails or other objects on the oral mucosa. The diagnosis of these conditions is simple and is often established from a careful history and examination of the physical findings.

The appearance of a mechanically induced traumatic ulcer varies according to the intensity and size of the agent. The ulcer usually appears slightly depressed and oval. An erythematous zone is initially found at the periphery; the zone progressively lightens because of the keratinization process. The center of the ulcer is usually yellow-gray. Chemically damaged mucosa, such as that seen with an aspirin burn, is less well defined and contains a loosely adherent, coagulated white surface slough. After removal of the traumatic influence, the ulcer should heal within 2 weeks; if healing does not occur, other causes should be suspected and a biopsy should be performed.

**Recurrent Aphthous Stomatitis (Minor Aphthae, Aphthous Ulcer) (Figs. 57.4–57.6)** Recurrent aphthous stomatitis is classified into three categories according to size: minor aphthae, major aphthae, and herpetiform ulcers. Approximately 20% of the population is afflicted with minor aphthae, or canker sores as they are commonly called. They may be seen in anyone, but females and young adults are slightly more susceptible. Familial patterns have been demonstrated, and persons who smoke are less frequently affected than nonsmokers. Factors that precipitate aphthae include atopy, trauma, endocrinopathies, menstruation, nutritional deficiencies, stress, and food allergies. Although the cause is unknown, studies suggest an immunopathic process involving cell-mediated cytolytic activity in response to human leukocyte antigen or foreign antigens. The L-form of streptococcus has been suggested to play a causal role, as has thinned mucosa for presentation of antigens to Langerhans' cells.

Minor aphthous ulcers have a propensity for movable mucosa that is situated over minor salivary gland tissue. The labial and buccal mucosa are frequently affected, whereas ulcers are rarely seen on heavily keratinized mucosa such as the gingiva and hard palate. Prodromal symptoms of paresthesia or hyperesthesia are sometimes reported.

Minor aphthae appear as shallow, yellow-gray, oval ulcers usually about 3–10 mm in diameter. A prominent erythematous border surrounds the fibrinous pseudomembrane. No vesicle formation is seen in this disease, a distinctive diagnostic feature. Ulcers that occur along the mucobuccal fold often appear more elongated.

Burning is a preliminary symptom that is followed by intense pain lasting a few days. Tender submandibular, anterior cervical, and parotid lymph nodes are often present, particularly when the ulcer becomes secondarily infected.

Aphthae are invariably recurrent, and the pattern of occurrence varies. Most persons exhibit single ulcers once or twice a year, beginning during childhood or adolescence. The ulcers occasionally appear in crops, but usually fewer than five occur at one time. The ulcers usually heal spontaneously without scar formation within 14 days. Some patients have multiple ulcers over a period of several months. In these cases, ulcers are in various stages of erupting and healing and produce constant pain.

Although no medication has been totally successful for treating aphthous stomatitis, patients have responded to topical corticosteroids and coagulating and cauterizing agents.

**Pseudoaphthous (Figs. 57.7 and 57.8)** Pseudoaphthae, a term coined by Binney, refers to recurrent, aphthous-like mucosal ulcers of the mouth that are associated with nutritional deficiency states. Studies indicate that 20% of patients with recurrent aphthous stomatitis are deficient in folic acid, iron, or vitamin $B_{12}$. Pseudoaphthae are frequently seen with inflammatory bowel disease, Crohn's disease, gluten intolerance, and pernicious anemia.

Pseudoaphthae resemble both minor and major aphthous ulcers but are characteristically more persistent. There is a slight predilection for women between the ages of 25 and 50 years. The ulcers are depressed, rounded, and painful and are sometimes multiple in number. The borders may be raised, firm, and irregular, but induration is seldom encountered. Alterations of the tongue papillae may suggest an underlying nutritional deficiency state. Healing is slow, and patients may report that they are rarely free of ulceration. Chronic and persistent presence of aphthous ulcers necessitates evaluation for nutritional deficiencies, including hematologic studies. If the laboratory results are abnormal, a medical referral is required.

# Ulcerative Lesions

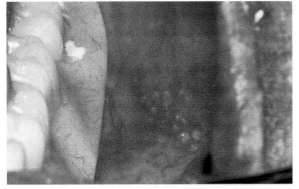

Figure 57.1. Traumatic ulcer: denture flange-induced.

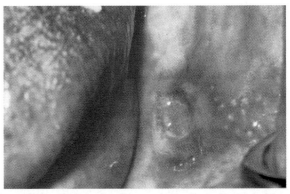

Figure 57.2. Traumatic ulcer: same patient shown in Figure 57.1.

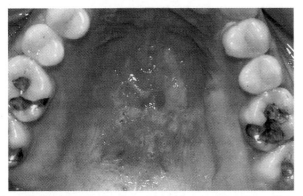

Figure 57.3. Traumatic ulcer caused by the ingestion of burning-hot food. (Courtesy Dr Donna Wood)

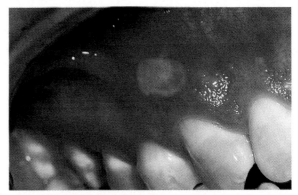

Figure 57.4. Aphthous: ulcer on the alveolar mucosa at the junction with the attached gingiva.

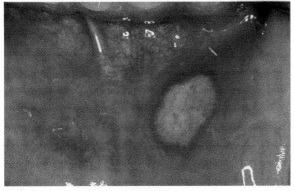

Figure 57.5. Aphthous: ulcer with prominent red border on labial mucosa. (Courtesy Dr Tom Schiff)

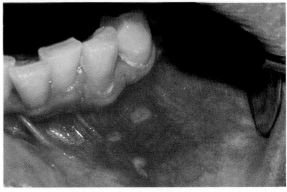

Figure 57.6. Aphthae: a clustering of ulcers with varying shapes.

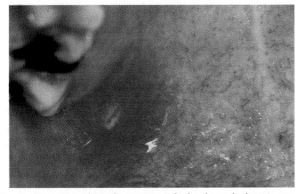

Figure 57.7. Pseudoapthous: irregularly shaped ulcer in a patient with Crohn's disease. (Courtesy Dr Donna Wood)

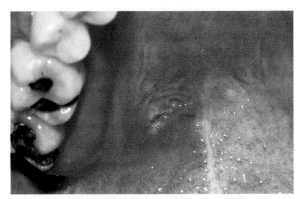

Figure 57.8. Pseudoaphthae: several ulcers with corrugations in a patient with Crohn's disease.

# Ulcerative Lesions

## Major Aphthous (Periadenitis Mucosa Necrotica Recurrens, Sutton's Disease, Scarifying Stomatitis, Recurrent Scarring Aphthous) (Figs. 58.1–58.4)

Major aphthous is an exaggerated variant of minor aphthous that produces larger (> 1 cm) and more destructive ulcers that last longer and recur more frequently. The cause is unknown; some suggest that an immune defect is involved. Others speculate that the large ulcer is a severe form of recurrent aphthous stomatitis that results from the coalescence of several smaller ulcers. Young women with anxious personality traits are most commonly affected.

Major aphthous ulcerations are often multiple. They involve the soft palate, tonsillar fauces, labial and buccal mucosa, and tongue and occasionally extend onto the attached gingiva. Characteristically, the ulcers are asymmetric and unilateral. The most prominent feature is the large size together with a depressed, necrotic center. A red raised inflammatory border is common. Depending on size, traumatic influences, and secondary infection, ulcers may last from several weeks to months. Because the ulcers erode deep into the connective tissue, they heal with scar formation and tissue distortion. Muscle destruction can result in tissue fenestration; if the periodontium is involved, loss of tissue attachment may occur. Extreme pain and lymphadenopathy are common symptoms.

Use of steroids can accelerate healing and reduce scarring. Ulcers similar to those of periadenitis mucosa necrotica recurrens are seen with some frequency in association with cyclic neutropenia, agranulocytosis, and gluten intolerance. Ulcers located on the tongue may strongly resemble carcinoma. The presence of scarring is of diagnostic importance to rule out a malignant condition.

## Herpetiform Ulceration (Figs. 58.5 and 58.6)

Herpetiform ulceration is a type of recurrent focal ulceration of the oral mucosa that clinically resembles the ulcers seen in primary herpes (hence the name herpetiform). This condition, however, is probably a variant form of recurrent aphthous ulceration. The prominent feature of the disease is the numerous, pinhead-sized, gray-white erosions that enlarge, coalesce, and become ill defined. The ulcers are initially 1–2 mm in diameter and occur in clusters of 10–100. The mucosa adjacent to the ulcer is erythematous, and pain is a predictable symptom.

Any part of the oral mucosa may be affected by herpetiform ulcerations, but the anterior tip of the tongue, margins of the tongue, and labial mucosa are particularly affected. The smaller size of these ulcerations distinguishes them from aphthae, and the absence of vesicles and gingivitis together with their frequent and recurrent nature distinguishes them from primary herpes and other oral viral infections. Virus cannot be cultured from these lesions, and the ulcers are not contagious.

The first episode of herpetiform ulceration usually occurs in patients in their late twenties and thirties, 10 years after the peak incidence of aphthae. The duration of recurrent attacks is variable and unpredictable; some patients have constant lesions for months. The cause has yet to be determined. Recurrent herpetiform ulcerations respond especially well to tetracycline suspensions, and the condition often regresses spontaneously after several years.

## Behçet's Syndrome (Oculo-Oral-Genital Syndrome) (Figs. 58.7 and 58.8)

Behçet's syndrome, named for the Turkish physician who first described the ulcerative disorder, principally involves the eye, oral cavity, and genitals. For this reason it has been categorized as a triple-symptom complex with ulcerative manifestations. In the disorder's fully developed state, cutaneous lesions, arthritis of the major joints, gastrointestinal ulcerations, neurologic manifestations, and thrombophlebitis can be seen, although rarely are all components present in the same patient. The syndrome appears to be the result of a delayed hypersensitivity reaction, immune complexes, and vasculitis triggered by the presentation of human leukocyte antigens or environmental antigens, such as viruses, bacteria, chemicals, and heavy metals.

Behçet's syndrome is two to three times more prevalent in males than in females and develops between the ages of 20 and 30 years. Persons from Asia, the Mediterranean coast, and Great Britain are most commonly affected.

Eye manifestations of Behçet's syndrome include photophobia, conjunctivitis, and chronic recurrent iritis with hypopyon that occasionally leads to blindness. Ocular manifestations may be concurrent with or occur years after oral and genital ulcers. Skin changes are characterized by subcutaneous nodules and macular and papular eruptions that vesiculate, ulcerate, and encrustate. Genital ulcers may involve the mucosa or skin and tend to be smaller and less common than the oral lesions.

Oral ulcers, the most prevalent lesion of Behçet's syndrome, may be the initial sign of the disease. One, a few, or crops of aphthous-like ulcers on the buccal or labial mucosa are characteristic, but any oral mucosal site may be involved. Similar to aphthous, the ulcers are flat, shallow, oval, and variable in size. Small lesions tend to occur more frequently than larger lesions. A serofibrinous exudate covers the surface, and the margins are red and well demarcated. Patients frequently report pain, and recurrent periods of exacerbation and remissions are characteristic. Topical and systemic steroids are used to treat the symptoms of patients with limited mucocutaneous involvement. Protracted disease involving the neuro-ocular structures requires the care of a physician. Azathioprine, cyclophosphamide, thalidomide, and colchicine have been used successfully in select cases. All of these agents have potentially serious side effects.

# Ulcerative Lesions

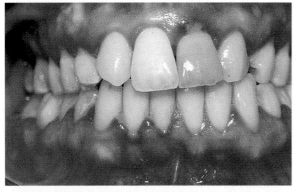

**Figure 58.1. Major aphthous:** persistent ulcers on the marginal and attached gingiva.

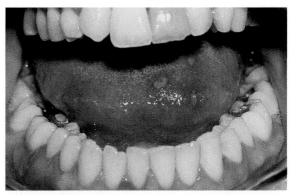

**Figure 58.2. Major aphthous:** multiple, irregular tongue ulcers.

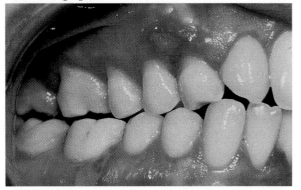

**Figure 58.3. Major aphthous:** deep, painful ulcers on the attached gingiva.

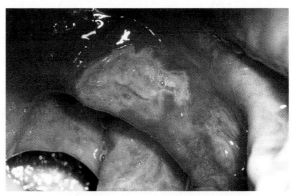

**Figure 58.4. Major aphthous:** large irregular ulcer of the soft palate (same patient shown in Figures 58.1–58.3).

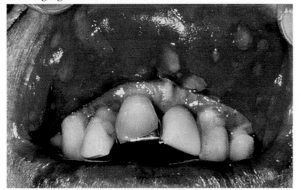

**Figure 58.5. Herpetiform ulceration:** hundreds of small and large ulcers of the labial mucosa and gingiva. (Courtesy Dr Geza Terezhalmy)

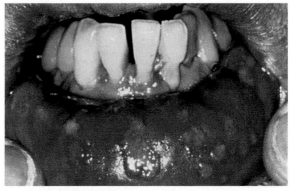

**Figure 58.6. Herpetiform ulcerations:** same patient shown in Figure 58.5. (Courtesy Dr. Geza Terezhalmy)

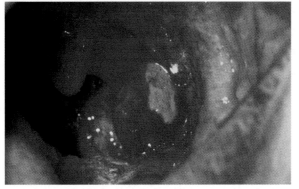

**Figure 58.7. Behçet's syndrome:** a 27-year-old man with tonsillar pillar ulceration. (Courtesy Dr Geza Terezhalmy)

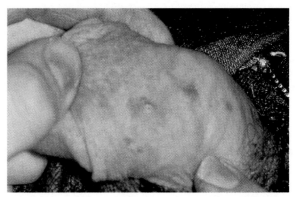

**Figure 58.8. Behçet's syndrome:** multiple genital ulcers in the same patient shown in Figure 58.7. (Courtesy Dr Geza Terezhalmy)

# Ulcerative Lesions

**Granulomatous Ulcer (Figs. 59.1 and 59.2)** Two common granulomatous infections that may produce oral ulcers are **tuberculosis** and **histoplasmosis**. These are rare lesions that are usually found in older adults after the disease is far advanced. Because of underlying disorders such as the acquired immune deficiency syndrome, a younger population group is affected. Pulmonary lesions often precede oral lesions; thus, the pulmonary symptom of persistent cough is an important historic finding.

Dissemination of organisms from the lungs to the mouth via infected sputum can result in oral infection. Oral tuberculosis and histoplasmosis infection are characterized by ulceration. These ulcers may occur on any mucosal surface; however, tuberculous lesions occur preferentially on the dorsum of the tongue and labial mucosa at the commissure. The clinical picture varies, and the ulcer may resemble a traumatic ulcer or epidermoid carcinoma, particularly when the lesion is located on the lateral border of the tongue. Lesions on the alveolar ridge often resemble a granulating extraction site. The center of the granulomatous ulcer is necrotic and yellow-gray or even bluish and is depressed several millimeters. The peripheral region of the ulcer is undulating or lumpy and has been described as cobblestoned. The margin of the lesion is irregular, well demarcated, and undermined. Nodular and vegetative components are often seen in conjunction with the ulcers of histoplasmosis. Cervical lymphadenopathy is a common finding. Depending on the location and irritating factors, some patients rarely report pain; in these patients the discovery may be an incidental finding. Other patients experience severe, unremitting discomfort. Tuberculous and histoplasmosis lesions are contagious, and active organisms can be transmitted under appropriate conditions.

A biopsy or culturing is required to confirm the diagnosis. Histologic features and special stains demonstrate the presence of the causative organisms. Treatment of the primary lung problem is with specific long-term antibiotics: for tuberculosis, isoniazid, rifampin, pyrazinamide for histoplasmosis, amphotericin B is administered. The primary lung problem should be treated before dental treatment.

**Squamous Cell Carcinoma (Figs. 59.3–59.6)** Squamous cell carcinoma often appears as an ulcer. In the early stages the condition is usually small, nonpainful, and nonulcerative; however, the persistent nature of the disease results in neoplastic proliferation that soon exhausts the blood supply, resulting in surface telangiectasia and eventual ulcer formation. Older ulcers tend to be large and crateriform, covered by a central yellow-gray necrotic slough. Red, raw foci are frequent; the borders are firm, raised, and sometimes fungating.

Carcinomas may occur anywhere in the mouth. The most common sites are the posterior third of the lateral margin of the tongue and the floor of the mouth. Associated features may include pain, numbness, leukoplakia, erythroplakia, induration, fixation, and lymphadenopathy. Metastatic lymphadenopathy is characterized by nonpainful rubbery or hard nodes that are fixed at the base and matted together. Excessive use of alcohol and tobacco by the patient should heighten the examiner's suspicion of oral carcinoma when a persistent ulcer does not heal within 14 days. Biopsy should be performed by the clinician, who provides the definitive treatment.

**Chemotherapeutic Ulcer (Figs. 59.7 and 59.8)** Patients receiving immunosuppressant drugs for a variety of serious illnesses, including organ transplantation, autoimmune conditions, and neoplasia, may develop oral ulcerations and stomatitis. Side effects of the chemotherapeutic drug may be directly or indirectly harmful to the oral mucosa. Antimetabolites such as methotrexate inhibit the replication of rapidly reproducing cells, including the oral epithelium, whereas alkaloids such as cyclophosphamide induce leukopenia and secondary ulcer formation.

The chemotherapeutic ulcer, an early sign of drug toxicity, appears during the second week of therapy and usually persists for 2 weeks. These ulcers may occur on any oral mucosal site. The lips, buccal mucosa, tongue, floor of the mouth, and palate are affected most frequently. The area is initially red and burns. The surface epithelium is lost and a large, deep, necrotic, and painful ulcer then forms. The margins of the ulcer are irregular, and the characteristic red inflammatory border is often not present because of the lack of an inflammatory response by the host. If the pain becomes severe and the intake of adequate nutrition and fluids is impaired, a reduction in drug dose may be necessary.

Culturing is highly recommended for all lesions because of their propensity for infection with Gram-negative organisms and fungi and because of the likelihood that the ulcers may represent recrudescence of latent herpes simplex virus. Topical anesthetics are used to minimize symptoms, whereas oral hygiene measures, including antimicrobial agents such as chlorhexidine, are critical to prevent secondary infection, soft tissue necrosis, and osseous necrosis. Consultation and open communication between the physician and the dentist can help reduce complications and promote oral comfort.

# Ulcerative Lesions

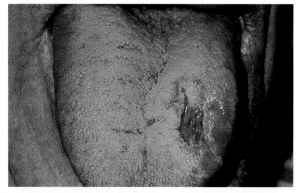

**Figure 59.1. Granulomatous ulcer** on anterior tongue caused by *Mycobacterium tuberculosis*. (Courtesy Dr Howard Birkholz)

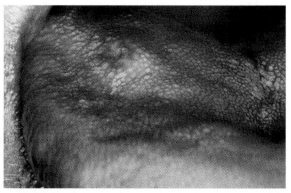

**Figure 59.2. Granulomatous ulcer** on the dorsum of the tongue: histoplasmosis. (Courtesy Dr Michael Huber)

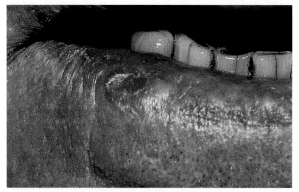

**Figure 59.3. Squamous cell carcinoma** of the lip: the margins are raised and the lesion is indurated.

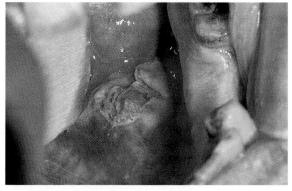

**Figure 59.4. Squamous cell carcinoma:** ulceration in the floor of the mouth. (Courtesy Dr Robert Craig)

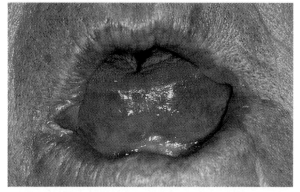

**Figure 59.5. Squamous cell carcinoma** at the labial commissure (Courtesy Dr Tom McDavid)

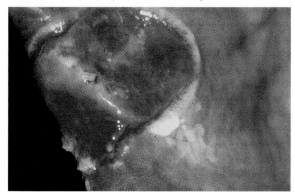

**Figure 59.6. Squamous cell carcinoma** in the same patient shown in Figure 59.5. (Courtesy Dr Tom McDavid)

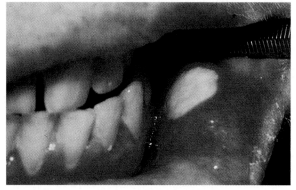

**Figure 59.7. Chemotherapy-induced ulceration** in a patient with leukemia. (Courtesy Dr Tom McDavid)

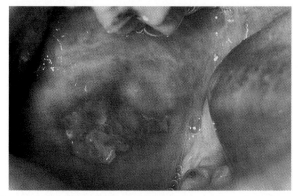

**Figure 59.8. Chemotherapy-induced ulceration** of the buccal mucosa associated with methotrexate therapy. (Courtesy Dr Jerry Cioffi)

# Section VII

# Sexually Related and Sexually Transmissible Conditions

# Sexually Related and Sexually Transmissible Conditions

**Traumatic Conditions (Figs. 60.1 and 60.2)** Injury to the lingual frenum and fellatio syndrome are common oral conditions associated with sexual activity. Ulceration of the lingual frenum may occur when the tongue is mechanically abraded against the incisal edge of the mandibular incisors during orogenital sexual activity. A white fibrinous exudate and an erythematous border are commonly seen. A history of cunnilinguis confirms the diagnosis and abstinence is recommended to permit healing. Chronic irritation may lead to secondary bacterial infection, development of leukoplakia, or a traumatic fibroma, or it may permit ingress of the human papillomavirus. Fellatio can traumatize oral soft tissues and produce erythema and submucosal hemorrhage of the soft palate. Isolated bright red petechiae initially appear, which eventually become a confluent patch that bridges the palatal midline. The purpuric lesion is painless and nonulcerative, does not blanch on diascopy, and clinically resembles the petechial patch produced by infectious mononucleosis; however, lymphadenopathy and fever are characteristically absent. Petechiae darken and fade away in about a week.

**Sexually Transmitted Pharyngitis (Figs. 60.3 and 60.4)** Venereal organisms such as herpes simplex virus type 2, *Neisseria gonorrhoeae*, and *Chlamydia trachomatis* may cause pharyngitis by transmission from direct contact with infected genital or oral secretions or lesions. Herpetic stomatitis (type II) is most prevalent after sexual activity begins, usually occurring in persons between the ages of 15 and 35 years. Limited reports indicate that primary herpes simplex virus type 2 infection produces a prominent pharyngotonsillitis and fever, whereas inflammation of the gingivae may be less severe than herpes simplex virus type 1 primary infection. Multiple small vesicles are usually apparent in the early stages; the vesicles collapse to form ulcers that resolve in 10–21 days.

Gonococcal pharyngitis may produce a diffuse erythematous throat; small pustules in the tonsillar area; or an erythematous and edematous patch involving the throat, tonsillar area, and uvula. Burning is the initial symptom, followed by increased salivary viscosity and halitosis. Other oral manifestations include painful, discrete ulcerations of the oral mucosa; fiery red and tender gingiva with or without necrosis of the interdental papilla; tongue ulcerations; and glossodynia. Penicillin G, tetracycline, and ceftriaxone regimens have been used effectively to treat this condition. *Chlamydia trachomatis* may also cause a sore, "lumpy" throat, mild pharyngitis, and tonsillar inflammation with pustule formation. The treatment of choice is tetracycline.

**Infectious Mononucleosis (Figs. 60.5 and 60.6)** Infectious mononucleosis is a relatively benign lymphocytic infection characterized by fatigue, fever, malaise, pharyngitis, stomatitis, and occasional hepatospleno-megaly. It is most commonly caused by the Epstein-Barr virus and occurs chiefly in adolescents and young adults. The disease is of low contagiousness and transmission is probably through exchange of virus-contaminated saliva during deep kissing. Oral lesions are often the earliest manifestations of infectious mononucleosis. Multiple red petechiae located at the junction of the hard and soft palate occur during the first few weeks of infection. These lesions turn brown and fade after several days. Acute ulcerative gingivitis, pharyngeal ulcerations, and erythematous exudative tonsillitis frequently develop during the acute phase of the infection. Bilateral, posterior, painful cervical lymphadenopathy is a consistent finding. Blood analysis reveals modest lymphocytosis, atypical lymphocytes, and the presence of heterophile antibiotics. Treatment is supportive and includes bed rest, soft diet, analgesics, and antipyretic agents. Recovery usually occurs within 1–2 months.

**Syphilis (Figs. 60.7 and 60.8)** Syphilis is a venereal disease caused by *Treponema pallidum*, an anareobic spirochete. The hallmark of primary oral syphilis is the nonpainful chancre, which represents a granulomatous reaction to vascular obliteration. Chancres may affect any oral soft tissue; however, the lips are the most common site of involvement, followed by the tongue, palate, gingiva, and tonsillar areas. Oral syphilis is usually observed in sexually active young men.

The syphilitic chancre initially appears as a small papule that elevates, enlarges, erodes, and becomes ulcerated. The lesion is usually punched-out, indurated, and 2 or 3 cm in diameter and lacks a red inflammatory border. The surface is covered by a yellowish, highly infectious serous discharge. Palatal erythema or an asymptomatic, reddish ulcer may be the initial lesions, along with swollen, nontender, firm, anterior cervical lymph nodes. Chancres typically persist for 2 to 4 weeks and heal spontaneously, causing patients to erroneously believe that no treatment is necessary. After a latent period of 4 weeks–6 months, the secondary stage of syphilis appears; during this stage, the patient may report headaches, lacrimation, nasal discharge, sore throat, and generalized arthralgia, together with lymphadenopathy, elevated temperature, and weight loss. A painless, symmetrical nonpruritic skin rash with notable maculo-papular palmar-plantar eruptions soon follows. Concurrent oral lesions of secondary syphilis appear as oval red macules, pharyngitis, or isolated or multiple mucous patches (painless, shallow, highly infectious ulcers surrounded by an erythematous halo). The borders are often irregular and resemble "snail tracks." Tertiary syphilis occurs in infected persons many years after nontreatment of secondary syphilis. It is primarily characterized by palatal perforation and neurologic symptoms. Parenteral penicillin G remains the drug of choice for treating all stages of syphilis.

# Sexually Related and Sexually Transmissible Conditions

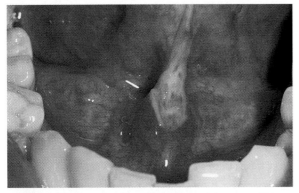

Figure 60.1. **Traumatic ulcer** of the lingual frenum. (Courtesy Dr James Cottone)

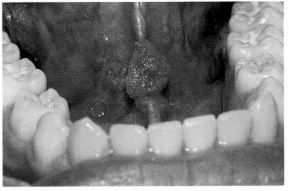

Figure 60.2. **Condyloma acuminatum** of the lingual frenum. (Courtesy Dr Marden Alder)

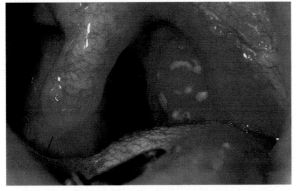

Figure 60.3. **Sexually transmitted pharyngitis:** primary herpes simplex virus type 2 infection. (Courtesy Dr James Cottone)

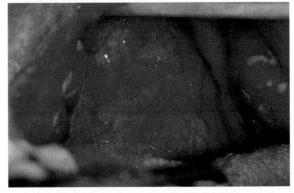

Figure 60.4. **Primary herpes virus type 2 infection:** same patient shown in Figure 60.3. Inflammation of lymphoid tissue comprising Waldyer's ring. (Courtesy Dr James Cottone)

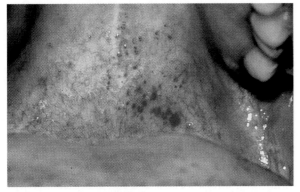

Figure 60.5. **Infectious mononucleosis:** palatal petechiae in the prodromal stage. (Courtesy Dr Geza Terezhalmy)

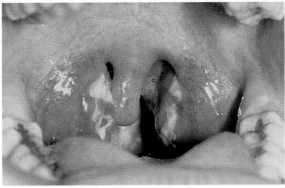

Figure 60.6. **Infectious mononucleosis:** exudative tonsillitis, same patient shown in Figure 60.5. (Courtesy Dr Geza Terezhalmy)

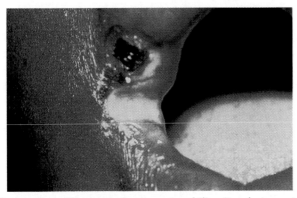

Figure 60.7. **Chancres of primary syphilis.** One lesion with hemorrhagic crust, the other with chamois-like covering without marginal inflammation. (Courtesy Dr Laurie Cohen and Dr John Coke)

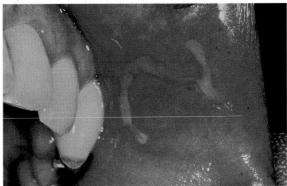

Figure 60.8. **Secondary syphilis:** mucus patch with a "snail track" pattern. (Courtesy Dr Laurie Cohen and Dr John Coke)

# HIV Infection and AIDS

Acquired immunodeficiency syndrome (AIDS) is a communicable disease caused by the human immunodeficiency virus (HIV) first reported by the Centers for Disease Control and Prevention in 1981. The virus is harbored in the blood, tears, saliva, breast milk, spinal fluid, vaginal secretions, and seminal fluid of infected persons and is predominantly spread by sexual contact, by blood or blood products, or perinatally. Infection may result by exposure to the virus through participation in high-risk activities such as sharing needles with injecting drug users; having unprotected sexual activity with several partners; receiving infected blood or blood products; or being accidentally exposed to infected materials.

In most instances, flu-like symptoms develop 2–6 weeks after the initial infection; persistent generalized lymphadenopathy then occurs, followed by a latent phase. Initially the latent phase is asymptomatic, later lymphadenopathy, weight loss, fever, diarrhea, fatigue, skin anergy, oral candidiasis, hairy leukoplakia, and herpes virus recrudescence develop. AIDS is defined as immune deficiency caused by HIV infection when CD4$^+$ T-cell counts decrease to less than 200 cells/mm$^3$ or when one of 30 opportunistic infections or certain forms of cancer develop. Treatment has focused on antiviral agents, such as nucleoside analogues and protease inhibitors, used in combination to block replication and maturation of HIV. These drugs have extended the lives of patients with HIV infection to more than 15 years.

Oral manifestations of HIV infection are often numerous and concurrent. Recognition of the oral features associated with HIV infection should warrant patient referral to a physician.

## Oral Bacterial Infections (Figs. 61.1–61.4)
Oral bacterial infections in patients infected with HIV often involve the periodontal tissue. Examples of these infections include acute necrotizing ulcerative gingivitis (ANUG), linear gingival erythema (previously called HIV gingivitis), and necrotizing ulceractive periodontitis (previously called HIV periodontitis).

## Nectrotizing Ulcerative Gingivitis (Figs. 61.1 and 61.2)
Necrotizing ulcerative gingivitis is common in HIV-infected and immunocompromised patients. It is characterized by sudden onset of fiery red, swollen, painful, bleeding gingiva and a fetor oris. The interdental papillae appear punched-out, ulcerated, and covered by a grayish necrotic slough. Treatment involves debridement alone or combined with metronidazole therapy if constitutional signs such as fever, malaise, anorexia, and lymphadenopathy are present.

## Linear Gingival Erythema (Fig. 61.3)
Linear gingival erythema is characterized by chronic gingival erythema in the absence of apparent local factors such as plaque. The maxilla and mandible are equally affected. Small, red, punctate, multifocal petechiae of the attached labial gingiva initially appear; these later form noncoalescing, distinctive red linear bands of the marginal and attached gingiva. Spontaneous gingival bleeding and lack of response to conventional therapy are common. The cause is uncertain, but it has been proposed that immune defects, in particular polymorphonuclear leukocyte abnormalities, may play a role.

## Necrotizing Ulcerative Periodontitis (Figs. 61.4)
Necrotizing ulcerative periodontitis is an extremely rapid and destructive process that produces loss of periodontal attachment within days. It initially manifests in the anterior periodontal tissues, radiates to the posterior areas with time, and has a distinct propensity for occurrence in the incisor and molar teeth. It is a bacterial infection characterized by pain and spontaneous gingival bleeding, interdental papilla necrosis and cratering, gingival edema and intense erythema, rapid gingival recession, extremely rapid and irregular bone loss (up to 10 mm in 6 months), delayed wound healing, and spread to adjacent mucosa. Aggressive periodontal measures and antibiotics are required to control this disease.

In HIV-infected patients, bacterial flora uncommon to the oral cavity can be found. The most commonly isolated bacteria are respiratory and coliform flora, *Klebsiella* species, and *Escherichia coli*. Infections by these organisms often produce diffuse, erythematous, and ulcerated changes of the tongue that result in symptoms of glossitis. Antibiotics are effective, but overgrowth of candidal organisms may occur as a result.

## Oral Fungal Infections (Figs. 61.5–61.8)
Candidiasis is the most common infection of the mouth affecting the mucosal surfaces of patients with AIDS and is often the first oral manifestation. Candidal infections are usually chronic and may appear red, white, flat, raised, or nodular. Any oral mucosal surface may be infected, but the palate, tongue, and buccal mucosa are the most frequent sites. Symptoms of infection include mild discomfort, burning, or altered taste. The different types of candidiasis are discussed below and in the section on Red/White Lesions.

## Pseudomembranous Candidiasis
Pseudomembranous candidiasis is characterized by creamy-white plaques that upon scraping reveal a red, raw, or bleeding mucosal surface. A potassium hydroxide-stained smear or fungal culture reveals the typical morphology of *Candida albicans*. The **erythematous (atrophic)** form of candidiasis clinically appears as a diffuse red area, usually located on the dorsum of the tongue. At this location the condition is associated with the loss of filiform papillae and is called **median rhomboid glossitis.** A diffuse, erythematous contact lesion corresponding in size and shape to the tongue lesion may be apparent on the palate. **Chronic hyperplastic candidiasis,** a late stage of candidal infection, clinically appears as diffuse white keratotic plaques on the buccal mucosa. These plaques cannot be wiped off. HIV-infected patients often require systemic therapy with antifungal drugs. The disease is often chronic and recurrent and may predict esophageal candidiasis. Infrequent oral fungal infections associated with AIDS are geotrichosis and histoplasmosis.

# HIV Infection and AIDS

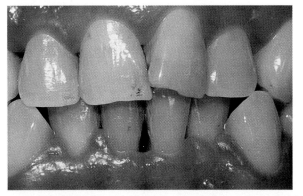

Figure 61.1. HIV-associated necrotizing ulcerative gingivitis: punched out interdental papillae.

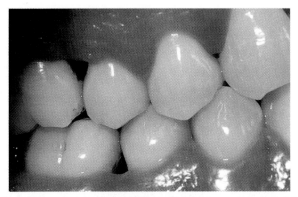

Figure 61.2. HIV-associated necrotizing ulcerative gingivitis: same patient shown in Figure 61.1.

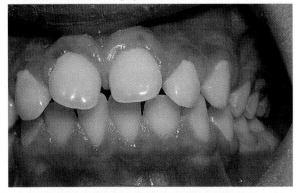

Figure 61.3. Linear gingival erythema: noncontinuous red band of attached gingiva not associated with plaque accumulation. (Courtesy Dr Michael Vitt)

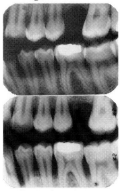

Figure 61.4. Necrotizing ulcerative peridontitis: rapid bone loss. Bottom film obtained 6 months after top film.

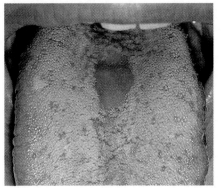

Figure 61.5. Median rhomboid glossitis: a form of HIV-associated candidiasis. (Courtesy Dr Ed Heslop)

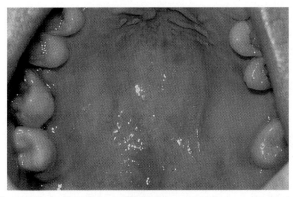

Figure 61.6. Atrophic candidiasis: contact lesion developing where infected tongue rests against palate (same patient shown in Figure 61.5).

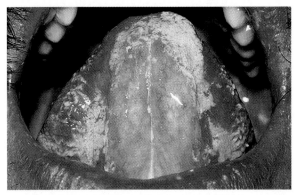

Figure 61.7. Acute pseudomembranous candidiasis in a patient with AIDS.

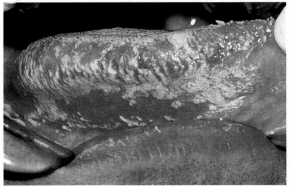

Figure 61.8. Acute pseudomembranous candidiasis in same patient shown in Figure 61.7.

# HIV Infection and AIDS

**Oral Viral Infections (Figs. 62.1–62.6)** There are eight human herpes viruses (herpes simplex virus types 1 and 2, varicella-zoster, cytomegalovirus, Epstein-Barr virus, human herpesvirus types 6, 7, and 8). These viruses figure prominently in acute and chronic oral disease in patients with AIDS. **Herpes simplex virus infections** usually appear on the lips as herpes labialis or in the mouth on keratinized epithelium. The recurrent infection forms small, round vesicles that rapidly erupt, leaving shallow yellow ulcers bordered by a red halo. Coalescence of adjacent vesicles into large ulcers is common. Unlike patients with normal immune function, patients with AIDS may have herpetic infections on mucosal surfaces typically ascribed to aphthous stomatitis such as the tongue and buccal mucosa. Recurrent infections are more frequent, more persistent, and more severe in patients immunosuppressed because of HIV infection.

**Varicella-Zoster Virus** Varicella-zoster virus recrudesces more frequently in HIV-infected persons than in the ordinary population. The clinical appearance is similar in both groups, but the prognosis is worse for patients with immune suppression. This virus produces multiple vesicles that are commonly located on the trunk or face and are usually self-limiting and unilateral. Cephalic vesicles are found along a branch of the trigeminal nerve, either inside or outside the mouth. Vesicle eruption, coalescence, ulcer formation and scabbing are characteristic of the condition. Deep searing pain is the premiere symptom and may persist as postherpetic neuralgia. The antiviral agent famciclovir is used to accelerate healing and alleviate symptoms.

**Cytomegalovirus** The prevalence of **cytomegalovirus** infection is nearly 100% in HIV-positive homosexual males and is approximately 10% in children with AIDS. The virus has a predilection for salivary tissue and, like herpes simplex virus, can be recovered from the saliva of persons infected with HIV. Inflammatory changes associated with cytomegalovirus and HIV infections include unilateral and bilateral parotid gland swelling and xerostomia. Cytomegalovirus-induced oral ulcerations resemble aphthous and herpes simplex virus ulcerations and can occur on periosteal-bound and non-periosteal-bound oral mucosa.

**Human Papillomavirus** Oral manifestations of **human papillomavirus** are frequently found in persons infected with HIV. So far, more than 85 serotypes of this virus have been identified. A variety of benign mucocutaneous lesions are induced by the virus, including squamous papilloma, verruca vulgaris, focal epithelial hyperplasia (Heck's disease), and condyloma acuminatum.

**Condyloma Acuminatum** The **condyloma acuminatum,** or venereal wart, usually appears as a small, soft, pink to dirty gray, exophytic growth that has a cauliflower-like surface. These lesions are often multiple and recurrent and coalesce to form large, sessile, pebbly growths. Condyloma acuminata can be found on any mucosal surface, particularly the ventral tongue, gingiva, labial mucosa, and palate. Transmission is by 1) direct contact that results in contagious spread from anal or genital sites or 2) self-inoculation. Treatment consists of local excision together with simultaneous eradication of all lesions of infected partners. See page 112 for more detail.

**Hairy Leukoplakia** Hairy leukoplakia is a raised, corrugated, poorly demarcated white lesion on the lateral border of the tongue that is associated with the Epstein-Barr virus and immunosuppression. Early lesions appear as discrete, white, vertical-oriented plaques on the lateral borders of both sides of the tongue. Mature lesions may cover the entire lateral and dorsal surface of the tongue and extend onto the buccal mucosa and palate. The lesions are asymptomatic, cannot be rubbed off, and may pose an esthetic problem to the patient. Histologic features are hyperkeratotic hairlike projections, koliocytosis, minimal inflammation, and candidal infection. Electronmicroscopic examination shows Epstein-Barr virus particles. Treatment is with antiviral agents.

**Oral Malignancies (Figs. 62.7 and 62.8)** Kaposi's sarcoma is the most common cancer associated with HIV infection. It is a tumor of vascular (endothelial) proliferation that affects the cutaneous and mucosal tissue. It is strongly associated with human herpes type 8, a virus capable of promoting angiogenesis. Approximately 20% of all patients with AIDS are affected; the prevalence is about 30% in HIV-infected homosexual males.

Kaposi's sarcoma is characterized by three stages. The disease initially appears an asymptomatic red macule. The tumor then enlarges into a red-blue plaque. Advanced lesions appear as lobulated, blue-violet nodules that ulcerate and cause pain. The hard palate is the most common location, followed by the gingiva and buccal mucosa. Lesions are frequently multifocal, uncomfortable, and esthetically displeasing. Similar-appearing lesions such as erythroplakia, hemangiomas, purpura, and bacillary angiomatosis should be ruled out by biopsy. Localized radiation therapy and direct injection of chemotherapeutic drugs (vinblastine) or sclerosing agents have proven beneficial.

**Non-Hodgkin's B-cell Lymphoma and Squamous Cell Carcinoma** Non-Hodgkin B-cell lymphoma and squamous cell carcinoma are associated with HIV infection, probably as a result of viral control over apoptosis and abnormal immune surveillance. Non-Hodgkin's lymphoma often appears as a diffuse, rapidly proliferating, purplish mass of the palatal-retromolar complex. Squamous cell carcinoma is most frequently found as a reddish-white or ulcerated lesion on the lateral border of the tongue. Although many of the usual cofactors, such as advanced age, alcohol abuse, and poor oral hygiene, are absent in HIV-infected persons with oral cancer, Epstein-Barr virus and human papillomavirus have been detected with increasing frequency in patients with B-cell lymphomas and patients with squamous cell carcinomas, respectively.

# HIV Infection and AIDS

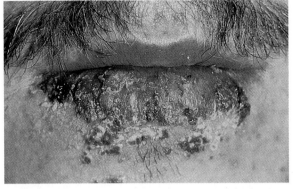

Figure 62.1. HIV-associated recurrent herpes labialis: lesions are more severe and last longer than occurs without HIV infection. (Courtesy Dr Jerry Cioffi)

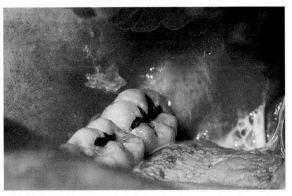

Figure 62.2. HIV-associated recurrent herpes simplex: unusual location in retromolar region.

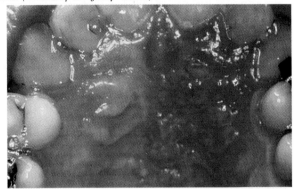

Figure 62.3. HIV-associated herpes zoster: longer-lasting and very painful lesions.

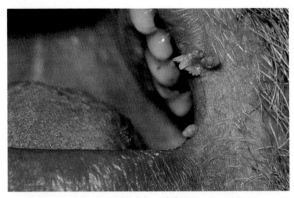

Figure 62.4. HIV-associated condyloma acuminata: partner had genital and anal lesions.

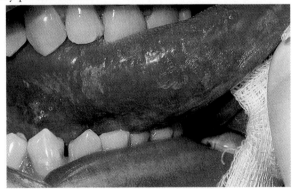

Figure 62.5. HIV-associated hairy leukoplakia: corrugated white patches on lateral tongue.

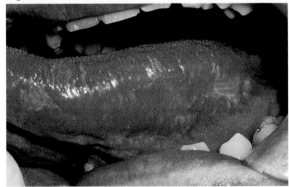

Figure 62.6. HIV-associated hairy leukoplakia: usual bilateral appearance on lateral tongue (same patient shown in Figure 62.5).

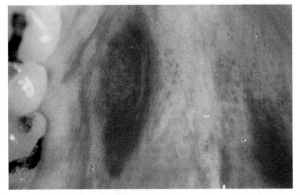

Figure 62.7. HIV-associated Kaposi's sarcoma: early purple macule. (Courtesy Dr Michael Huber)

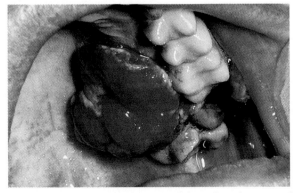

Figure 62.8. HIV-associated non-Hodgkin's lymphoma: nodular mass of palate. (Courtesy Dr George Kaugers)

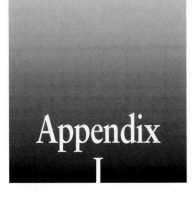

# Appendix I

# Rx Abbreviations

| ABBREVIATION | ENGLISH | LATIN DERIVATIVE |
| --- | --- | --- |
| ad lib | at pleasure | ad libitum |
| a.c. | before meals | ante cibum |
| p.c. | after meals | post cibum |
| aq. | water | aqua |
| d. | a day, daily | dies |
| b.i.d | twice a day | bis in die |
| t.i.d. | three times a day | ter in die |
| q.i.d | four times a day | quater in die |
| h. | hour | hora |
| h.s. | at bedtime | hora somni |
| q.h. | every hour | quaque hora |
| q.3h. | every three hours | quaque tertia hora |
| q.4h. | every four hours | quaque quarta hora |
| q.6h. | every six hours | quaque sexta hora |
| n.r. | do not repeat | non repetatur |
| p.r.n. | as needed | pro re nata |
| stat. | immediately | statim |
| Sig. | label | signetur |
| c. | with | cum |
| gtt. | drops | guttae |
| tab | tablet | tabella |
| caps. | capsule | capsula |
| q.d. | every day | quaque die |
| p.o. | orally | per os |

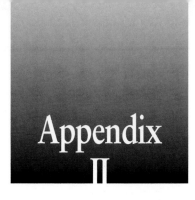

Appendix
II

# Therapeutic Protocols

# ANALGESICS
FOR RELIEF OF MILD TO MODERATE PAIN

| | |
|---|---|
| **Rx** | Acetaminophen 325 mg |
| | Tylenol (McNeil) |
| **Disp.:** | 25 Tablets |
| **Sig:** | Take 2 tablets q.4h. p.r.n.; pain not to exceed 12 tablets in 24 hours. |

| | |
|---|---|
| **Rx** | Aspirin 325 mg |
| | Bayer Aspirin (Glenbrook) |
| **Disp.:** | 25 Tablets |
| **Sig:** | Take 2 tablets q.4h. p.r.n for pain. |

| | |
|---|---|
| **Rx** | Ibuprofen |
| | Motrin 400 mg (Upjohn) |
| **Disp.:** | 25 Tablets |
| **Sig:** | Take 2 tablets q.4h. p.r.n for pain. |

| | |
|---|---|
| **Rx** | Propoxyphene napsylate 50 mg, and acetaminophen, 325 mg |
| | Darvocet-N 50 (Eli Lilly) |
| **Disp.:** | 25 Tablets |
| **Sig:** | Take 2 tablets q.4h. p.r.n. for pain. |

| | |
|---|---|
| **Rx** | Naproxen sodium |
| | Alleve (Procter & Gamble) 220 mg, and Naprosyn® 375 mg (Syntex) |
| **Disp.:** | 50 Tablets |
| **Sig:** | Take 2 tablets b.i.d p.r.n. for pain. |

# ANALGESICS
FOR RELIEF OF MODERATE PAIN

| | |
|---|---|
| **Rx** | Acetaminophen 300 mg, with codeine 30 mg |
| | Tylenol with Codeine No.3 (McNeil Pharm) |
| **Disp.:** | 30 Tablets |
| **Sig:** | Take 2 tablets q.4h. p.r.n. for pain. |

| | |
|---|---|
| **Rx** | Aspirin 325 mg, with codeine 30 mg |
| | Empirin with Codeine No.3 (Burroughs Wellcome) |
| **Disp.:** | 30 Tablets |
| **Sig:** | Take 2 tablets q.4h. p.r.n. for pain. |

| | |
|---|---|
| **Rx** | Aspirin 325 mg, butalbital 50 mg, caffeine 40 mg |
| | Fiorinal (Sandoz) |
| **Disp.:** | 40 Tablets |
| **Sig:** | Take 1 to 2 tablets q.4h. p.r.n. for pain. |

| | |
|---|---|
| **Rx** | Aspirin 325 mg, butalbital 50 mg, caffeine 40 mg, codeine 30 mg |
| | Fiorinal with codeine 30 mg (Sandoz) |
| **Disp.:** | 30 Tablets |
| **Sig:** | Take 1 to 2 tablets q.4h. p.r.n. for pain. |

| | |
|---|---|
| **Rx** | Acetaminophen 650 mg, with codeine 30 mg |
| | Margesic No. 3 (McNeil) |
| **Disp.:** | 30 Tablets |
| **Sig:** | Take 1 to 2 tablets q.4h. p.r.n. for pain. |

| | |
|---|---|
| **Rx** | Hydrocodone bitartrate 5 mg, with acetaminophen 500 mg |
| | Lortab 5 (Whitby), Anexsia 5/500 (Boehringer Mannheim), Bancap-HC (Forest), Vicodin (Knoll), Zydone (DuPont) |
| **Disp.:** | 30 Tablets |
| **Sig:** | Take 1 tablet q.4h. p.r.n. for pain. |

(ALL DOSAGES ARE ADULT DOSAGES UNLESS OTHERWISE NOTED)

FOR RELIEF OF MODERATE PAIN

| Rx | Dihydrocodeine bitartrate 16 mg, aspirin 356.4 mg, caffeine 30 mg |
|---|---|
| | Synalgos-DC Capsules (Wyeth-Ayerst) |
| Disp.: | 40 Tablets |
| Sig: | Take 1 to 2 tablets q.4h. p.r.n. for pain. |

# ANALGESICS
## FOR RELIEF OF MODERATE TO SEVERE PAIN

| Rx | Hydrocodone bitartrate 7.5 mg, with acetaminophen 500 mg |
|---|---|
| | Lortab 7.5/500 (Pharma) |
| Disp.: | 30 Tablets |
| Sig: | Take 1 tablet q.6h. p.r.n. for pain. |

| Rx | Hydrocodone bitartrate 7.5 mg, with acetaminophen 650 mg |
|---|---|
| | Lorcet Plus (Whitby) |
| Disp.: | 30 Tablets |
| Sig: | Take 1 tablet q.6h. p.r.n. for pain. |

| Rx | Hydrocodone bitartrate 10 mg, with acetaminophen 650 mg |
|---|---|
| | Lorcet 10/650 (UAD) |
| Disp.: | 30 Tablets |
| Sig: | Take 1 tablet q.6h. p.r.n. for pain. |

| Rx | Oxycodone HCl 5 mg, with acetaminophen 325 mg |
|---|---|
| | Percocet (Dupont), Roxicet (DuPont) |
| Disp.: | 25 Tablets |
| Sig: | Take 1 tablet q.6h. p.r.n. for pain. |

| Rx | Oxycodone HCl 5 mg, with acetaminophen 500 mg |
|---|---|
| | Tylox (McNeil) |
| Disp.: | 25 Tablets |
| Sig: | Take 1 tablet q.6h. p.r.n. for pain. |

| Rx | Oxycodone HCl 4.5 mg, oxycodone terephthalate 0.38 mg, aspirin 325 mg |
|---|---|
| | Percodan Tablets (Dupont) |
| Disp.: | 25 Tablets |
| Sig: | Take 1 tablet q.4h. p.r.n. for pain. |

(ALL DOSAGES ARE ADULT DOSAGE UNLESS OTHERWISE NOTED)

## FOR RELIEF OF MODERATE TO SEVERE PAIN

| | |
|---|---|
| **Rx** | Meperidine HCl 50 mg, with promethazine HCl 25 mg |
| | Mepergan Fortis Capsules (Wyeth-Ayerst) |
| **Disp.:** | 25 Tablets |
| **Sig:** | Take 1 tablet q.4 to 6h. p.r.n. for pain. |

# ANTIBIOTIC THERAPY
## TO ELIMINATE PATHOGENIC BACTERIAL ORGANISMS THAT CAUSE ORAL INFECTION

| | |
|---|---|
| **Rx** | Phenoxymethyl penicillin |
| | Penicillin V 500 mg tablets (Goldline) |
| **Disp.:** | 40 Tablets |
| **Sig:** | Take 2 tablets immediately and then 1 tablet q.6h. 1 hour a.c. |

| | |
|---|---|
| **Rx** | Penicillin V potassium liquid |
| | Penicillin VK liquid, 125 mg/5 mL |
| **Disp.:** | 200 mL |
| **Sig:** | Children should take 1 teaspoonful q.6h. |

| | |
|---|---|
| **Rx** | Amoxicillin |
| | Amoxil 500 mg (Beecham Labs) |
| **Disp.:** | 40 Tablets |
| **Sig:** | Take one 500-mg tablet t.i.d. |

| | |
|---|---|
| **Rx** | Dicloxacillin sodium |
| | Dynapen 500 mg (Bristol) |
| **Disp.:** | 40 Tablets |
| **Sig:** | Take one 500-mg tablet q.8 h. |
| **Note:** | For penicillinase-resistant infection. |

| | |
|---|---|
| **Rx** | Trimethoprim 80 mg, with sulfamethoxazole 400 mg |
| | Bactrim (Roche) |
| **Disp.:** | 40 Tablets |
| **Sig:** | Take 1 tablet q.12 h. |
| **Note:** | For infections with *Escherichia coli*, *Haemophilus influenzae*, and *Klebsiella* and *Enterobacter* species. |

| | |
|---|---|
| **Rx** | Metronidazole |
| | Flagyl 500 mg (Searle) |
| **Disp.:** | 40 Tablets |
| **Sig:** | Take 2 tablets immediately, then 1 tablet q.6h. until gone. |
| **Note:** | For febrile patients with acute necrotizing ulcerative gingivitis involving anaerobic bacteria. |

(ALL DOSAGES ARE ADULT DOSAGES UNLESS OTHERWISE NOTED)

| Rx | Erythromycin ethylsuccinate |
|---|---|
| | EES 400 mg (Abbott) |
| Disp.: | 56 Tablets |
| Sig: | Take one 400-mg tablet q.6h. Continue for 7 days. |

| Rx | Tetracycline HCl |
|---|---|
| | Achromycin V 250 mg (Lederle) |
| Disp.: | 56 Tablets |
| Sig: | Take 1 tablet q.i.d. Continue for 7 days. |

| Rx | Cephalexin |
|---|---|
| | Keflex 250 mg (Dista) |
| Disp.: | 56 Tablets |
| Sig: | Take 2 tablets q.6h. Continue for 7 days. |

# ANTIBIOTIC THERAPY—BACTERIAL ENDOCARDITIS PROPHYLAXIS

TO PREVENT INFECTIVE ENDOCARDITIS IN PATIENTS WITH RHEUMATIC, CONGENITAL, OR OTHER ACQUIRED VALVULAR HEART DISEASE WHO ARE UNDERGOING INVASIVE DENTAL PROCEDURES

## ADULT

| Rx | Amoxicillin 500 mg |
|---|---|
| Disp.: | 4 Tablets (2 g) |
| Sig: | Take 4 tablets (2 g) p.o. 1 h. before dental procedure.* |
| Note: | Standard regimen for preventing bacterial endocarditis in adults and children >66 lbs (30 kg). |

## ADULT UNABLE TO TAKE ORAL MEDICATIONS

| Rx | Ampicillin |
|---|---|
| Disp.: | 2-g vial, dissolve in sterile saline |
| Sig: | Administer 2.0 g IM or IV within 30 minutes of procedure.* |

## ADULT ALLERGIC TO PENICILLIN

| Rx | Clindamycin 300 mg |
|---|---|
| Disp.: | 2 Tablets |
| Sig: | Take 2 tablets p.o., 1 h. before dental treatment.* |

### OR

| Rx | Cephalexin or cefadroxil 500 mg |
|---|---|
| Disp.: | 4 Tablets |
| Sig: | Take 2 g p.o. 1 h. before dental treatment.* |
| Note: | Avoid in patients who are allergic to penicillins. |

### OR

*For patients in the high-risk category for endocarditis, half the dose may be repeated 6 hours after the initial dose (the exception is azithromycin, for which a second dose is not necessary).

(ALL DOSAGES ARE ADULT DOSAGE UNLESS OTHERWISE NOTED)

| Rx | Azithromycin or clarithromycin 500 mg |
|---|---|
| Disp.: | 1 Tablet |
| Sig: | Take 1 tablet p.o. 1 h. before dental treatment.* |

## ADULT ALLERGIC TO PENICILLIN AND UNABLE TO TAKE ORAL MEDICATIONS

| Rx | Clindamycin 600 mg |
|---|---|
| Disp.: | 600-mg vial |
| Sig: | Administer 600 mg IM or IV within 30 minutes of procedure.* |

### OR

| Rx | Cefazolin |
|---|---|
| Disp.: | 1-g vial |
| Sig: | Administer 1 g IM or IV within 30 minutes of procedure.* |

## CHILD

| Rx | Amoxicillin 250 mg/5 mL elixir |
|---|---|
| Disp.: | 10 mL |
| Sig: | Take 50 mg/kg p.o. 1 h. before dental treatment.* |
| Note: | Standard regimen for preventing infective endocarditis in children < 66 lbs (30 kg). The following weight ranges may also be used for the initial pediatric dose of amoxicillin: < 15 kg, 750 mg; 15–30 kg, 1000 mg; and > 30 kg, 2000 mg. |

## CHILD ALLERGIC TO PENICILLIN

| Rx | Clindamycin, 75 mg |
|---|---|
| Disp.: | By weight |
| Sig: | Take 20 mg/kg 1 h. before dental treatment.* |

### OR

| Rx | Cephalexin or cefadroxil 125 mg/5 mL |
|---|---|
| Disp.: | By weight |
| Sig: | Take 50 mg/kg p.o. 1 h. before dental treatment.* |
| Note: | Avoid in patients who are allergic to penicillins. |

### OR

| Rx | Azithromycin or clarithromycin 125 mg |
|---|---|
| Disp.: | By weight |
| Sig: | Take 15 mg/kg p.o. 1 h. before dental treatment.* |

## CHILD ALLERGIC TO PENICILLIN AND UNABLE TO TAKE ORAL MEDICATIONS

| Rx | Clindamycin |
|---|---|
| Disp.: | 600-mg vial |
| Sig: | Administer 25 mg/kg IM or IV within 30 minutes of procedure.* |

### OR

| Rx | Cefazolin |
|---|---|
| Disp.: | 500-mg vial |
| Sig: | Administer 25 mg/kg IM or IV within 30 minutes of procedure.* |

## HIGH-RISK ADULT PATIENT

| Rx | Ampicillin |
|---|---|
| Disp.: | 2 g |
| Sig: | 2 g IM or IV 30 minutes before dental treatment. |

### PLUS

| Rx | Gentamycin |
|---|---|
| Disp.: | By weight |
| Sig: | 1.5 mg/kg (not to exceed 120 mg) IM or IV 30 minutes before dental treatment |

### SIX HOURS LATER

Ampicillin, 1 g IM or IV, or amoxicillin, 1 g p.o.

(ALL DOSAGES ARE ADULT DOSAGES UNLESS OTHERWISE NOTED)          **149**

## HIGH-RISK ADULT PATIENT ALLERGIC TO AMPICILLIN OR AMOXICILLIN

| | |
|---|---|
| **Rx** | Vancomycin |
| | Vancocin (Lilly) in parenteral solution |
| **Disp.:** | 1 g |
| **Sig:** | 1 g IV delivered over 1–2 h. |

### PLUS

| | |
|---|---|
| **Rx** | Gentamycin |
| **Disp.:** | By weight |
| **Sig:** | 1.5 mg/kg (not to exceed 120 mg) IM or IV. Complete injection or infusion within 30 minutes of starting procedure. |

## MEDIUM-RISK ADULT PATIENT

| | |
|---|---|
| **Rx** | Amoxicillin |
| **Disp.:** | 2 g |
| **Sig:** | 2 g p.o. 1 h. before dental treatment. |

### OR

| | |
|---|---|
| **Rx** | Ampicillin |
| **Disp.:** | 2 g |
| **Sig:** | 2 g IM or IV within 30 minutes of starting procedure. |

## MEDIUM-RISK ADULT PATIENT ALLERGIC TO AMPICILLLIN OR AMOXICILLIN

| | |
|---|---|
| **Rx** | Vancomycin |
| | Vancocin (Lilly) in parenteral solution |
| **Disp.:** | 1 g |
| **Sig:** | Slowly administer 1 g over 1–2 h. IV; complete infusion within 30 minutes of starting procedure. |

## HIGH-RISK CHILD

| | |
|---|---|
| **Rx** | Ampicillin |
| **Disp.:** | 2-g vial |
| **Sig:** | 50 mg/kg IM or IV (not to exceed 2.0 g) within 30 minutes of starting procedure. |

### PLUS

| | |
|---|---|
| **Rx** | Gentamycin |
| **Disp.:** | By weight |
| **Sig:** | 1.5 mg/kg (not to exceed 120 mg) IM or IV within 30 minutes of starting procedure‡ |

### SIX HOURS LATER

| |
|---|
| Ampicillin 25 mg/kg IM or IV, or amoxicillin, 25 mg/kg p.o. |

## HIGH-RISK CHILD ALLERGIC TO AMPICILLIN OR AMOXICILLIN

| | |
|---|---|
| **Rx** | Vancomycin |
| | Vancocin (Lilly) in parenteral solution |
| **Disp.:** | 500 mg |
| **Sig:** | 20 mg/kg IV delivered over 1–2 h. |

### PLUS

| | |
|---|---|
| **Rx** | Gentamycin |
| **Disp.:** | By weight |
| **Sig:** | 1.5 mg/kg (not to exceed 120 mg) IM or IV. Complete injection or infusion within 30 minutes of starting procedure.‡ |

## MEDIUM-RISK ADULT PATIENT

| | |
|---|---|
| **Rx** | Amoxicillin |
| **Disp.:** | 1 g/50 mL |
| **Sig:** | 50 mg/kg p.o. 1 h. before dental treatment. |

### OR

‡Total child's dose should not exceed adult dose.

(ALL DOSAGES ARE ADULT DOSAGE UNLESS OTHERWISE NOTED)

| Rx | Ampicillin |
|---|---|
| Disp.: | 1-g vial |
| Sig: | 50 mg/kg IM or IV within 30 minutes of starting procedure.‡ |

## MEDIUM-RISK ADULT PATIENT ALLERGIC TO AMPICILLLIN OR AMOXICILLIN

| Rx | Vancomycin |
|---|---|
| | Vancocin (Lilly) in parenteral solution |
| Disp.: | 1-g vial |
| Sig: | Slowly administer 20 mg/kg IV over 1–2 h. Complete infusion within 30 minutes of starting procedure.‡ |

# ANTIMICROBIAL TOPICAL AGENTS AND RINSES
TO REDUCE THE PATHOGENIC MICROBIAL FLORA OFTEN ASSOCIATED WITH THE INFLAMMATORY ORAL DISEASE

| Rx | Chlorhexidine gluconate 0.12% |
|---|---|
| | Peridex 0.12% Oral Rinse (Procter & Gamble) |
| Disp.: | 480-mL |
| Sig: | Swish 1 teaspoonful for 1 minute, then expectorate. Perform twice daily (morning and evening) after brushing teeth. Avoid eating or drinking for 30 minutes. |

| Rx | Tetracycline HCl 250 mg |
|---|---|
| | Tetracyn 250 mg (Pfizer) |
| Disp.: | 40 Capsules |
| Sig: | Dissolve 1 capsule in 1 teaspoon of warm water, then swish the solution for 3 to 5 minutes and swallow. Repeat q.i.d. |

| Rx | Tetracycline HCl 125 mg/5 mL |
|---|---|
| | Achromycin V 125 mg/5 mL (Lederle) |
| Disp.: | 60-mL (also available in 16 fluid oz.) |
| Sig: | Rinse with 2 teaspoonfuls for 3 minutes and swallow. Repeat q.i.d. |

| Rx | Tetracycline HCl 12.7 mg, in ethylene/vinyl acetate copolymer |
|---|---|
| | Actisite (Procter & Gamble) |
| Disp.: | Box of 100 fibers |
| Sig: | Place in gingival sulcus with cyanoacrylate for 10 days, then remove. |

‡Total child's dose should not exceed adult dose.

(ALL DOSAGES ARE ADULT DOSAGES UNLESS OTHERWISE NOTED)

# ANTIFUNGAL THERAPY
TO ELIMINATE PATHOGENIC FUNGAL
ORGANISMS AND REESTABLISH THE NORMAL
ORAL FLORA

| | |
|---|---|
| **Rx** | Nystatin vaginal tablets 100,000 IU. |
| | Nilstat 100,000 IU (Lederle) |
| **Disp.:** | 90 Tablets |
| **Sig:** | Dissolve 1 tablet as a lozenge 5 times d. for 14 consecutive days. |

| | |
|---|---|
| **Rx** | Nystatin 200,000 U |
| | Mycostatin Pastilles 200,000 U (Squibb) |
| **Disp.:** | 60 Tablets |
| **Sig:** | Dissolve 1 pastille in mouth q.i.d. as a lozenge for 14 consecutive days. |

| | |
|---|---|
| **Rx** | Clotrimazole 10 mg |
| | Mycelex Troches 10 mg (Miles Pharm) |
| **Disp.:** | 60 Tablets |
| **Sig:** | Dissolve 1 tablet as a lozenge 5 times d. for 14 consecutive days. |

| | |
|---|---|
| **Rx** | Ketoconazole 200 mg |
| | Nizoral 200 mg (Janssen Pharm) |
| **Disp.:** | 14 Tablets |
| **Sig:** | Take 1 tablet q.d. for 2 weeks. |

| | |
|---|---|
| **Rx** | Fluconazole 50 or 100 mg |
| | Diflucan 100 mg (Roerig) |
| **Disp.:** | 60 Tablets |
| **Sig:** | Take 1 tablet q.d. for 14 consecutive days. |

| | |
|---|---|
| **Rx** | Itraconazole 100 mg |
| | Sporanox 100 mg  (Janssen) |
| **Disp.:** | 60 Tablets |
| **Sig:** | Take 1 tablet q.d. for 14 consecutive days. |

| | |
|---|---|
| **Rx** | Nystatin topical powder |
| | Mycostatin® topical powder 100,000 IU (Squibb) |
| **Disp.:** | 15-g squeeze bottle |
| **Sig:** | Apply liberally to tissue side of clean denture p.c. Soak the clean denture in a suspension of 1 teaspoon of powder and 8 oz. of water overnight. |

| | |
|---|---|
| **Rx** | Nystatin ointment |
| | Mycostatin ointment 100,000 IU (Squibb) |
| **Disp.:** | 15-g (30-g) tube |
| **Sig:** | Apply liberally to affected area 4–6 times d. |

| | |
|---|---|
| **Rx** | Betamethasone dipropionate 0.05% and clotrimazole 1% |
| | Lotrisone (Schering) |
| **Disp.:** | 15-g (30-g) tube |
| **Sig:** | Apply liberally to affected area 4 or 5 times d. |

| | |
|---|---|
| **Rx** | Iodoquinol 10 mg, and hydrocortisone 10 mg ointment |
| | Vytone Ointment (Dermik) |
| **Disp.:** | 15-g (30-g) tube |
| **Sig:** | Apply liberally to affected area 4 or 5 times d. |

| | |
|---|---|
| **Rx** | Nystatin 100,000 U and triamcinolone acetomide 0.1% |
| | Tri-Statin II (Rugby) |
| **Disp.:** | 15-g (30-g, 60-g) tube |
| **Sig:** | Apply liberally to affected area t.i.d. to q.i.d. |

**Note:** These drugs are most effective when dentures are removed and treated if applicable, and when intake of fermentable carbohydrates is reduced.

(ALL DOSAGES ARE ADULT DOSAGE UNLESS OTHERWISE NOTED)

# ANTIVIRAL THERAPY
## TO PREVENT OR TREAT ORAL HERPETIC INFECTIONS

| | |
|---|---|
| **Rx** | Acyclovir ointment |
| | Zovirax ointment 5% (Glaxo Wellcome) |
| **Disp.:** | 15 g |
| **Sig:** | Apply to oral lesions with a cotton tip applicator 6 times d. |
| **Note:** | Treatment should begin during the early (prodromal) stage of the recurrence. |

| | |
|---|---|
| **Rx** | Acyclovir |
| | Zovirax 200 mg (Glaxo Wellcome) |
| **Disp.:** | 50 Capsules |
| **Sig:** | 1 capsule 5 times d. for at least 4 days. |
| **Note:** | Treatment should begin during the early stage of the recurrence. |

| | |
|---|---|
| **Rx** | Acyclovir |
| | Zovirax 400 mg (Glaxo Wellcome) |
| **Disp.:** | 50 Capsules |
| **Sig:** | 1 capsule t.i.d. for at least 4 days. |
| **Note:** | Treatment should begin during the early stage of the recurrence. |

| | |
|---|---|
| **Rx** | Acyclovir |
| | Zovirax 800 mg (Glaxo Wellcome) |
| **Disp.:** | 50 Capsules |
| **Sig:** | 1 capsule b.i.d. for at least 4 days. |
| **Note:** | Treatment should begin during the early stage of the recurrence. |

| | |
|---|---|
| **Rx** | Valacyclovir |
| | Valtrex 500 mg (Glaxo Wellcome) |
| **Disp.:** | 50 Capsules |
| **Sig:** | 1 capsule b.i.d. for at least 4 days. |
| **Note:** | Treatment should begin during the early stage of the recurrence. |

| | |
|---|---|
| **Rx** | Famciclovir |
| | Famvir 500 mg (Smith-Kline-Beecham) |
| **Disp.:** | 50 Capsules |
| **Sig:** | 1 capsule t.i.d. for at least 4 days. |
| **Note:** | Treatment should begin during the early stage of the recurrence. |

| | |
|---|---|
| **Rx** | L-Lysine |
| | Enisyl 500 mg (Person & Covey) |
| **Disp.:** | 100 Tablets |
| **Sig:** | Take 4 tablets q.4h. until symptoms subside. |
| **Note:** | Treatment should begin during the early stage of the recurrence. Most effective if foods containing high content of arginine are avoided. |

| | |
|---|---|
| **Rx** | Penciclovir ointment |
| | Denavir 1% (Smith-Kline-Beecham) |
| **Disp.:** | 15 g |
| **Sig:** | Apply to lesions with a cotton tip applicator at least 5 times daily. |
| **Note:** | Treatment should begin during the early (prodromal) stage of the recurrence. |

(ALL DOSAGES ARE ADULT DOSAGES UNLESS OTHERWISE NOTED)

# ANTIANXIETY AGENTS
## TO MANAGE AND PROVIDE SHORT-TERM RELIEF OF THE SYMPTOMS OF ANXIETY

| | |
|---|---|
| **Rx** | Alprazolam |
| | Xanax 0.25 mg (Upjohn) |
| **Disp.:** | 20 Tablets |
| **Sig:** | Take 1 tablet b.i.d. |

| | |
|---|---|
| **Rx** | Chlordiazepoxide |
| | Librium 10 mg (Roche) |
| **Disp.:** | 20 Tablets |
| **Sig:** | Take 1 tablet b.i.d. |

| | |
|---|---|
| **Rx** | Diazepam |
| | Valium 5 mg (Roche) |
| **Disp.:** | 20 Tablets |
| **Sig:** | Take 1 tablet b.i.d. or t.i.d. and 1 tablet 1 h. before dental appointments. |

| | |
|---|---|
| **Rx** | Oxazepam |
| | Serax 10 mg (Wyeth-Ayerst) |
| **Disp.:** | 20 Tablets |
| **Sig:** | Take 1 tablet q.d. |

| | |
|---|---|
| **Rx** | Buspirone |
| | Buspar 5 mg (Mead Johnson) |
| **Disp.:** | 20 Tablets |
| **Sig:** | Take 1 tablet b.i.d. |

# ANTIHISTAMINES
## TO RELIEVE SYMPTOMS OF ANXIETY AND ANXIETY-RELATED SKIN ERUPTIONS

| | |
|---|---|
| **Rx** | Hydroxyzine |
| | Atarax 25 mg (Roerig) |
| **Disp.:** | 50 Tablets |
| **Sig:** | Take 2 tablets q.i.d. p.r.n. |

| | |
|---|---|
| **Rx** | Hydroxyzine |
| | Atarax syrup 10 mg/5 mL (Roerig) |
| **Disp.:** | 50 mL |
| **Sig:** | Take 2 teaspoonsful 1 h. before dental appointment |

| | |
|---|---|
| **Rx** | Diphenhydramine hydrochloride |
| | Benadryl 25 mg (Parke-Davis) |
| **Disp.:** | 25 Tablets |
| **Sig:** | Take 1 tablet q.i.d. |

(ALL DOSAGES ARE ADULT DOSAGE UNLESS OTHERWISE NOTED)

# ANTIHISTAMINES
TO REDUCE THE EFFECTS OF HISTAMINE-MEDIATED HYPERSENSITIVITY AND TEMPORARILY RELIEVE SYMPTOMS ASSOCIATED WITH MINOR ORAL IRRITATIONS

| | |
|---|---|
| **Rx** | Diphenhydramine HCl |
| | Benadryl 25 mg (Parke-Davis) |
| **Disp.:** | 40 Tablets |
| **Sig:** | Take 1 tablet q.6h. p.r.n. |

| | |
|---|---|
| **Rx** | Brompheniramine maleate HCl |
| | Dimetane 4 mg (Robins) |
| **Disp.:** | 40 Tablets |
| **Sig:** | Take 1 or 2 tablets q.6h. p.r.n. |

| | |
|---|---|
| **Rx** | Phenylpropanolamine HCI 25 mg, and brompheniramine maleate HCl 4 mg |
| | Dimetapp (Robins) |
| **Disp.:** | 40 Tablets |
| **Sig:** | Take 1 tablet q.4h. p.r.n. |

| | |
|---|---|
| **Rx** | Terfenadine |
| | Seldane 60 mg (Merrell Dow) |
| **Disp.:** | 30 Tablets |
| **Sig:** | Take 1 tablet b.i.d. |

| | |
|---|---|
| **Rx** | Astemizole |
| | Hismanal 10 mg (Janssen) |
| **Disp.:** | 25 Tablets |
| **Sig:** | Take 1 tablet q.d. |

| | |
|---|---|
| **Rx** | Loratadine |
| | Claritin 10 mg (Schering) |
| **Disp.:** | 25 Tablets |
| **Sig:** | Take 1 tablet q.d. |

| | |
|---|---|
| **Rx** | Cetirizine |
| | Reactine 5 mg (Prizer) |
| **Disp.:** | 25 Tablets |
| **Sig:** | Take 1 or 2 tablets q.d. |

# TOPICAL ORAL ANESTHETICS
TO RELIEVE SYMPTOMS ASSOCIATED WITH MINOR IRRITATIONS OF THE MOUTH

| | |
|---|---|
| **Rx** | Diphenhydramine HCl |
| | Benadryl elixir 12.5 mg/5 mL (Parke-Davis) |
| **Disp.:** | 4 fluid oz. |
| **Sig:** | Rinse with 1 tablespoonful a.c. and p.r.n. for pain. |

| | |
|---|---|
| **Rx** | Benadryl elixir, 12.5 mg/5 mL (Parke-Davis) and Kaopectate (Upjohn), 50% mixture by volume |
| **Disp.:** | 4 fluid oz. of each; mix equal parts |
| **Sig:** | Rinse with 1 tablespoonful for 2 minutes a.c. and p.r.n. for pain. |

| | |
|---|---|
| **Rx** | Lidocaine HCl 2% |
| | Xylocaine 2% viscous solution (Astra) |
| **Disp.:** | 4 fluid oz. |
| **Sig:** | Rinse with 1 teaspoonful a.c. and p.r.n. for pain. Expectorate after rinsing. |

| | |
|---|---|
| **Rx** | Orabase with Benzocaine (Colgate-Hoyt) |
| **Disp.:** | 5 g (15 g) |
| **Sig:** | Apply to affected area a.c. and p.r.n. for pain. |

| | |
|---|---|
| **Rx** | Dyclonine 0.5% |
| | Dyclone (Astra) |
| **Disp.:** | 30 mL |
| **Sig:** | Apply to affected area a.c. and p.r.n. pain. |

(ALL DOSAGES ARE ADULT DOSAGES UNLESS OTHERWISE NOTED)

# CORTICOSTEROIDS
ADJUNCTIVE TREATMENT FOR AND
TEMPORARILY RELIEF OF SYMPTOMS
ASSOCIATED WITH ORAL INFLAMMATORY
AND ULCERATIVE LESIONS

## LOW POTENCY

| | |
|---|---|
| **Rx** | Hydrocortisone acetate ointment 0.5% |
| | Orabase HCA 0.05% (Colgate-Hoyt) |
| **Disp.:** | 5-g tube |
| **Sig:** | Apply to oral lesions p.c. and h.s. |

## MEDIUM POTENCY

| | |
|---|---|
| **Rx** | Triamcinolone acetonide ointment 0.1% |
| | Kenalog in Orabase 0.1% (Squibb) |
| **Disp.:** | 5-g tube |
| **Sig:** | Apply to ulcerated area p.c. and h.s. |

| | |
|---|---|
| **Rx** | Betamethasone valerate ointment 0.1% |
| | Valisone 0.1% (Schering) |
| **Disp.:** | 15-g (45-g) tube |
| **Sig:** | Apply to mouth sores p.c. and h.s. |

| | |
|---|---|
| **Rx** | Betamethasone syrup 0.1% |
| | Celestone 0.1% (Schering) |
| **Disp.:** | 50 mL |
| **Sig:** | Rinse with 1 teaspoonful q.i.d, p.c. and h.s. |

| | |
|---|---|
| **Rx** | Triamcinalone |
| | Kenalog-40 (Westwood-Squibb) |
| **Disp.:** | 5-mL injectable vials |
| **Sig:** | Mix 1 mL of steroid with 0.5 mL of anesthetic. Inject 0.25 mL at four locations around border of ulcer. Total 1 mL injected. |

## HIGH POTENCY

| | |
|---|---|
| **Rx** | Augmented betamethasone dipropionate ointment 0.05% |
| | Diprolene 0.05% (Schering) |
| **Disp.:** | 15-g (45-g) tube |
| **Sig:** | Apply to mouth sores p.c. and h.s. |

| | |
|---|---|
| **Rx** | Fluocinonide gel 0.05% |
| | Lidex 0.05% (Syntex) |
| **Disp.:** | 15-g (30-g) tube |
| **Sig:** | Apply to mouth sores p.c. and h.s. |

| | |
|---|---|
| **Rx** | Dexamethasone elixir 0.5% |
| | Decadron 0.5% (Merck-Sharp-Dohme) |
| **Disp.:** | 100-mL bottle |
| **Sig:** | Rinse with 1 teaspoonful q.i.d. for 2 minutes, then expectorate. |

## VERY HIGH POTENCY*

| | |
|---|---|
| **Rx** | Dexamethasone elixir 0.75% |
| | Decadron 0.75% (Merck-Sharp-Dohme) |
| **Disp.:** | 100-mL bottle |
| **Sig:** | Rinse with 1 teaspoonful q.i.d. for 2 minutes, then swallow. |

| | |
|---|---|
| **Rx** | Dexamethasone elixir |
| | Decadron 0.75% elixir (Merck-Sharp-Dohme) |
| **Disp.:** | 100-mL bottle |
| **Sig:** | Rinse with 1 teaspoonful q.i.d. for 2 minutes, then swallow. |

| | |
|---|---|
| **Rx** | Clobetasol 0.05% ointment |
| | Temovate (Glaxo) 0.05% ointment |
| **Disp.:** | 15 g |
| **Sig:** | Apply to affected area q.i.d. |

| | |
|---|---|
| **Rx** | Halbetasol propionate 0.05% ointment |
| | Ultravate (Westwood-Squibb) 0.05% ointment |
| **Disp.:** | 15 g |
| **Sig:** | Apply to affected area q.i.d. |

*High-potency steroids should be avoided in patients with gastrointestinal ulcers, diabetes, hematologic malignancy, and hepatitis and in women who are pregnant or nursing. Imuran can be prescribed with prednisone to reduce the prednisone dose.

(ALL DOSAGES ARE ADULT DOSAGE UNLESS OTHERWISE NOTED)

| **Rx** | Halcinonide 0.1% ointment |
| | Halog (Princeton) 0.1% ointment |
| **Disp.:** | 15 g |
| **Sig:** | Apply to affected area q.i.d. |

| **Rx** | Methylprednisolone |
| | Medrol 4 mg Dosepak 21s (Upjohn) |
| **Disp.:** | 1 dosepak (21 tablets) |
| **Sig:** | Take graduated daily doses according to the manufacturer's directions listed on the dosepak. |

| **Rx** | Prednisone 10 mg |
| **Disp.:** | 36 Tablets |
| **Sig:** | Take 4 tablets in a.m. for 4 days. |

| **Rx** | Azathioprine[a] |
| | Imuran 50 mg (Burroughs Wellcome) |
| **Disp.:** | 30 Tablets |
| **Sig:** | Take one 50-mg dose q.d. (Patients not improved in 12 weeks may be refractory to this drug). |
| **Caution:** | Chronic immunosuppression with azathioprine increases the risk for neoplasia. Doctors prescribing this drug should be familiar with this risk and the serious mutagenic and hematologic consequences to both men and women. |

# FLUORIDE THERAPY
## TO PREVENT DENTAL CARIES IN SUSCEPTIBLE PATIENTS

| **Rx** | Stannous fluoride 0.4% |
| **Disp.:** | 4.3 fluid oz. |
| **Sig:** | Apply 5–10 drops in a carrier and place carrier on teeth daily for 5 minutes. |

| **Rx** | Oral fluoride |
| | Luride 0.125 mg per drop (Colgate Hoyt) |
| **Disp.:** | 60-mL bottle with dropper |
| **Sig:** | Birth–2 years of age: apply 2 drops q.d.*; 2–3 years: 4 drops q.d.; 3–12 years: 8 drops q.d.* |

[a]Often used in combination with systemic steroids.

*In the mouth of the child.

(ALL DOSAGES ARE ADULT DOSAGES UNLESS OTHERWISE NOTED)

# NUTRIENT DEFICIENCY THERAPY
TO REPLACE DEFICIENT NUTRIENTS NECESSARY FOR HOMEOSTASIS

| | |
|---|---|
| **Rx** | Ferrous sulfate 250 mg |
| **Disp.:** | 100 Tablets |
| **Sig:** | Take 1 tablet q.d. for 1 month, then reassess patient's hemoglobin level. |

| | |
|---|---|
| **Rx** | Folic acid 0.4 mg |
| **Disp.:** | 30 Tablets |
| **Sig:** | Take 1 tablet q.d. for 1 month, then reassess patient's folic acid level. |
| **Caution:** | Medical supervision is advised. |

| | |
|---|---|
| **Rx** | Cyanocobalamin (vitamin $B_{12}$) |
| **Disp.:** | 1000 $\mu$g/mL; 10-mL vial |
| **Sig:** | Inject 0.1–1 mL IM in deltoid; reassess patient's symptoms and blood profile monthly. |

| | |
|---|---|
| **Rx** | Water-soluble bioflavinoids 200 mg, with ascorbic acid 200 mg<br>Peridin-C 400 mg (Beutlich) |
| **Disp.:** | 100 Tablets |
| **Sig:** | Take 1 tablet t.i.d. |

# SALIVA SUBSTITUTE
TO RELIEVE DRY MOUTH

| | |
|---|---|
| **Rx** | Carboxymethyl cellulose 0.5% aqueous solution. |
| **Disp.:** | 8 fluid oz. |
| **Sig:** | Use as a rinse p.r.n. |

| | |
|---|---|
| **Rx** | Carboxymethyl cellulose sprays<br>Moi-stir[a] (KingsWood), Salivart[b] (Gebauer Company),<br>Xerolube (Veterans Administration) |
| **Disp.:** | [a]120 mL with pump spray; [b]75 mL with pump spray |
| **Sig:** | Use as a rinse p.r.n. |

| | |
|---|---|
| **Rx** | Hydroxyethylcellulose, xylitol, citric acid |
| **Disp.:** | Optimoist spray 9 mL |
| **Sig:** | Spray in mouth p.r.n. for dry mouth |

| | |
|---|---|
| **Rx** | Glucose oxidase and lactoperoxidase |
| **Disp.:** | Biotene 120 mL |
| **Sig:** | Rinse in mouth for 1 minute p.r.n. for oral dryness. |

| | |
|---|---|
| **Rx** | Pilocarpine, 5 mg<br>Salagen 5 mg (MGI Pharma) |
| **Disp.:** | 100 |
| **Sig:** | Take 1 tablet t.i.d. or q.i.d. |

| | |
|---|---|
| **Rx** | Bethanechol, 25 mg<br>Urecholine 25 mg (Bolar) |
| **Disp.:** | 100 |
| **Sig:** | Take 1 or 2 tablets up to t.i.d. p.r.n. for oral dryness. |

(ALL DOSAGES ARE ADULT DOSAGE UNLESS OTHERWISE NOTED)

## SEDATIVE/HYPNOTICS
TO PRODUCE A "SLEEP-LIKE" STATE FOR THE EFFECTIVE MANAGEMENT OF AN ORAL DISEASE OR CONDITION

| | |
|---|---|
| **Rx** | Triazolam |
| | Halcion 0.25 mg (Upjohn) |
| **Disp.:** | 30 Tablets |
| **Sig:** | Take 1 tablet h.s. |
| **Note:** | Not to exceed nightly use for more than 2 weeks. |

| | |
|---|---|
| **Rx** | Flurazepam |
| | Dalmane 15 mg (Roche) |
| **Disp.:** | 30 Tablets |
| **Sig:** | Take 1 tablet h.s. |

| | |
|---|---|
| **Rx** | Temazepam |
| | Restoril 15 mg (Sandoz) |
| **Disp.:** | 30 Tablets |
| **Sig:** | Take 1 tablet h.s. |

| | |
|---|---|
| **Rx** | Chloral hydrate |
| | Noctec 500 mg/5 mL (Squibb) |
| **Disp.:** | 1 pint |
| **Sig:** | Take 1 teaspoonful before bedtime or 30 minutes before surgery. |

(ALL DOSAGES ARE ADULT DOSAGES UNLESS OTHERWISE NOTED)

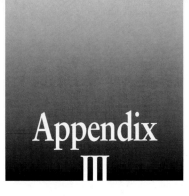

# Appendix III

# Guide to Diagnosis and Management of Common Oral Lesions

## WHITE LESIONS

| Disease | Age | Sex | Race/Ethnicity | Clinical Characteristics | Treatment |
|---|---|---|---|---|---|
| Fordyce's granules | Any | M-F | Any | Whitish-yellow granules clustered in plaques located on buccal mucosa (bilaterally), labial mucosa, retromolar pad, lip, attached gingiva, tongue, and frenum. Lesions are nontender and rough to palpation and do not rub off. Onset after puberty; persists for life. | None required. |
| Linea alba buccalis | Any | M-F | Any | White wavy line of varying length located on buccal mucosa, bilaterally. Lesions are nontender and smooth to palpation and do not rub off. Variable onset, persists with oral habits. | Eliminate bruxism and clenching. |
| Leukoedema | Any | M-F | Melanoderms | Grayish-white patch of variable size located on buccal mucosa (bilaterally), labial mucosa, and soft palate. Lesions are nontender and smooth to palpation and disappear when the mucosa is stretched. Leukoedema becomes more evident with increasing age. | None required. |
| Morsicatio buccarum | Any | M-F | Any | Asymmetric white plaque located on buccal mucosa and labial mucosa, often bilaterally. Lesions are nontender and rough to palpation and peel slightly when rubbed. Variable onset; persists with cheek or lip biting habit. | Eliminate cheek/lip chewing habit |
| White sponge nevus | Any | M-F | Any | Solitary or confluent raised white plaques that may appear on buccal mucosa, labial mucosa, alveolar ridge, floor of the mouth, or soft palate. Lesions are nontender and rough to palpation and do not rub off. Onset at birth; persists for life. | None required. |
| Traumatic white lesions | Any | M-F | Any | White surface slough (eschar) usually located on the less-keratinized alveolar mucosa. Palate common for food "burns." Lesions are tender to palpation and rub off, leaving a raw or bleeding surface. Onset within hours of trauma; regression in 1–2 weeks. | Eliminate irritant; topical anesthetics and analgesics. |

| Disease | Age | Sex | Race/Ethnicity | Clinical Characteristics | Treatment |
|---|---|---|---|---|---|
| Leukoplakia | 45–65 | 2:1 (M:F) | Any | White patch that varies in size, homogeneity, and texture. High-risk locations include floor of the mouth, ventral tongue, lateral tongue, and uvulo-palatal complex. Lesions do not rub off and usually are nontender. Onset occurs after prolonged contact with an inducing agent, persists as long as the inducing agent is present. | Biopsy and histologic examination. Close follow-up mandatory |
| Cigarette keratosis | Elderly | M | Any | White pebbly circular patches located on upper and lower lips (kissing lesions). Keratoses are firm and nontender and do not rub off. Onset in conjunction with a prolonged cigarette smoking habit; persists with habit. | Use filtered cigarettes, or stop smoking. Biopsy if lesion becomes ulcerated or indurated |
| Nicotine stomatitis | 40–70 | M | Any | White cobblestoned papules located on hard palate, excluding the anterior third. Papules have red centers, are nontender, and do not rub off. Onset varies according to degree of smoking; lesions are long-standing. | Stop pipe, cigar, or reverse smoking habit. |
| Snuff dipper's patch | Teenagers and adult | M | Any | Corrugated whitish-yellow patch located on mucobuccal fold, most prominent unilaterally. Patch is rough and nontender and does not rub off. Long-standing habit precedes lesion; patch persists with continuation of habit. | Discontinue tobacco use. Biopsy color changes or if lesion becomes ulcerated or indurated. |
| Verrucous carcinoma | Over 60 | M | Any | Papulonodular whitish-red mass located on buccal mucosa, alveolar ridge, gingiva. Lesion is firm, nontender, and rough to palpation and does not rub off. Long-standing tobacco habit precedes onset; human papillomavirus present in 30%; lesion enlarges unless treated. | Biopsy to confirm diagnosis, then surgical excision. AVOID RADIATION THERAPY. |
| Squamous cell carcinoma (see Red and/or Red-White Lesions) | | | | | |

## RED LESIONS

| Disease | Age | Sex | Race/Ethnicity | Clinical Characteristics | Treatment |
|---------|-----|-----|----------------|--------------------------|-----------|
| Purpura | Any | M-F | Any | Red spot or patch consisting of extravasated blood that develops soon after trauma. Lesions do not blanch upon diascopy and size varies (petechiae < ecchymosis < hematoma). Petechiae are common on soft palate; other purpurae typically occur on buccal or labial mucosa, depending on site at which blood pools. Lesions fade away. | Eliminate underlying problem. |
| Varicosity | Over 55 | F | Any | Reddish-purple papule or nodule located on ventral tongue, lip, or labial mucosa. Lesions are asymptomatic and blanch upon diascopy. Varicosities increase in size and number with increasing age and are persistent. | None necessary. Surgery for esthetics. |
| Thrombus | Over 30 | M-F | Any | Red to blue-purple nodule located on labial mucosa, lip, or tongue. Lesions are firm and may be tender to palpation. Onset after traumatic bleeding; lesion is negative on diascopy and persists until treatment. Thrombi sometimes spontaneously regress. | Surgical removal and histologic examination, if persistent or symptomatic. |
| Hemangioma | Child-adolescent | F | Any | Red to purple, soft, smooth-surfaced, or multinodular exophytic mass located on dorsal tongue, buccal mucosa, or gingiva. Lesions are positive on diascopy. Develops early in life, persists until treated. Hemangiomas sometimes spontaneously regress. | No treatment is necessary if present since youth, no functional disability and no changes in size, shape, or color. Otherwise, surgery or histologic examination. |
| Hereditary hemorrhagic telangiectasia | Post-puberty | M-F | Any | Multifocal red macules located on palms, fingers, nail beds, face, neck, conjunctiva, nasal septum, lips, tongue, hard palate, and gingiva. Lesions are present at birth, become more visible at puberty, and increase in number with age. Telangiectasias lack central pulsation and blanch upon diascopy; if they rupture, severe bleeding may result. | Avoid trauma. Monitor for hemorrhage or anemia. |

| Disease | Age | Sex | Race/Ethnicity | Clinical Characteristics | Treatment |
|---------|-----|-----|----------------|--------------------------|-----------|
| Sturge-Weber syndrome | Birth | M-F | Any | Syndrome associated with seizures, mental deficits, gyriform calcifications, and a red to purple flat or slightly raised facial hemangioma. Vascular lesion often affects lips, labial or buccal mucosa, and gingiva along branches of trigeminal nerve. Abnormal oral enlargements may be concurrent. | None required. Elective surgery for esthetics. |
| Kaposi's sarcoma | 20–45 and Over 60 | M | Jewish, Mediterranean or HIV-infected | Asymptomatic red macule of mucocutaneous structures that enlarges and becomes raised and then darkens in color. Advanced lesions are red-blue-violet nodules that ulcerate and cause pain. The hard palate, gingiva, and buccal mucosa are the most common oral locations. | Palliative, consisting of radiation therapy, laser surgery, chemotherapy, sclerosing agents, or a combination thereof. |

## RED AND RED-WHITE LESIONS

| Disease | Age | Sex | Race/Ethnicity | Clinical Characteristics | Treatment |
|---|---|---|---|---|---|
| Erythroplakia | Over 50 | M>F | Any | Red patch of variable size located on any oral mucosal site. High-risk areas include floor of the mouth, soft palate-retromolar trigone, lateral border of tongue. Erythroplakias do not rub off and are usually asymptomatic. Lesions develop after prolonged contact with carcinogens; duration varies. Regression is rare. | Biopsy and histologic examination. Close follow-up. |
| Erythroleukoplakia and speckled erythroplakia | Over 50 | M | Any | Red patch with multiple foci of white. Nontender, do not rub off, often superficially infected with candida. Common locations include lateral tongue, buccal mucosa, soft palate, and floor of the mouth. Onset after prolonged exposure to carcinogens. Regression unlikely even if inducing agent is removed. | Biopsy and histologic examination. Examine for candidiasis. Close follow-up. |
| Squamous cell carcinoma | Over 50 | 2:1 M:F | Any | Red or red and white lesion or ulcer commonly located on lateral tongue, ventral tongue, oropharynx, floor of the mouth, gingiva, buccal mucosa, or lip. Carcinoma often asymptomatic until it becomes large, indurated or ulcerated. Onset after prolonged exposure to carcinogens. Persistence results in metastasis, usually apparent as painless, firm, matted, fixed lymph nodes. | Biopsy and histologic examination. Complete surgical removal, radiation therapy, chemotherapy, or photodynamic therapy. Close follow-up. |
| Lichen planus | Over 40 | F | Any | Purple, polygonal, pruritic papules on flexor surfaces of skin; finger nails are sometimes affected. Intraoral lesions are often symptomatic and consist of white linear papules, reddish patches and ulcerated regions of mucosa. Affected surfaces are often bilateral. Most common locations include buccal mucosa, tongue, lips, palate, gingiva, and the floor of the mouth. Lesions develop with stress and liver disese, they persist for many years with periods of remission and exacerbation. | Rest, anxiolytic agents, topical corticosteroids. Evaluate for liver disease, close follow-up for occasional malignant transformation in the erosive type. |

# Appendix III • Guide to Diagnosis and Management of Common Oral Lesions

| Disease | Age | Sex | Race/Ethnicity | Clinical Characteristics | Treatment |
|---|---|---|---|---|---|
| Electrogalvanic white lesion | Over 30 | F | Any | Reddish-white patches that resemble lichen planus located on buccal mucosa adjacent to metallic restorations. Lesions do not rub off and are usually tender or cause a burning sensation. Onset after weeks to years of exposure to metallic restoration; duration varies depending on the persistence of the allergen. | Replace metallic restoration or clasp that is causing the hypersensitive response. |
| Lupus erythematosus | Over 35 | F | Any | Reddish butterfly rash on bridge of nose. Maculopapular eruption with atrophic central areas may involve the lower lip, buccal mucosa, tongue, and palate. Intraoral lesions invariably have red and white radiating lines emanating from the lesion. Lesions do not rub off but are tender to palpation. Lesions often develop after short-term sun exposure. Lesions persist and require drug treatment. | Topical and systemic steroids; antimalarial agents in conjunction with adequate medical treatment. |
| Lichenoid and lupus-like drug eruption | Adult | M-F | Any | Red-white patches that resemble lichen planus and lupus. The lesions are often atrophic or ulcerated centrally. Buccal mucosa, bilaterally, is the most common site. Onset varies and may be weeks or years after an allergic medication is begun. Regression occurs when the offending drug is eliminated. | Withdraw offending drug and substitute medication. |
| Candidiasis | Newborns, adults | M-F | Any | Variable appearance; white curds, red patches, white patches with red margins. Any oral soft tissue site is susceptible, but the attached gingiva is rarely affected. Onset often coincides with neutropenia, or immune suppression. Lesions persist until adequate antifungal therapy is provided. | Antifungal therapy. Eliminate diabetes, endocrinopathy, immunosuppression |

## PIGMENTED LESIONS

| Disease | Age | Sex | Race/Ethnicity | Clinical Characteristics | Treatment |
|---------|-----|-----|----------------|--------------------------|-----------|
| Melanoplakia | Any | M-F | Melanoderms | Generalized constant dark patch located on attached gingiva and buccal mucosa. Pigmentation varies from light brown to dark brown and is often diffuse, curvilinear, and asymptomatic and does not rub off. Melanoplakia present at birth and persists for life. | None required. |
| Tattoo | Teenagers adults | M-F | Any | Amalgam tattoo is the most common type of intraoral tattoo. Appears as a blue-black macule on gingiva, edentulous ridge, vestibule, palate, or buccal mucosa. Radiographs may demonstrate radiopaque foci. Lesions are asymptomatic, do not blanch, and persist for life. | None required. |
| Ephelis | Any | M-F | Light-skinned persons | Light to dark brown macule that appears on facial skin, extremities, or lip after sun exposure. Ephelides are initially small but may enlarge and coalesce. Lesions are nontender and do not blanch or rub off. | None required. |
| Smoker's melanosis | Older adult | M-F | Any | Diffuse brown patch with diameter of several centimeters, usually on posterior buccal mucosa and soft palate. History of heavy tobacco smoking precedes development of the lesion. Features may decrease with discontinuation of the habit. Melanosis is asymptomatic and nonpalpable. | Diminish or stop smoking. |
| Oral melanotic macule | 24–45 | Slight male predilection | Any | Asymptomatic brown to black macule usually located on lower lip near midline; also occurs on palate, buccal mucosa, and gingiva. Onset is post-inflammatory and the lesion persists until treatment. | Biopsy and histologic examination to rule out other similar-appearing pigmented lesions. |
| Nevus | Any | F | Any | Nevi vary greatly in appearance. They may be pink, blue, brown, or black but do not blanch on diascopy. They usually appear as a bluish or brownish smooth-surfaced papule located on the palate. Other common sites include the buccal mucosa, face, neck, and trunk. Many lesions are present at birth. They increase in size and number with increased age. | Excisional biopsy and histologic examination. |

| Disease | Age | Sex | Race/Ethnicity | Clinical Characteristics | Treatment |
|---------|-----|-----|----------------|--------------------------|-----------|
| Melanoma | 25–60 | M | White persons, especially light-skinned persons | Painless, slightly raised plaque or patch that has many colors, especially foci of brown, black, gray, or red. Ill-defined margins, satellite lesions, and inflammatory borders are characteristic. They are usually located on the maxillary alveolar ridge, palate, anterior gingiva, and labial mucosa. Thirty percent arise from pre-existing pigmentations. A recent change in size, shape, or color is particularly ominous. | Excisional biopsy, surgical removal, and referral for complete medical work-up to rule out metastasis. |
| Peutz-Jeghers syndrome | Child, young adult | M-F | Any | Multiple, asymptomatic melanotic oval macules, prominently located on the skin of the palmar or plantar surfaces of the hands and feet, around the eyes, nose, mouth, lips, and perineum. In the mouth, brown discolorations occur on the buccal mucosa, labial mucosa, and gingiva. Lesions do not increase in size, but cutaneous lesions often fade with age; mucosal pigmentation persists for life. Colicky intestinal symptoms are probable. | Oral: none required. Gastrointestinal evaluation and genetic counseling. |
| Addison's disease | Adult | M-F | Any | Diffuse intraoral hypermelanotic patches occurring in conjunction with bronzing of the skin, especially of the knuckles, elbows, and palmar creases. Patches are nontender and nonraised and vary in shape. The buccal mucosa and gingiva are most commonly affected. Onset of the disorder is insidious and associated with adrenal gland hypofunction. Patient may report gastrointestinal symptoms and fatigue. | Systemic corticosteroids. |
| Heavy metal pigmentation | Adult | M-F | Any | Blue-black linear pigmentation of marginal gingiva, prominently viewed along anterior gingiva. Spotty gray macules may be apparent on buccal mucosa. Neuralgic symptoms, headache, and hypersalivation are common. Argyria: Blue-gray skin pigmentation, especially in sun-exposed areas. | Terminate exposure to heavy metal, medical referral. Oral lesions require no treatment. |

## PAPULES AND NODULES

| Disease | Age | Sex | Race/Ethnicity | Clinical Characteristics | Treatment |
|---|---|---|---|---|---|
| Retrocuspid papilla | Child, young adult | M-F | Any | Smooth-surfaced pink papule. 1–4 mm in diameter, located on the lingual attached gingiva apical to the marginal gingiva of the mandibular cuspids. These papules appear early in life, are often found bilaterally, and regress as the patient ages. The retrocuspid papilla is firm to palpation, asymptomatic, and nonhemorrhagic. | None required. |
| Lymphoepithelial cyst | Child, young adult | M-F | Any | Well-circumscribed, soft, fluctuant yellowish swelling that ranges in size from a few millimeters to 1 cm. Common locations for this nontender cyst include the lateral neck just anterior to the sternocleidomastoid muscle, floor of the mouth, lingual frenum, and ventral tongue. Lesion develops during childhood or adolescence and persists until treatment. | Excisional biopsy and histologic examination. |
| Torus, exostosis, and osteoma | Adult | F | Any | Torus: bony hard nodule or multinodular mass located on the palate at the midline, or mandibular lingual alveolar ridge. Exostosis: bony hard nodule, often multiple, located on buccal or labial alveolar ridge. Osteoma: bony hard nodule located adjacent to the jaws, often embedded in soft tissue. All 3 types of lesions are firm, asymptomatic (unless traumatized), slow growing, and long-standing. Osteomas have the greatest growth potential. | Torus and exostosis: none required unless functional problems arise. Osteomas: gastrointestinal evaluation to rule out Gardner's syndrome: if test results are positive, then gastrointestinal surgery and genetic counseling. |
| Fibroma | Adult | M-F | Any | Irritation fibroma: smooth-surfaced, pink, firm, symmetric papule or nodule that arises at a site of chronic irritation, such as the buccal mucosa, labial mucosa, and tongue. The gingiva is the common location for the peripheral odontogenic fibroma. Both lesions have sessile bases and are nontender and nonhemorrhagic. | Excisional biopsy and histologic examination. |

| Disease | Age | Sex | Race/Ethnicity | Clinical Characteristics | Treatment |
|---|---|---|---|---|---|
| Lipoma | Over 30 | M-F | Any | Well-circumscribed, smooth-surfaced, dome-shaped, yellowish to pink nodule commonly located on buccal mucosa, lip, tongue, floor of the mouth, soft palate, or muco-buccal fold. Lesion is slightly doughy upon palpation and grows slowly. | Excisional biopsy and histologic examination. |
| Lipofibroma | Over 30 | M-F | Any | Well-circumscribed, smooth-surfaced, dome-shaped, pinkish nodule commonly located on buccal or labial mucosa. Lesion is painless, movable, and rather firm. Slow growth and persistence are characteristic. | Excisional biopsy and histologic examination. |
| Traumatic neuroma | Over 25 | M-F | Any | Small, slightly raised, firm, pressure-sensitive papule that is commonly located in the mandibular mucobuccal fold near the mental foramen, facial to mandibular incisors, lingual retromolar regions, and ventral tongue. Visualization of the lesion may be difficult if the neuroma is subjacent to normal-appearing mucosa. Palpation elicits an electric shock sensation Onset occurs after trauma; lesions persist until treated. | Excisional biopsy and histologic examination; if lesion recurs, corticosteroid injections may be effective. |
| Neurofibroma | Childhood | M-F | Any | Firm pink nodules that are often deep-seated. These tumors are located in skin, bones, buccal mucosa, tongue, or lips. Lesions are nontender but movable. Continued enlargement can lead to deformity. Multiple lesions and skin pigmentations are associated with von Recklinghausen's disease (neurofibromatosis). | Excisional biopsy, histologic examination, and follow-up for malignant transformation in cases of neurofibromatosis |
| Papilloma | 30s | M | Any | Small, pink, pebbly, slow-growing papule located on uvula, soft palate, tongue, frenum, lips, buccal mucosa, or gingiva. The base is pedunculated and well circumscribed, whereas the surface is most often rough to palpation. | Excisional biopsy and histologic examination |
| Verruca vulgaris | Child-hood young adult | M-F | Any | Rough, whitish-pink papule located on the skin of the hands and perilabially on the lips, labial and buccal mucosa, and attached gingiva. Lesions are slow growing and have a sessile base. Verrucae may regress spontaneously or spread to adjacent mucocutaneous surfaces. | Excisional biopsy and histologic examination |

| Disease | Age | Sex | Race/Ethnicity | Clinical Characteristics | Treatment |
|---|---|---|---|---|---|
| Condyloma acuminatum | 20–45 | M | Any | Small, pink-to-dirty gray papule with rough, papillary surface that resembles a cauliflower. Base of condyloma is sessile, and the borders are raised and rounded. Lesions occur in multiples and onset rapidly occurs after inoculation from affected sexual partner. Most common location is genitalia, labial mucosa, labial commissure, attached gingiva, and soft palate. Lesions can spread and coalesce into extensive clusters. | Excisional biopsy and histologic examination. |
| Lymphangioma | Childhood, adolescent | M-F | Any | Soft, compressible, pinkish-white swelling that may be superficial or deep-seated. Superficial lesions resemble papillomas; deep-seated lesions cause diffuse enlargement. Lymphangiomas may occur in neck (cystic hygroma), dorsal or lateral tongue, lip, or labial mucosa. Long-standing lesions can cause functional problems or regress spontaneously. | Surgical excision; depending on size and location, surgery may require general anesthesia. |

## VESICULOBULLOUS DISEASES

| Disease | Age | Sex | Race/Ethnicity | Clinical Characteristics | Treatment |
|---------|-----|-----|----------------|--------------------------|-----------|
| Primary herpetic gingivostomatitis | Infant, child, young adult | M-F | Any | Multiple vesicles that rupture, coalesce, and form ulcers of the lip, buccal and labial mucosa, gingiva, palate, and tongue. Ulcers are painful and initially are small and yellow, and have red inflammatory borders. Onset is rapid, several days after contact with person harboring the virus. Lesions persist for 12–20 days. | Fluids, antipyretic agents, antibiotics to prevent secondary infection, oral anesthetic rinses, analgesics. |
| Recurrent herpes simplex | Adult | M-F | Any | Multiple small vesicles that rupture and ulcerate. These lesions occur repeatedly at same site: usually the lip, hard palate, and attached gingiva. Onset is rapid and is preceded by prodromal burning or tingling. Lesions last 5–12 days and heal spontaneously. | Bioflavanoids, sunscreens (lip), lysine. Acyclovir in severe cases or for immuno-suppressed patients. |
| Herpangina | Child, young adult | M-F | Any | Light gray papillary vesicles that rupture and form many discrete shallow ulcers. Lesions have erythematous border and are limited to the anterior pillars, soft palate, uvula, and tonsils. Pharyngitis, headache, fever, and lymphadenitis are often concurrent. Lesions heal spontaneously in 1–2 weeks. | Palliative; vesicles heal spontaneously. |
| Chicken pox | Child | M-F | Any | Vesicles on skin and face that, after rupturing, resemble a "dew drop." Ulcers may be seen on soft palate, buccal mucosa, and mucobuccal fold. Skin lesions crust over and heal without scar formation. Condition often accompanied by chills, fever nasopharyngitis, and malaise. Spontaneous healing occurs in 7–10 days. | Palliative; vesicles heal spontaneously. Avoid scratching to limit scar formation. |
| Herpes zoster | Over 55, over 35 in HIV-positive | M-F | Any | Unilateral vesicular and pustular eruptions that develop over 1–3 days. Lesions occur along dermatomes and especially along the trigeminal nerve tract. Lesions are vesicular, ulcerative, and intensely painful and commonly affect the lip, tongue, and buccal mucosa extending up to the midline. Neuralgia may persist after healing. | Palliative; lesions heal spontaneously. Famciclovir in severe cases or immunosuppressed patients. |

| Disease | Age | Sex | Race/Ethnicity | Clinical Characteristics | Treatment |
|---|---|---|---|---|---|
| Hand-foot-and-mouth disease | Child, young adult | M-F | Any | Crops of multiple small yellowish ulcers that occur on palm and sole of hand and foot. The tongue, hard palate, and buccal and labial mucosa are affected. Total number of lesions may approach 100. Healing occurs spontaneously in about 10 days. | Palliative; ulcers heal spontaneously. |
| Allergic reactions immediate | Any | M-F | Any | Red swellings or wheals that occur periorally or on lips, buccal mucosa, gingiva, lips, and tongue. Contact with allergen usually precedes episode by a few minutes to hours. Warmth, tenseness, and itchiness are concurrent. Lesions regress if the allergen is withdrawn. | Remove allergen; antihistamines. |
| Allergic reactions delayed | Any | M-F | Any | Itchy erythematous lesions that may eventually ulcerate. May occur on any cutaneous or mucocutaneous surface. The lips, gingiva, alveolar mucosa, tongue, and palate are affected. Erythema develops slowly over 24–48 hours. Fissuring and ulceration may result. | Remove allergen; corticosteroids. |
| Erythema multiforme | Young adult | M | Any | Skin—target lesions. Oral—hemorrhagic crust of the lips, painful ulcerations of the tongue and buccal mucosa. Attached gingiva rarely affected. Headache, low-grade fever, and previous respiratory infection often precede lesions. | Topical analgesics, antipyretic agents, fluids, corticosteroids, antibiotics to prevent secondary infection. |
| Stevens-Johnson syndrome | Child, young adult | Slight preference for males | Any | Skin—target lesions. Eye—conjunctivitis. Genital—balanitis. Oral—hemorrhagic crust of the lips, painful ulcerations, and weeping bullae of the tongue and buccal mucosa. Attached gingiva rarely affected. Stevens-Johnson syndrome is the fulminant form of erythema multiforme. Eating and swallowing are often impaired. | Topical analgesics, antipyretic agents, fluids, corticosteroids, antibiotics to prevent secondary infection; hospitalization. |
| Toxic Epidermal Necrolysis | Older adults | Women | Any | Severe large coalescing bullae | IV fluids corticosteroids |

| Disease | Age | Sex | Race/Ethnicity | Clinical Characteristics | Treatment |
|---|---|---|---|---|---|
| Pemphigus vulgaris | 30–50 | M-F | Light skinned persons, Jewish and Mediterranean persons | Multiple skin and mucosal bullae that rupture, hemorrhage, and crust. Lesions tend to recur in the same area, have circular or serpiginous borders, and tend to spread to adjacent areas. Nikolsky's sign positive. Collapsed bullae are a common sign. Dehydration can occur if lesions are extensive. | Medical referral, systemic steroids, and oral topical steroids. |
| Benign mucous membrane pemphigoid | Over 50 | 2.1 F:M | Any | Bullae on skin folds and inguinal and abdominal areas. Corneal lesions can lead to scarring. Bullae are often hemorrhagic and persist for days, then desquamate. Lesions occur on the gingiva, palate and buccal mucosa. | Oral topical steroids. Medical referral and systemic steroids if severe; rule out corneal involvement and internal malignancy. |

ULCERATIVE LESIONS

| Disease | Age | Sex | Race/Ethnicity | Clinical Characteristics | Treatment |
|---|---|---|---|---|---|
| Traumatic ulcer | Any | M-F | Any | Symptomatic, yellow-gray ulcer of variable size and shape, depending on inducing agent. Ulcers are often depressed and usually oval in shape, with erythematous border. Commonly located on labial and buccal mucosa, tongue at the borders, and hard palate. Ulcer lasts 1–2 weeks. | Palliative; remove traumatic influence. |
| Recurrent aphthous stomatitis | Young adult | F | Any | Small yellowish oval ulcer with red border, located on movable nonkeratinized mucosa. Common sites include labial mucosa, buccal mucosa, floor of the mouth, tongue, and occasionally soft palate. Ulcers are tender and may be associated with a tender lymph node. Lesions develop rapidly and disappear in 10–14 days without scar formation. | Spontaneous healing in 10–14 days. If acute symptoms or recurrent and symptomatic, topical anesthetics, coagulating agents, or topical steroids may be used. |
| Pseudoaphthous | 25–50 | F | Any | Depressed yellowish round or oval ulcer located on movable nonkeratinized mucosa. Common sites include labial mucosa, buccal mucosa, floor of the mouth, tongue, and occasionally soft palate. Tongue may demonstrate atrophied papillae. Ulcers are tender, develop during deficiency state, and disappear with replacement therapy within 20 days. | Evaluate for deficiency state. If patient is deficient, then nutritional supplements (e.g., iron, vitamin $B_{12}$, folate) are recommended. Gluten abstinence may be required. |
| Major aphthous stomatitis | Young adult | F | Any | Asymmetric unilateral ulcer with necrotic and depressed center. Ulcers have a red inflammatory border and are extremely painful. Located on soft palate, tonsillar fauces, labial mucosa, buccal mucosa, and tongue; may extend onto attached gingiva. Rapid onset. Underlying tissue is often destroyed. Lesions heal in 15–30 days with scar formation. Recurrences are common. | Spontaneous healing, sometimes with scar formation. Topical anesthetics, topical steroids, stress management; identify allergens. |

| Disease | Age | Sex | Race/Ethnicity | Clinical Characteristics | Treatment |
| --- | --- | --- | --- | --- | --- |
| Herpetiform ulceration | Late 20s | M | Any | Multiple pinhead-sized yellowish ulcers located on movable nonkeratinized mucosa. Common sites include anterior tip of tongue, labial mucosa, and floor of the mouth. No vesicle formation. Ulcers are painful and may be associated with several tender lymph nodes. Lesions develop rapidly and disappear in 10–14 days without scar formation. | Tetracycline rinses. |
| Behçet's syndrome | 20–30 | 3:1 (M:F) | Asian, Mediterranean, Anglo | Eye: conjunctivitis, iritis; Genital: ulcers; Oral: painful aphthous-like ulcers on labial and buccal mucosa; Skin: maculopapular rash and nodular eruptions. Oral ulcers are often an initial sign of the disease onset. Arthritis and gastrointestinal symptoms may be concurrent. Recurrences, exacerbations, and remissions are likely. | Topical and systemic steroids. |
| Granulomatous ulcer (Tuberculosis, Histoplasmosis) | Older adult | M-F | Any | Asymptomatic, cobblestoned ulcer that usually occurs on dorsum of tongue, or labial commissure. Cervical lymphadenopathy and primary respiratory symptoms often are concurrent. Onset of oral disease follows lung infection lasting several weeks to months. Oral ulcer may persist for months to years if underlying disease not treated. | Biopsy, histologic examination. Tuberculosis—streptomycin and isoniazid Histoplasmosis—Amphotencin B. |
| Squamous cell carcinoma | Over 50 | 2:1 (M:F) | Any | Nonpainful yellowish ulcer with red indurated borders commonly located on posterior third of the lateral border of tongue, ventral tongue, lips, and floor of the mouth. Associated features may include numbness, leukoplakia, erythroplakia, induration, fixation, fungation, and lymphadenopathy. Carcinoma has a slow onset and is often noticed after a recent increase in size. | Surgery, radiation therapy, or chemotherapy; smoking and alcohol cessation. |
| Chemotherapeutic ulcer | 15–30 and older adult | M-F | Any | Irregular ulcerations of the lips, labial and buccal mucosa, tongue, and palate. Red inflammatory border is often lacking. Hemorrhage is likely when ulcers are deeply situated. Lesions are extremely painful and usually limit mastication and swallowing. Develops during second week of chemotherapy. Secondary infection with oral microorganisms is likely. | Antimicrobial rinses to prevent secondary infection. Topical anesthetics, intravenous fluids |

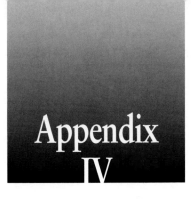

Appendix
IV

# Self-Assessment Quiz

1. **(Fig. 63.1)** This soft tissue swelling was observed on the gingiva of a 7-month-old infant. The infant's mother states that during the past several days the lesion has slowly increased in size. Aspiration yielded a straw-colored fluid. This lesion is most likely a:

   A. congenital epulis of the newborn
   B. congenital lymphangioma
   C. mucus-retention phenomenon
   D. gingival eruption cyst
   E. traumatic hyperplasia

2. **(Fig. 63.2)** This dome-shaped papule on the ventral surface of the tongue is soft and fluctuant. Although the lesion is painless, the lesion occasionally fluctuates in size. A history of trauma was confirmed. The most likely diagnosis for this lesion is a(n):

   A. fibroma
   B. lymphoepithelial cyst
   C. mucus-retention phenomenon
   D. accessory salivary gland tumor
   E. bulla of pemphigoid

3. **(Fig. 63.3)** A 34-year-old man who is a member of the wind section of the symphony arrives at the dental clinic for evaluation of a sore lump on his palate. He states that he was unaware of the swelling until 4 days ago, when the reed of his clarinet contacted the lesion. Palpation reveals the mass to be very firm. This patient most likely has a(n):

   A. periapical abscess
   B. incisive canal cyst
   C. necrotizing sialometaplasia
   D. adenocarcinoma of the palate
   E. traumatic ulcer of the palatal torus

4. **(Fig. 63.4)** A healthy 9-year-old boy appears at the dental clinic with this soft tissue mass. It has been present for 3 weeks and has progressively increased in size. The patient claims that moderate bleeding occurs every time he brushes his teeth, so he has avoided brushing that area for the last several days. All the adjacent teeth are asymptomatic and test vital. Periapical radiographs of the area reveal no abnormalities. This lesion shows features of malignancy.

   A. true
   B. false

5. **(Fig. 63.4)** The most likely diagnosis for the lesion described in question 4 is:

   A. irritation fibroma
   B. peripheral odontogenic fibroma
   C. peripheral giant cell granuloma
   D. peripheral fibroma with ossification
   E. pyogenic granuloma

6. **(Fig. 63.5)** This raised soft tissue lesion is located on the patient's lower lip. In the central region of the lesion it appears translucent. Palpation reveals the lesion to be soft and fluctuant. The differential diagnosis for this lesion should include:

   A. lymphangioma
   B. hemangioma
   C. varix
   D. mucocele

7. **(Fig. 63.5)** The most likely diagnosis of this lesion is:

   A. lymphangioma
   B. hemangioma
   C. varix
   D. mucocele

8. **(Fig. 63.6)** A 45-year-old woman appears at the dental clinic with this pink smooth-surfaced papule. It is 7 mm in diameter, firm, and nonfluctuant. The swelling has been present for several years and has slowly increased in size. The lesion is most likely a(n):

   A. irritation fibroma
   B. peripheral odontogenic fibroma
   C. parulis
   D. pyogenic granuloma
   E. lipoma

9. **(Fig. 63.7)** This asymptomatic, speckled-red and white patch of the tongue was found in an elderly man who admitted to heavy alcohol and tobacco use. The patient was aware of the lesion's presence but was uncertain of the duration. The lesion was firm to palpation. The most likely diagnosis of this lesion is:

   A. an accessory salivary gland tumor
   B. traumatic erythema
   C. candidiasis
   D. squamous cell carcinoma
   E. lichen planus

10. **(Fig. 63.8)** This asymptomatic lesion was discovered in a 45-year-old woman who has had several moles removed from her trunk over the last several years. The term that best describes this lesion is:

    A. macule
    B. papule
    C. plaque
    D. patch

11. **(Fig. 63.8)** The most likely diagnosis of this lesion is:

    A. melanoplakia
    B. melanotic macule
    C. blue nevus
    D. intramucosal nevus
    E. malignant melanoma

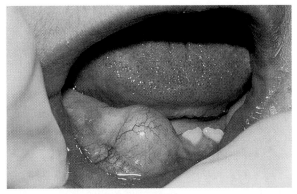

Figure 63.1. Courtesy Dr Barney Olsen

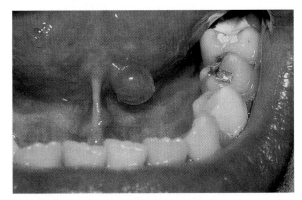

Figure 63.2.

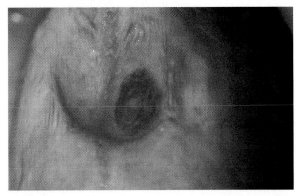

Figure 63.3.

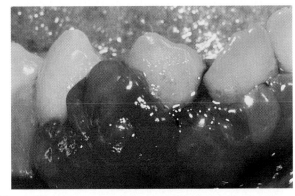

Figure 63.4.

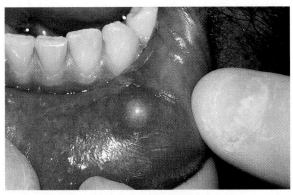

Figure 63.5. Courtesy Dr Nancy Mantich

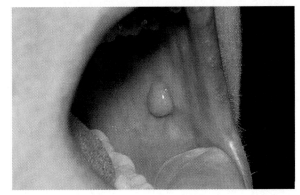

Figure 63.6. Courtesy Dr Curt Lundeen

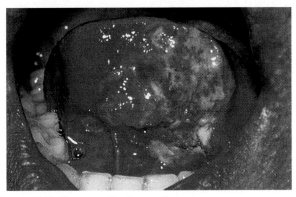

Figure 63.7. Courtesy Dr James Cottone

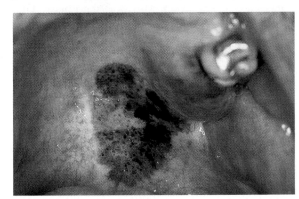

Figure 63.8. Courtesy Dr Michael Vitt

12. **(Fig. 64.1)** A 66-year-old man presents to the dental clinic with pain associated with these lesions on his tongue. He states that the lesions cropped up overnight and the discomfort he is experiencing is limiting his ability to swallow. Although the patient has had a history of intraoral ulcerations, he says that he has never before had one in this location. The most likely diagnosis for this condition is:

A. recurrent herpes simplex
B. aphthous stomatitis
C. traumatic ulceration
D. herpangina
E. pemphigoid

13. **(Fig. 64.2)** This ulcer appeared 8 days ago in a 31-year-old homosexual man after a vacation in the Caribbean. He claims that the lesion began as a vesicle but enlarged over the last several days; it is now quite painful. The regional lymph nodes on that side are tender to palpation. This lesion is most likely a:

A. traumatic ulcer
B. recurrent aphthous ulcer
C. recurrent herpetic ulcer
D. syphilitic ulcer
E. granulomatous ulcer

14. **(Fig. 64.3)** Two months after you treated the patient shown in Figure 64.2, he returns to the dental clinic for a surgical appointment. Your examination reveals scattered white plaques on the lateral border of the tongue and persistent anterior and posterior cervical lymphadenopathy. A low-grade fever is also concurrent. This patient demonstrates clinical features most consistent with:

A. lichen planus
B. lupus erythematosus
C. infectious mononucleosis
D. syphilis
E. HIV infection

15. **(Fig. 64.3)** The condition affecting this patient's tongue is most likely:

A. coated tongue
B. hairy tongue
C. hairy leukoplakia
D. leukoplakia
E. erythroleukoplakia

16. **(Fig. 64.4)** A 34-year-old HIV-positive man appears at the dental clinic reporting a burning tongue. Clinical examination reveals an isolated area on the dorsal surface of the tongue that is red and denuded. Bacterial and fungal cultures are obtained. Forty-eight hours later the fungal cultures are reported to be negative; the bacterial cultures are positive for gastrointestinal flora. The most likely causative organism is:

A. *Escherichia coli*
B. *Streptococcus mutans*
C. *Streptococcus viridans*
D. *Actinomyces viscosus*
E. *Treponema pallidum*

17. **(Fig. 64.5)** This 28-year-old woman presents to the dental clinic with the chief symptom of a "burning sensation in my mouth and throat." She does not report dryness. Review of her medical history reveals a recent upper respiratory infection that was treated with a 14-day course of amoxicillin. Intraorally one finds multiple red patches on buccal mucosa, soft palate, and posterior pharyngeal wall that are tender to palpation. This condition is most likely:

A. lichen planus
B. pemphigoid
C. pemphigus
D. acute atrophic candidiasis
E. chronic atrophic candidiasis

18. **(Fig. 64.6)** These bilateral linear white plaques were discovered in a 50-year-old woman during a routine dental examination. The patient claims she has been under a lot of stress lately because of family problems. The plaques are asymptomatic and do not rub off. The most likely diagnosis is:

A. lupus erythematosus
B. lichen planus
C. candidiasis
D. frictional keratosis
E. none of the above

19. **(Fig. 64.7)** A 45-year-old woman appears at the dental clinic with a swelling of the palate that has been slowly enlarging over the past several months. The lesion is painless but firm to palpation. The condition is most likely a:

A. periodontal abscess
B. palatal abscess
C. palatal torus
D. pleomorphic adenoma
E. malignant accessory salivary gland tumor

20. **(Fig. 64.8)** This 53-year-old woman came to the dental clinic because of burning, painful gingiva. An incisional biopsy was performed, and during the initial incision the gingiva began to slough. The biopsy report indicated that the epithelium was separating from the lamina propria below the basal cell layer. The most likely diagnosis is:

A. pemphigus
B. pemphigoid
C. lichen planus
D. lupus erythematosus
E. erythema multiforme

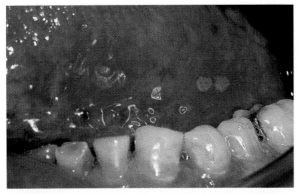

Figure 64.1.

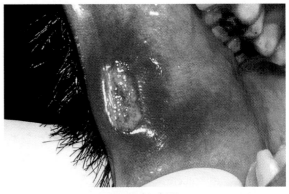

Figure 64.2. Courtesy Dr Michael Vitt

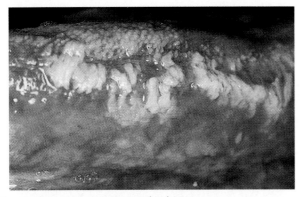

Figure 64.3. Courtesy Dr Michael Vitt

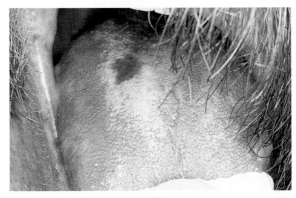

Figure 64.4. Courtesy Dr Sol Silverman

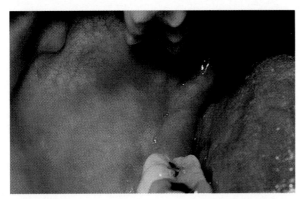

Figure 64.5.

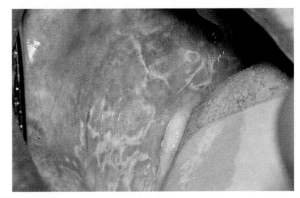

Figure 64.6.

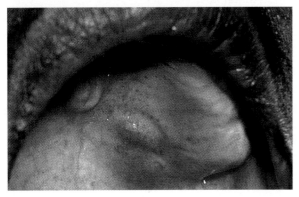

Figure 64.7.

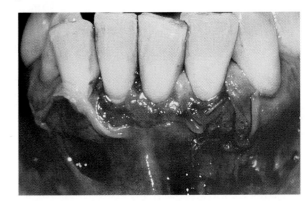

Figure 64.8. Courtesy Dr Nancy Mantich

ANSWERS TO SELF-ASSESSMENT

| | |
|---|---|
| 1. D | 11. E |
| 2. C | 12. B |
| 3. E | 13. C |
| 4. B | 14. E |
| 5. E | 15. C |
| 6. E | 16. A |
| 7. D | 17. D |
| 8. A | 18. B |
| 9. D | 19. D |
| 10. D | 20. B |

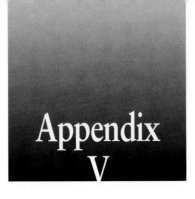

# Appendix
# V

# Glossary

**Abdomen:** The part of the body lying between the thorax (chest) and pelvis.

**Acute:** Having severe symptoms and a short course.

**Adrenal gland:** A small endocrine gland located near the kidney that secretes 1) endogenous glucocorticosteroids, which control digestive metabolism; 2) mineralocorticoids, which control sodium and potassium balance; 3) sex hormones; and 4) catecholamines (epinephrine and norepinephrine), which alter blood pressure and heart function.

**Adrenalectomy:** Surgical removal of the adrenal gland.

**Afunctional:** Not functioning or working.

**Agenesis:** Complete absence of a structure or part of a structure caused by an absence of the tissue of origin in the embryo.

**AIDS:** Acronym for acquired immune deficiency syndrome, reserved for patients infected with HIV (human immunodeficiency virus). It also refers to the terminal stage of the disease.

**Allergen:** A substance that induces hypersensitivity or an allergic reaction.

**Amalgam:** An alloy used to restore teeth, composed mainly of silver and mercury.

**Amelogenesis:** The formation of the enamel portion of the tooth.

**Amputation:** Strictly, this term refers to the removal of a limb such as an arm or of an appendage such as a finger. With reference to a neuroma, however, amputation means a tumor of nerve tissue that results from severing of a nerve.

**Analgesic:** A drug or substance used to relieve pain.

**Analogous:** Having similar properties.

**Anaplastic:** Pertaining to adult cells that have changed irreversibly toward more primitive cell types. Such changes are often malignant.

**Anergy:** A total loss of reactivity to specific antigens.

**Angioma:** A tumor made up of blood or lymph vessels.

**Anodontia:** Congenital condition in which all the teeth fail to develop.

**Anomaly:** Deviation from normal.

**Anorexia:** A lack or loss of appetite for food.

**Anterior:** Located toward the front (opposite of posterior).

**Antibiotic:** A chemical compound that inhibits the growth or replication of certain forms of life, especially pathogenic organisms such as bacteria or fungi. Antibiotics are classified as either biostatic or biocidal.

**Antibiotic sensitivity:** Testing a suspected organism to see whether it is sensitive to destruction by one or more specific antibiotics.

**Antibody:** A protein produced in the body in response to stimulation by an antigen. Antibodies react specifically to antigens in an attempt to neutralize these foreign substances.

**Antigen:** A substance, usually a protein, that is recognized as foreign by the body's immune system and stimulates formation of a specific antibody to the antigen.

**Antipyretic:** A drug or substance used to relieve fever.

**Aplasia:** Absence of an organ or organ part resulting from failure of development of the embryonic tissue of origin.

**Arthralgia:** Pain in one or more joints.

**Aspiration:** The withdrawal of fluid, usually into a syringe.

**Asymptomatic:** A lack of symptoms in the patient.

**Atherosclerosis:** A condition consisting of degeneration and hardening of the walls of arteries caused by fat deposition.

**Atopy:** Hypersensitivity or allergy caused by hereditary influences.

**Atrophic:** A normally developed tissue that has decreased in size.

**Atypical:** Pertaining to a deviation from the normal or typical state.

**Autoinoculation:** To inoculate with a pathogen such as a virus from one's own body. An example would be to spread herpesvirus from one's own mouth or lips to one's finger.

**Autosomal dominant:** The appearance in offspring of one of two mutually antagonistic features in association with one of the 22 pairs of chromosomes in humans that is not concerned with sexual determination.

**Bacterial plaque:** A collection of bacteria, growing in a deposit of material on the surface of a tooth, that can cause disease.

**Bilateral:** On both sides of the body, or mouth.

**Biopsy:** Excision of living tissue for the purpose of examination by a pathologist.

**Bosselated:** Covered with bosses or bumps.

**Bruxism:** A habit related to stress or a sleep disorder, characterized by grinding one's teeth.

**Bulimia:** An eating disorder characterized by frequent periods of excessive food consumption followed by the purging of the ingested food by vomiting or the use of laxatives.

**Bulla:** A circumscribed, fluid-containing, elevated lesion of the skin that is more than 1 cm in diameter.

**Carcinogen:** An agent that induces cancer.

**Carcinoma:** A malignant growth made up of epithelial

cells that are capable of infiltration and metastasis. Carcinoma is a specific form of cancer.

**Cellulitis:** A spreading, diffuse, edematous, and sometimes suppurative (pus-producing) inflammation in cellular tissues.

**Cervical lymphadenopathy:** Abnormally large lymph nodes in the neck, often caused by lymphocyte replication in response to a disease state.

**Chemotaxis:** Taxis or movement of cells in response to chemical stimulation.

**Chemotherapy:** Treatment by chemical substances that have a specific effect on the microorganisms causing the disease. This term is usually reserved for the treatment of cancer with the use of drugs that inhibit rapidly reproducing cells. Side effects are possible.

**Chronic:** Persisting over a long time; when applied to a disease, chronic means that there has been little change or extremely slow progression over a long period.

**Cirrhosis:** A chronic disease of the liver characterized by degenerative changes in the liver cells, the deposition of connective tissue, and other changes. The result is that the liver cells stop functioning and the flow of blood through the liver decreases. There are many causes of cirrhosis, including infection, toxic substances, and long-term alcohol abuse.

**Clavicle:** The collar bone, connecting the shoulder bone (scapula) to the chest bone (sternum).

**Coagulation:** The process of clotting, usually of blood. Clotting is the natural means by which bleeding ceases when a vessel has been severed.

**Collagen:** A protein present in the connective tissue of the body.

**Coloboma:** A developmental defect that may affect various parts of the eye, characterized by a missing part of the structure affected. For example, a coloboma of the lower eyelid means a missing part of the lower eyelid.

**Commissure:** The junction of the upper and lower lips at the corner of the mouth.

**Complement:** A series of enzymatic proteins in normal serum that, in the presence of a specific sensitizer, can destroy bacteria and other cells. C1 through C9 are the nine components of complement that combine with the antigen-antibody complex to produce lysis.

**Concretion:** A hardened mass such as calculus.

**Concurrent:** One or more conditions, events, or findings occurring at the same time.

**Congenital:** Present at or existing from the time of birth.

**Constitutional symptoms:** Symptoms affecting the whole body, such as fever, malaise, anorexia, nausea, and lethargy.

**Cornified:** A process whereby a tissue, usually epithelium, becomes rough and thickened in its outer coating.

**Culture:** The propagation of an organism in a medium conducive to growth.

**Cyst:** A pathologic epithelium-lined cavity, usually containing fluid or semisolid material.

**Cytologic:** Pertaining to the scientific study of cells.

**Cytopathic:** Pertaining to or characterized by pathologic changes in cells.

**Debilitation:** The process of becoming weakened.

**Deciduous tooth:** The primary dentition, or baby teeth. The normal number is 20.

**Deglutition:** The process of taking a substance through the mouth and throat into the esophagus. Deglutition is a stage of swallowing.

**Dehydration:** The removal of water from a substance. Prolonged fever and diarrhea cause dehydration.

**Dental lamina:** The embryonic tissue of origin of the teeth.

**Developmental:** Pertaining to growth to full size or maturity.

**Diascopy:** The examination of tissue under pressure through a transparent medium. For example, suspected vascular lesions are examined by pressing a glass slide over an abnormality to see if the reddish tissue turns white. Because blood flows through vascular lesions, pressure causes them to turn white and thus helps to confirm the diagnosis.

**Distal:** Furthest from a point of reference. In dentistry, distal describes the surface furthest from the midline of the patient.

**Dorsal:** Directed toward or situated on the back surface (opposite of ventral).

**Dysplasia:** An abnormality of development and maturation characterized by the loss of normal cellular architecture.

**Dysplastic:** Pertaining to an abnormality of development. This term is often used to describe the appearance of abnormal, premalignant cells under the microscope. The cells begin to lose their normal maturation pattern and have abnormally shaped, hyperchromatic nuclei.

**Dyspnea:** Labored or difficult breathing.

**Ecchymoses:** Large reddish-blue areas caused by the escape of blood into the tissues, commonly referred to as a bruise. Ecchymoses do not blanch on diascopy.

**Ecosystem:** The interaction of living organisms and nonliving elements in a defined area.

**Ectodermal:** Pertaining to the outermost of the three primitive germ layers of an embryo. The middle layer is the mesoderm and the innermost layer is the endoderm. Ectodermal structures include the skin, hair, nails, oral mucous membrane, and the enamel of the teeth.

**Ectopic:** Located in an abnormal place. The ectopic tissue or structure may or may not be normal.

**Edema:** Abnormal amounts of fluid in the intercellular spaces, resulting in visible swelling.

**Emanate:** To give off or flow away from.

**Embryonic:** Pertaining to the earliest stage of development of an organism.

**Encephalitis:** Inflammation of the brain.

**Endocrinopathy:** A disease or abnormal state of an endocrine gland.

**Endodermal:** Pertaining to the innermost of the three primitive germ layers of an embryo. Endodermal structures include the epithelium of the pharynx, respiratory tract (except the nose), and the digestive tract.

**Epistaxis:** Bleeding from the nose.

**Epithelium:** The cellular makeup of skin and mucous membranes.

**Epulis:** A nodular of tumorous enlargement of the gingiva.

**Erosion:** The wearing away of teeth through the action of chemical substances, or a denudation of epithelium above the basal cell layer.

**Eruption:** An emergence from beneath a surface. For teeth, eruption means their growth into the oral cavity; it may also refer to the development of skin lesions.

**Erythematous:** Characterized by a redness of the tissue due to engorgement of the capillaries in the region. Erythematous lesions blanch on diascopy.

**Erythroplastic:** Characterized by a reddish appearance. This term implies abnormal tissue proliferation in the reddish area.

**Eschar:** A slough of epithelium often caused by disease, trauma, or chemical burn.

**Esthetic:** Pertaining to the appearance of oral or dental structures or the pleasing effect of dental restorations or procedures.

**Everted:** Folded or turned outward.

**Exacerbation:** An increase in severity.

**Exanthematic:** Characterized by the development of an eruption or rash.

**Excisional biopsy:** To completely remove a mass of tissue for the purpose of scientific analysis.

**Exophytic:** An outwardly growing lesion.

**Extensor surface:** Because the arms and legs can be extended or tensed by the appropriate extensor or tensor muscles, the anterior surface is referred to as the extensor surface and the posterior surface is referred to as the tensor surface.

**Extirpate:** To completely remove or eradicate.

**Extremity:** A limb of the body, such as an arm or leg.

**Exudate:** Material that has escaped from blood vessels into tissue or onto the surface of a tissue, usually because of inflammation.

**Factitial:** Self-induced, as in factitial injury.

**Fascial plane:** Spaces between adjacent bundles of fascia that cover muscles. Infection often spreads along these planes.

**Fenestration:** A perforation or opening in a tissue.

**Fetor oris:** An unpleasant or abnormal odor emanating from the oral cavity.

**Field cancerization:** Malignant growths occurring in multiple sites of the oral cavity. The oral tissues have often been exposed to a carcinogen for a long time.

**Fissure:** A narrow slit or cleft.

**Fluctuant:** Strictly, this term describes a palpated, wavelike motion that is felt in a fluid-containing lesion. In this text, the term is frequently used to describe a soft, readily yielding mass on palpation.

**Fontanelle:** One of several soft spots on the skull of infants and children in which the bones of the skull have not yet completely united. In these areas, the brain is covered only by a membrane beneath the skin.

**Frenum:** A fold of mucous membrane that limits the movement of an organ or organ part. For example, the lingual frenum limits tongue movement, and the labial frenuli limit lip movements.

**Frontal bone:** This bone forms the part of the skull consisting mainly of the forehead. The frontal bone corresponds to the front part of the skull and contains an air space called the frontal sinus.

**Furcal:** Pertaining to or associated with the part of a multirooted tooth where the roots join the crown.

**Ganglion:** A collection of cell bodies of neurons outside of the central nervous system. A ganglion is essentially a terminal through which many peripheral circuits connect with the central nervous system.

**Gastroenterologist:** A medical specialist whose field is disorders of the stomach and intestines.

**Gastrointestinal:** Pertaining to the stomach and intestine.

**Genetic counseling:** A form of patient counseling in which the transmission of inherited traits is discussed.

**Genodermatosis:** a hereditary skin disease.

**Gingivectomy:** Surgical removal of gingival tissue.

**Glaucoma:** A disease of the eye characterized by increased intraocular pressure. This condition is often asymptomatic and, if not recognized or treated, leads to blindness.

**Glossal:** Pertaining to or associated with the tongue.

**Glucose:** A form of sugar that is the most important carbohydrate in the body's metabolism.

**Glucosuria:** The presence of an abnormal quantity of glucose in the urine. A sign of diabetes mellitus.

**Granulomatous:** Pertaining to a well-defined area that has developed as a reaction to the presence of living organisms or a foreign body. The tissue consists primarily of histiocytes.

**Gravid:** Pregnant.

**Halitosis:** An unpleasant odor of the breath or expired air.

**Hamartoma:** A tumor-like nodule consisting of a mixture of normal tissue usually present in an organ but existing in an unusual arrangement or an unusual site.

**Hapten:** An incomplete allergen. When combined with another substance to form a molecule, a hapten may stimulate a hypersensitivity or allergic reaction.

**Hematopoietic:** Pertaining to the production of blood or of its constituent elements. Hematopoiesis is the main function of the bone marrow.

**Hematoma:** A large ecchymosis or bruise caused by the escape of blood into the tissues. Hematomas are blue on the skin and red on the mucous membranes. As hematomas resolve they may turn brown, green, or yellow.

**Hematuria:** The presence of blood in the urine.

**Hemihypertrophy:** The presence of hypertrophy on one side only of a tissue or organ. In facial hemihypertrophy, for example, one half of the face is visibly larger than the other.

**Hemoglobin:** The iron-containing pigment of the erythrocytes. Its function is to carry oxygen to the tissues. One of the causes of anemia is a deficiency of iron, causing patients to look pale and feel tired.

**Hemolysis:** Generally speaking, this term refers to the disintegration of elements in the blood. A common form of hemolysis occurs during anemia and involves lysis or the dissolution of erythrocytes.

**Hemorrhage:** Bleeding; the escape of blood from a severed blood vessel.

**Hemostasis:** The stoppage of blood flow. This can occur naturally by clotting or artificially by the application of pressure or the placement of sutures.

**Hereditary:** Transmitted or transmissible from parent to offspring; determined genetically.

**Hiatal hernia:** Protrusion of any structure through the hiatus of the diaphragm. Affected patients are prone to indigestion.

**Histiocyte:** A large phagocytic cell from the reticuloendothelial system. The reticuloendothelial system is a network made up of all of the phagocytic cells in the body, which include macrophages, Kupffer cells in the liver, and the microglia of the brain.

**Histology:** The microscopic study of the structure and form of the various tissues making up a living organism.

**Hyperdontia:** A condition or circumstance characterized by one or more extra, or supernumerary teeth.

**Hyperemia:** The presence of excess blood in a tissue area.

**Hyperglycemia:** The presence of excessive sugar or glucose in the bloodstream.

**Hypermenorrhea:** Excessive uterine bleeding of unusually long duration at regular intervals.

**Hyperorthokeratosis:** Keratin is the outermost layer of epithelium as seen under the microscope and is seen in two forms: orthokeratin and parakeratin. Orthokeratin has no visible nuclei within the outer layer, whereas nuclei are present in parakeratin. Hyperorthokeratosis is the presence of excess orthokeratin.

**Hyperplasia:** An increase in the size of a tissue or organ caused by an increase in the number of constituent cells.

**Hypersensitivity:** Generally, this term means an abnormal sensitivity to a stimulus of any kind. The term, however, is often used with specific reference to some form of allergic response.

**Hypertension:** High blood pressure.

**Hypertrophy:** An increase in the size of a tissue or organ caused by an increase in the size of constituent cells.

**Hypocalcification:** Less than normal amount of calcification.

**Hypodontia:** The congenital absence of one or several teeth as a result of agenesis.

**Hypoplasia:** Incomplete development of a tissue or organ; a tissue reduced in size because of a decreased number of constituent cells.

**Hypopyon:** Pus in the anterior chamber of the eye.

**Hypotension:** Low blood pressure.

**Ileum:** The distal or terminal portion of the small intestine, ending at the cecum, which is a blind pouch forming the proximal or first part of the large intestine.

**Ilium:** The lateral or flaring part of the pelvic bone, otherwise known as the hip.

**Incisional biopsy:** The removal of a portion of suspected abnormal tissue for microscopic study.

**Incisive papilla:** A slightly elevated papule of normal tissue on the palate in the midline immediately posterior to the central incisors. Immediately beneath this structure lies the incisive canal.

**Induration:** Characterized by being hard; an abnormally hard portion of a tissue with respect to the surrounding similar tissue; often used to describe the feel of locally invasive malignant tissue on palpation.

**Infant:** A human baby from birth to 2 years of age.

**Infarct:** A localized area of ischemic necrosis resulting from a blockage of the arterial supply or the venous drainage of tissue. Ischemic necrosis is dead tissue resulting from an inadequate blood supply. An example is a heart attack, which is an infarct of heart muscle.

**Insulin:** A protein hormone secreted by the islets of Langerhans of the pancreas; insulin deficiency produces hyperglycemia, otherwise known as diabetes mellitus.

**Invaginate:** To fold and grow within, in the manner of a pouch.

**Iris:** The part of the eye that is blue, gray, green, or brown. It is a muscular tissue and its function is to constrict and dilate the pupil. The pupil is the black portion in the middle of the iris that allows light into the eye.

**Iritis:** Inflammation of the iris that is often caused by viral infection or rheumatoid disease. The main symptom of iritis is photophobia (aversion to light).

**Ischemia:** A deficiency of blood to a body part, usually caused by constriction or blockage of a blood vessel.

**Kaposi's sarcoma:** A malignant tumor of vascular tissue. Once rare in the Americas, it is now seen frequently in patients with AIDS. The lesions are red-purple in appearance and may be seen anywhere on the skin, especially on the face and in the oral cavity.

**Keratinization:** The formation of microscopic fibrils of keratin in the keratinocytes (keratin-forming cells). In the oral cavity, the term is used to describe changes in the outer layer of the epithelium.

**Keratotic:** A condition of the skin characterized by the presence of horny growths. On the oral mucous membrane, keratotic tissue usually looks white; the term implies a thickening of the outer layer of the oral epithelium.

**Lamina propria:** The layer of connective tissue immediately beneath the epithelium of the oral mucosa.

**Laryngeal:** Pertaining to the larynx, which is a part of the airway. It is located between the pharynx at the back of the oral cavity and the trachea at the beginning of the lungs. The larynx contains the vocal cords, which make audible sounds.

**Lateral:** Pertaining to or situated at the side.

**Leptomeninges:** The two more delicate components of the meninges, the pia mater and the arachnoid.

**Lesion:** A site of structural or functional change in body tissues that is produced by disease or injury.

**Leukoplakia:** A white patch that cannot be rubbed off and that does not clinically represent any other condition.

**Lipid:** Fat or fatty; a naturally occurring substance made up of fatty acids.

**Lobulated:** Made up of lobules, which are smaller divisions of lobes. Many structures are divided into lobes and lobules, such as the brain, lung, and salivary glands. Some pathologic lesions are described as lobulated when the lesion is divided into smaller parts.

**Lymphadenitis:** Inflammation of lymph nodes generally resulting in enlargement and tenderness.

**Lymphoblastic:** Pertaining to a cell of the lymphocytic series; the term implies proliferation. Lymphoblastic is one of the forms of leukemic cancer of the leukocytes characterized by the presence of malignant lymphoblasts or immature lymphocytes.

**Lymphocyte:** A variety of leukocyte that is important to the immune response and that arises in the lymph nodes. Lymphocytes can be large or small; they are round and nongranular and are classified as either T or B lymphocytes.

**Macrocheilia:** Abnormally large lips.

**Macrodontia:** Teeth that are considerably larger than normal.

**Macule:** A spot or stain on the skin or mucous membrane that is neither raised nor depressed. Some examples of macules include café au lait spots, hyperemia, erythema, petechiae, ecchymoses, purpura, oral melanotic macules, and many others illustrated in this atlas.

**Malaise:** A constitutional symptom that describes a feeling of uneasiness, discomfort, or indisposition.

**Malignant:** A neoplastic growth that is not usually encapsulated, grows rapidly, and can readily metastasize.

**Mastication:** Chewing.

**Medial:** Situated toward the midline (opposite of lateral).

**Melena:** Darkened or black feces that are caused by the presence of blood pigments; a sign of intestinal bleeding.

**Meningitis:** Inflammation of the meninges, which are the three membranes covering the brain and spinal cord (the dura mater, arachnoid, and pia mater). Meningitis produces both motor and mental signs, such as difficulty in walking and confusion.

**Mesenchymal:** The meshwork of embryonic connective tissue in the mesoderm that gives rise to the connective tissue of the body, blood vessels, and lymph vessels.

**Mesial:** Toward the front, anterior, or midline. The mesial surface of teeth is the side of the tooth closest to the midline. The five surfaces of teeth are mesial, distal, occlusal or incisal, labial or facial, and lingual or palatal.

**Metastasize:** To spread or travel from one part of the body to another; a term usually reserved to describe the spread of malignant tumors.

**Microdontia:** Teeth that are considerably smaller than normal.

**Mineralized:** Characterized by the deposition of mineral, often calcium and other organic salts in a tissue. The term "calcified" is used when the mineral content is known to be calcium, whereas the term "mineralized" is more general and does not specify the exact nature of the mineral.

**Monocytic leukemia:** Leukemia is cancer of the leukocytes; in this condition the predominating leukocytes are monocytes.

**Morphology:** Descriptive of shape, form, or structure, or the science thereof.

**Mucopurulent:** Consisting of both mucous and pus.

**Mutagenesis:** The induction of genetic mutation.

**Myelogenous leukemia:** Leukemia is cancer of the leukocytes; in this instance the predominating leukocytes are myeloid or granular (polymorphonuclear leukocytes).

**Nasopharyngitis:** Inflammation of the nasopharynx (the back of the nasal complex and upper throat). Sore throat, postnasal drip, and fever are common signs.

**Neocapillary:** New growth of capillaries, which are the smallest blood vessels and connect small arterioles to small venules.

**Necrosis:** The death of a cell as a result of injury or disease.

**Neoplasia:** Characterized by the presence of new and uncontrolled cellular growth.

**Neoplasm:** A mass of newly formed tissue; a tumor.

**Neurogenic:** Originating in or from nerve tissue.

**Neuropathy:** Any abnormality of nerve tissue.

**Neutrophil:** A medium-sized leukocyte with a nucleus consisting of three–five lobes and a cytoplasm containing small granules; one of a group of leukocytes is called granulocytes, and the others are eosinophils and basophils. Neutrophils make up about 65% of the leukocytes in normal blood. Also known as polymorphonuclear leukocyte, PMN, or "poly."

**Neutrophil chemotaxis:** Taxis or movement of neutrophils in response to chemical substances or agents.

**Nevus:** A small tumor of the skin containing aggregations or theques of nevus cells; a mole. It may be flat or elevated and pigmented or nonpigmented; it may or may not contain hair.

**Nodule:** A circumscribed, usually solid lesion having the dimension of depth. Nodules are less than 1 cm in diameter.

**Noncaseating:** A tissue-degenerative process that forms a dry, shapeless mass resembling cheese.

**Occipital bone:** One of the bones that make up the skull; a thick bone at the back of the head.

**Oligodontia:** Presence of fewer than the normal number of teeth.

**Oncogenic:** Capable of causing tumor formation.

**Opportunistic microorganism:** Microorganisms that usually are not pathogenic but become so under certain circumstances, such as an environment altered by the action of antibiotics or long-term steroid therapy. Opportunistic microorganisms cause opportunistic infections.

**Organism:** Any viable life form, such as animals, plants, and microorganisms, including bacteria, fungi, and viruses.

**Otorhinolaryngologist:** An ear, nose, and throat specialist.

**Palliative:** Treatment or the relief of symptoms, not of the cause of a condition.

**Pallor:** Paleness of the skin or mucous membrane; an absence of a healthy color. This sign often accompanies constitutional symptoms and anemia.

**Palpate:** To feel with the fingers or hand.

**Papule:** A small mass, without the dimension of depth, that is smaller than 1 cm in diameter. When described as pedunculated, a papule is on a stalk; when described as sessile, a papule is attached at its base and does not have a stalk.

**Parturition:** The delivery of the fetus from the mother; to give birth.

**Patch:** Similar to a macule but larger; a large stain or spot, usually neither raised or depressed, which may be textured.

**Patent:** The condition of being open; this term is often applied to ducts, vessels, and passages to indicate that they are not blocked.

**Pathognomonic:** Uniquely distinctive of a specific disease or condition; usually consists of signs or findings that, when present and recognized, enable the diagnosis to be made.

**Pathologic:** Pertaining to or caused by disease.

**Pathosis:** An abnormal state or condition.

**Parietal bone:** One of the bones that makes up the skull; there is one parietal bone on each side of the skull, forming the skull's top and upper sides.

**Pedunculated:** A tissue mass originating by a stalk from its base.

**Periapical:** Pertaining to or located at the apex (root end) of a tooth.

**Perifurcal:** Pertaining to or located at the furcum of a tooth; below the cementoenamel junction where the roots fuse together.

**Perilabial:** Pertaining to the region around or near the lips.

**Perineum:** The lower surface of the trunk; when a patient is lying down with legs spread apart, the perineum is the area from the base of the spine to the anal region to the genital area and, finally, to the crest of the mons pubis.

**Perioral:** In the proximity of or around the oral cavity.

**Periorbital:** In the proximity of or around the orbit, which is the bony socket of the eye.

**Peripheral:** Pertaining to the outer part, such as the edge or margin.

**Permanent dentition:** Succedaneous (adult) teeth, which follow the primary teeth. Because there are no replacements for the permanent teeth, they must last a lifetime. There are 32 permanent teeth.

**Petechiae:** Little red spots, ranging in size from pinpoint to several millimeters in diameter. Petechiae consist of extravasated blood.

**Physiologic:** Refers to normal body function (opposite of pathologic).

**Pilocarpine:** A drug used to stimulate salivary flow or to produce constriction of the pupil of the eye.

**Plaque:** An area with a flat surface and raised edges.

**Platelet:** One of the elements found in circulating blood. A platelet has a circular or disk-like shape and is small; hence the term platelet. Platelets aid in blood coagulation and clot retraction.

**Polydipsia:** Excessive thirst. A sign of disease.

**Polypoid:** A polyp-like protruding growth with a base that is equal in diameter to the surface of the mucosal lesion.

**Polyuria:** Excessive amounts of urine. A sign of disease.

**Posterior:** Directed toward or situated at the back (opposite of anterior).

**Primary tooth:** Deciduous (baby) tooth; there are 20 primary teeth.

**Prognathism:** A developmental deformity of the mandible that causes it to protrude abnormally.

**Pruritis:** Itching.

**Pseudohyphae:** Long, filamentous forms that can be seen under the microscope when *Candida albicans*, a fungal microorganism, assumes its pathogenic form.

**Pulse:** A patient's heartbeat, as felt through palpation of a blood vessel.

**Punctate:** Spotted; characterized by small points or punctures.

**Purpuric:** Pertaining to purpura, which are large bruises consisting of blood extravasated into the tissues. Bruises are bluish-purple in color.

**Purulent:** Containing pus.

**Pustule:** A well-circumscribed, pus-containing lesion, usually less than 1 cm in diameter.

**Qualitative:** Of or pertaining to quality; descriptive information about what something looks and feels like.

**Quantitative:** Of or pertaining to quantity; descriptive information about how much of something there is or how big something is.

**Radiation:** In dentistry, electromagnetic energy or x-rays transmitted through space. Radiation also means divergence from a common center; one of the properties of x-rays is that, like a beam of light, they diverge from their source.

**Radiotherapy:** Radiation therapy; the use of radiation from various sources to treat or cure malignant disorders.

**Recrudescence:** Recurrence of signs and symptoms of a disease after temporary abatement.

**Refractory:** Not readily responsive to treatment.

**Remission:** Improvement or abatement of the symptoms of a disease; the period during which symptoms abate.

**Retinopathy:** A disease or abnormality of the retina of the eye. The retina cannot be seen without special instruments and is the part of the eye which receives and transmits visual information coming in from the pupil and lens onto the brain via the optic nerve.

**Renal failure:** Inability of the kidneys to function properly. A patient whose kidneys fail completely will die without renal dialysis or a kidney transplantation. One of the causes of kidney failure is prolonged hypertension (high blood pressure).

**Sarcoma:** A malignant growth of cells of embryonic connective tissue origin. This condition is highly capable of infiltration and metastasis.

**Sarcomatous:** Pertaining to sarcoma, which is a malignant tumor of mesenchymal tissue origin.

**Scar:** A mark or cicatrix remaining after the healing of a wound or other morbid process.

**Sclera:** The strong outer tunic of the eye, or whites of the eyes. When the sclera turns blue or yellow, it is a sign of systemic abnormality.

**Sepsis:** A morbid state resulting from the presence of pathogenic microorganisms, usually in the bloodstream.

**Septicemia:** The presence of pathogenic bacteria in the blood.

**Sequestration:** Abnormal separation of a part from the whole, such as when a piece of bone sequestrates from the mandible because of osteomyelitis; the act of isolating a patient.

**Serpiginous:** Characterized by a wavy or undulating margin.

**Serum:** The watery fluid remaining after coagulation of the blood. If clotted blood is left long enough, the clot shrinks and the fibrinogen is depleted, the remaining fluid is the serum.

**Sessile:** Attached to a surface on a broad base; does not have a stalk.

**Sign:** An objective finding or observation made by the examiner that the patient may be unaware of or does not report.

**Sinus:** An airspace inside the skull, such as the maxillary sinus; an abnormal channel, fistula, or tract allowing the escape of pus.

**Supernumerary:** In excess of the regular number.

**Splenic:** Of or pertaining to the spleen, which is a structure in the upper left abdomen just behind and under the stomach. The spleen contains the largest collection of reticuleondothelial cells in the whole body; its functions include blood formation, blood storage, and blood filtration.

**Spontaneous:** Occurring unaided or without apparent cause; voluntary.

**Superficial:** Located on or near the surface.

**Symptom:** A manifestation of disease that the patient is usually aware of and frequently reports.

**Syndrome:** A combination of signs and symptoms occurring commonly enough to constitute a distinct clinical entity.

**Taurodont:** A malformed multirooted tooth characterized by an altered crown-to-root ratio, the crown being of normal length, the roots being abnormally short, and the pulp chamber being abnormally large.

**Telangiectasia:** The formation of capillaries near the surface of a tissue. Telangiectasia may be a sign of hereditary disorder, alcohol abuse, or malignancy in the region.

**Template bleeding time:** The amount of time necessary for bleeding to stop, following a skin incision of consistent length and depth.

**Texture:** Pertains to the characteristics of the surface of an area or lesion. Some descriptions of texture are as follows: smooth, rough, lumpy, and vegetative. The tiny bumps on the surface of a wart cause it to have a vegetative texture.

**Therapeutic:** Of or pertaining to therapy or treatment; beneficial. Therapy has as its goal the elimination or control of a disease or other abnormal state.

**Thorax:** That part of the body between the neck and abdomen, enclosed by the spine, ribs, and sternum. In the vernacular, the thorax is referred to as the chest. The main contents of the thorax are the heart and lungs.

**Thrombophlebitis:** The development of venous thrombi in the presence of inflammatory changes in the vessel wall.

**Thrombosis:** Formation of thrombi within the lumen of the heart or a blood vessel. A lumen is the space within a passage; a thrombus is a solid mass that can form within the heart or blood vessels from constituents in the circulating blood. Patients prone to the formation of thrombi should receive anticoagulant therapy.

**Tooth bud:** The embryonic tissue of origin of the teeth; tooth buds develop from the more primitive tissue of the dental lamina.

**Torus:** A bony nodule on the hard palate or on the lingual aspect of the premolars.

**Tourniquet test:** When pressure is applied to the blood vessels of the upper arm using a blood pressure cuff, a bleeding tendency is detected when petechiae develop in the region.

**Transient:** Temporary; of short duration.

**Translucent:** Somewhat penetrable by rays of light.

**Trauma:** A wound or injury; damage produced by an external force.

**Trismus:** Tonic contraction of the muscles of mastication; commonly referred to as lockjaw. Trismus is caused by oral infections, salivary gland infections, tetanus, trauma, and encephalitis.

**Trunk:** The main part of the body, to which the limbs are attached. The trunk consists of the thorax and abdomen and contains all of the internal organs. This term is also used to describe the main part of a nerve or blood vessel.

**Tumor:** A solid, raised mass that is larger than 1 cm in diameter and has the dimension of depth. This term also describes a mass consisting of neoplastic cells.

**Ulcer:** Loss of surface tissue caused by a sloughing of necrotic inflammatory tissue; the defect extends into the underlying lamina propia.

**Unilateral:** Affecting only one side of the body.

**Uremia:** A toxic condition caused by the accumulation of nitrogenous substances in the blood that are normally eliminated in the urine.

**Urticaria:** A vascular reaction of the skin characterized by the appearance of slightly elevated patches that are either more red or paler than the surrounding skin. Urticaria is also known as hives and may be caused by allergy, excitement, or exercise. These patches are sometimes intensely itchy.

**Vasoconstriction:** To decrease the diameter or caliber of a blood vessel.

**Ventral:** Directed toward or situated on the belly surface (opposite of dorsal).

**Vermilion:** That part of the lip which has a naturally pinkish red color and is exposed to the extraoral environment. The vermilion contains neither sweat glands nor accessory salivary glands.

**Vermilion border:** The mucocutaneous margin of the lip.

**Vermilionectomy:** Surgical removal of the vermilion border of the lip.

**Vertigo:** An unpleasant sensation characterized mainly by a feeling of dizziness or that one's surroundings are spinning or moving.

**Vesicle:** A well-defined lesion of the skin and mucous membranes that resembles a sac, contains fluid, and is less than 1 cm in diameter.

**Visceral:** Pertaining to body organs.

**Viscous:** Thick or sticky.

**Wheal:** A localized area of edema on the skin. The area is usually raised and smooth-surfaced and is often very itchy.

**Xerostomia:** Dry mouth.

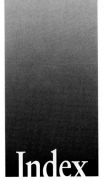

# Index

References in italics denote figures

# Index

# Index